From the reviews of *Spastic D*

Full reviews available at www.Gillett<

This book provides the answers we have all been looking for ... the perfect balance of science and practical knowledge ...With a resource of this quality, the future is bright for all of us.

DR. LINDA A HALLMAN, parent of teenager with spastic diplegia, Director of Orthodontics, MedStar Washington Hospital Center and Children's National Medical Center, Washington DC, USA

This co-developed parent–professional book on the focused topic of spastic diplegia is a must-read for professionals, parents, and the individual with cerebral palsy (CP). The range of the book is "real-world focused" with the latest accurate literature incorporated ... It serves a unique educational niche ... I am recommending it already!

DR. DEBORAH GAEBLER-SPIRA, Director Cerebral Palsy Program, Shirley Ryan AbilityLab, Professor of Pediatrics and Physical Medicine and Rehabilitation, Northwestern Feinberg School of Medicine, Past President, American Academy for Cerebral Palsy and Developmental Medicine, Illinois, USA

This book is excellent, insightful, and educational: it will open minds and touch hearts. It is very clear and easy to read. As an adult with spastic diplegia, I have learned many new things about my condition from reading it.

SAMANTHA MARIE LADEMANN, adult with spastic diplegia, Minnesota, USA

This book provides a comprehensive overview of all aspects of living with bilateral spastic CP ...The combination of evidence-based information and personal experience ensures that this book is an engaging and thought-provoking read, which families and health professionals would benefit from owning.

DR. JENNIFER RYAN, Research Lecturer, Royal College of Surgeons in Ireland (RCSI), Dublin, Ireland

I met Lily Collison for the first time in mid-September 2001, when I was lecturing at a cerebral palsy seminar held at the Central Remedial Clinic in Dublin, Ireland. Lily later brought Tommy to Gillette ... for treatment. That began a doctor-patient relationship that lasted up until my retirement in 2008, and a friendship that has lasted to this present day. Lily wrote a book for parents, much as I did for orthopedic surgeons back in 1991. This book, Spastic Diplegia—Bilateral Cerebral Palsy ... is a must-read for parents of children with spastic diplegia, and if its guiding principles are followed, it will do much to ensure that their particular child reaches maturity with an optimal outcome.

DR. JAMES R. GAGE, Medical Director Emeritus, Gillette Children's Specialty Healthcare, Past President, American Academy for Cerebral Palsy and Developmental Medicine, Professor of Orthopedics Emeritus, University of Minnesota, USA

*Lily Collison and the staff at Gillette have taken a very complex disorder—spastic diplegia—and made it comprehensible to the lay reader. CP is a disorder that many clinicians do not fully understand either. As a pediatric orthopedic surgeon who specializes in the care of children and adults with CP, as well as being the father of a 37-year-old man who has CP, I highly recommend this book to people who have CP, parents, family members, **and** medical professionals. It is a fantastic overview of the subject with many insightful passages by those who have taken the journey.*

DR. HANK CHAMBERS, Professor of Clinical Orthopedic Surgery, University of California, San Diego, Director of the Southern Family Cerebral Palsy Center at Rady Children's Hospital, San Diego, Past President, American Academy for Cerebral Palsy and Developmental Medicine, California, USA

This book is beautifully balanced—from references and information, to the heart of a mom lighting the way for other parents struggling to filter an overload of information … I would have loved to have had this book at the time of our son's diagnosis, and would recommend any family members to also read it for a much deeper understanding of CP and how to help the family and child with CP … What a gift you have written.

CARY SOMMER, parent of an eight-year-old with spastic diplegia, Minnesota, USA

Health care is at its best when the patient is at the heart of health services. One of the fundamental components in this process of patient participation is sufficient knowledge about the disease and its treatments. This will allow good communication and making informed choices about treatment. This book provides that knowledge … For patients with spastic diplegic CP and their families this book provides a perfect start to become equal partners in their health care decisions.

DR. ANJA VAN CAMPENHOUT, Pediatric Orthopedic Surgeon, University Hospital Leuven, Belgium

As I read this book I found myself changing hats; one minute I was reading it as a GP, the next minute I was reading it as the mum of a son with a disability. The scientific and medical content of the book is excellent, and I learnt a lot by reading it … For a parent of a child with spastic diplegia, this book is an incredible resource. I would have loved one about spina bifida 21 years ago.

DR. SIOBHÁN TEMPANY, GP, parent of son with spina bifida, Ireland

This book is a valuable addition to the CP literature … A particular strength of the book is the road map that is outlined as the child with CP grows from infancy to adulthood … The addition of reliable and user-friendly web links is very helpful for the reader.

DR. OWEN HENSEY, Medical Director, Central Remedial Clinic, Dublin, Ireland

This is a wonderful resource for people with spastic diplegia and their families, which draws robust scientific information together in a clear and accessible way ... Teamwork between health professionals, the person with CP, and their family is essential to achieve the best management plan ...This book supports the voice of the person and parents in the team, empowering shared decision-making ... a must-read for people with CP, families, health professionals, and students alike.

DR. CATHERINE BLAKE, Dean and Head, UCD School of Public Health, Physiotherapy and Sport Science, Dublin, Ireland

I needed this book when my son was born almost 15 years ago and didn't meet his developmental milestones ... I needed it when I was conducting my own research without the skill set on what intervention he needed when he was seven years old. I need it now as he ages and has growth spurts and we are researching orthopedic procedures. I will need it when he becomes an adult and lives independently.

LORI POLISKI, parent of teenager with spastic diplegia, Marketing Manager, Cerebral Palsy Research Network, Washington, USA

Although we are in a low-resource setting, the team working with children and families ... strives to provide the best care possible. Much of what has been described in this book is not yet available here, but the desire to improve options for care is honest and committed. This book, although written for families, has the potential to have a great impact on health care professionals and other stakeholders who have the ability to work on improvements at a more global level.

SUE MURR, Physiotherapist, Uganda

Thank you, Lily, for providing such an accessible resource for so many people, the person with spastic diplegia, their parents and families, medical professionals, and education professionals like me who prepare teachers to work with children with CP. I will certainly be using it to inform my practice with my students. This book should be on so many people's reading list!

DR. ANNE O'BYRNE, Lecturer in Inclusive Education for Children with Special Educational Needs, Mary Immaculate College, parent of adult with disability, Limerick, Ireland

As a personal trainer who has multiple clients with physical challenges and CP, this book brought a whole new level of insight into what my clients have experienced ... Rich in encouragement, scientific knowledge, practical advice, and personal stories, it will deepen your empathy and drive to achieve fitness for clients with physical disabilities.

VANESSA LIU, Personal Trainer whose father has CP, California, USA

A must-read for anyone working with young athletes with CP. This masterfully written book weaves together a wonderful spirit of optimism with practical tools for parents, educators, coaches, and medical professionals. As we look to grow the Paralympic movement in the United States, Lily's work is critical to elevating the level of development programs available to young Paralympic hopefuls.

KARA BUCKLEY, Director, U.S. Olympic and Paralympic Properties (USOPP), California, USA

This is a unique book which gives an excellent insight into and holistic understanding of ... spastic diplegia ... from birth to adulthood ...This book will assist any parent or relative of a child ... or indeed a young person themselves in understanding their condition ... and, most importantly, what they themselves can do to influence outcome ... This book should also be read by all professionals working with persons impacted by disability and specifically CP.

MIKE WALSH, Head of Specialist Services and Research, Central Remedial Clinic, Dublin, Ireland

This book ... is a fantastic resource for parents and professionals alike ... I wish that an equivalent book might soon be written for hemiplegia.

EIMEAR GABBETT, parent of an eight-year-old with hemiplegia, Ireland

I compliment the author of this amazing "sat nav" for parents, siblings, families, carers, and teachers who may be setting out on a care journey of a young person with ... spastic diplegia ... I don't think there is anyone who wouldn't benefit from reading this book.

UNA COLLINS, teacher of children aged four to 13, whose sister has a disability, Ireland

When someone important to us is living with a long-term health condition, we often want to know what we can do to help. However, locating accurate, easy-to-understand information, specific to our needs, is not always easy. Parents and caregivers of children living with spastic diplegia will find this book provides them with such information.

DR. DÉSIRÉE B. MALTAIS, Associate Professor, Rehabilitation Department, Université Laval, Researcher, Centre for Interdisciplinary Research in Rehabilitation and Social Integration, Quebec City, Canada

SPASTIC DIPLEGIA

BILATERAL CEREBRAL PALSY

SPASTIC DIPLEGIA

BILATERAL CEREBRAL PALSY

Understanding the motor problems,
their impact on walking,
and management throughout life:
a practical guide for families

Lily Collison MA, MSc
PARENT

Edited by
Jean Stout, PT, MS
Amy Schulz, PT, NCS
Candice Johnson, OTD, OTR/L
Tom F. Novacheck, MD
GILLETTE CHILDREN'S SPECIALTY HEALTHCARE

Gillette Children's Healthcare Press
200 University Avenue East
St Paul, MN 55101
www.GilletteChildrensHealthcarePress.org

ISBN 978-1-952181-00-9 (paperback)
ISBN 978-1-952181-01-6 (ebook)

For information about special discounts for bulk purchases, please contact HealthcarePress@gillettechildrens.com

COPYEDITED BY Joan McGarry Moore and Rebecca Hiscott
ORIGINAL ILLUSTRATIONS BY Olywn Roche
COVER AND INTERIOR DESIGN BY Jazmin Welch
PROOFREAD BY Ruth Wilson
INDEX BY Stephen Ullstrom
PROJECT MANAGEMENT BY Carra Simpson

Printed and bound in the United States of America

All proceeds from sales of this book will be donated to CP research.

Contents

Author and Editors ··· xi

Foreword by Dr. Tom F. Novacheck ··· xiii

Preface ··· xv

1 CEREBRAL PALSY (CP) ·· 1

    1.1   Introduction ··· 2
    1.2   Causes, risk factors, and prevalence ································· 7
    1.3   Diagnosis ·· 12
    1.4   The International Classification of Functioning,
           Disability and Health (ICF) ·· 16
    1.5   Motor function, gross motor milestones ························· 22
    1.6   Classification of CP ·· 27
    Key points Chapter 1 ··· 44

2 SPASTIC DIPLEGIA—BILATERAL CP ··· 47

    2.1   Introduction ··· 48
    2.2   The brain injury ·· 53
    2.3   Growth ·· 56
    2.4   Bones, muscles, joints, and movements ·························· 62
    2.5   Normal walking ·· 69
    2.6   Primary abnormalities ·· 72
    2.7   Secondary abnormalities ·· 80
    2.8   Tertiary abnormalities ·· 94
    2.9   Walking in individuals with spastic diplegia ······················ 96
    Key points Chapter 2 ··· 104

3 MANAGEMENT AND TREATMENT OF
SPASTIC DIPLEGIA—BILATERAL CP TO AGE 20 ············ 107

3.1 Introduction ··· 108
3.2 What does best practice look like? ······································· 111
3.3 Therapies ··· 123
3.4 The home program ··· 144
3.5 Orthoses ··· 158
3.6 Tone reduction ··· 166
3.7 Orthopedic surgery ··· 178
3.8 The overall musculoskeletal management plan to age 20 ············· 193
3.9 Alternative and complementary treatments ···················· 197
3.10 What the parent can do to help the child, what the
     adolescent can do to help themselves ······························ 201
Key points Chapter 3 ·· 214

4 THE ADULT WITH SPASTIC DIPLEGIA—BILATERAL CP ··· 217

4.1 Introduction ··· 218
4.2 Aging in the typical population ··· 222
4.3 Aging with spastic diplegia ··· 228
4.4 Management and treatment of spastic diplegia in adulthood ······· 240
Key points Chapter 4 ·· 253

5 LIVING WITH SPASTIC DIPLEGIA—BILATERAL CP ········ 255

6 FURTHER READING ·· 269

Epilogue by Tommy Collison ·· 277

Acknowledgments ··· 281

APPENDICES ·· 285

Appendix 1   Dealing with a diagnosis ·················· 286
Appendix 2   Gross motor function ······················ 290
Appendix 3   Measurement tools ························ 291
Appendix 4   Positioning ······························· 293
Appendix 5   Exercise and physical activity ············· 297
Appendix 6   Rehabilitation post-selective dorsal rhizotomy (SDR) ······· 300
Appendix 7   Gait analysis ···························· online

Glossary ··· 303

References ·· 309

Index ··· 335

Author and Editors

Lily Collison, MA, MSc, parent of a 25-year-old with spastic diplegia. She worked in industry and education.

Jean Stout, PT, MS, Research Physical Therapist at the James R. Gage Center for Gait and Motion Analysis, Gillette Children's Specialty Healthcare, St. Paul, Minnesota, USA.

Amy Schulz, PT, NCS, Physical Therapist and Clinical Educator at Gillette Children's Specialty Healthcare.

Candice Johnson, OTD, OTR/L, Rehabilitation Therapies Administrative Supervisor–CORE (Clinical Outcomes, Research, and Education) at Gillette Children's Specialty Healthcare and Gillette Phalen Clinic.

Tom F. Novacheck, MD, Associate Medical Director at Gillette Children's Specialty Healthcare, Professor of Orthopedics at the University of Minnesota, and Vice-President, American Academy for Cerebral Palsy and Developmental Medicine.

Foreword

I have known Lily Collison since 2010. I first knew her as a concerned and dedicated parent of a child with spastic diplegia seeking advice about the best treatment approaches. She had sought care at Gillette Children's a few years earlier; now her adolescent son, Tommy, was having intractable knee pain and she hadn't found answers closer to home. Thankfully, we were able to work through that problem. We stayed connected as I continued to see Tommy through to the present day. During that time, Lily has applied her knowledge and experience to firmly advocating for the development of resources for and the dissemination of knowledge to families and patients. She and I have worked together on projects that have supported our gait lab, Gillette-based research, and the communication of awareness and knowledge.

When Lily first mentioned that she thought there should be a book like this for spastic diplegia—bilateral cerebral palsy (CP) and that she was willing to write it, I was unsure and skeptical. However, she made a strong case for it. After investigating the resources available to parents whose child has been diagnosed with CP, I found that she was indeed right. Parents are left mainly to self-educate from various piecemeal resources—books (limited in number), websites, pamphlets, handouts, etc. The variability of the condition and its causes, delayed diagnosis, and misinformation litter the playing field, causing bewilderment and frustration.

Lily's background as both a parent and medical sciences graduate made her an ideal person to write this book for families. She has been dedicated to understanding this condition and the treatment options available since her son was first diagnosed. She dearly wants others to have an easier path than the one she experienced as she gained the knowledge to advocate for her child. Through what she learned over the years and her detailed research, and with support and editorial review from staff at Gillette, she has delivered this comprehensive and comprehensible book, which you will be able to use as your child grows right through to adulthood. She has balanced the scientific information with personal anecdotes and stories from a variety of others whose lives have been affected by CP.

This is a unique book; it tells not only the detailed technical story of spastic diplegia but also the human story of the condition. This is a valuable book; in fact, it is so well done that it could be a resource not only for parents but also for health professionals in the field. I have learned much by listening to Lily and other parents like her ... and to their children. Lily's experience was of spastic diplegia, and this is what she has written about. Although spastic diplegia is only part of the spectrum of CP, it is one of the most common forms. In addition, many of the principles in this book can be applied more broadly to other forms of CP because the child's growing body can be similarly affected.

As you read this book, you will wonder how a parent could write such a comprehensive book about this medical condition, but Lily has skillfully done so. When I first read the full book, my reaction was, wow! This is a unique gem; it hits a target that has not been struck before.

Dr. Tom F. Novacheck

Preface

*Education is the most powerful weapon
which you can use to change the world.*
Nelson Mandela

If you are reading this book, most likely you are the parent of a child with spastic diplegia or you yourself have the condition. You may have a family member, friend, or student with spastic diplegia, or you may be a professional working with people with the condition. Spastic diplegia, also known as bilateral spastic cerebral palsy (CP) or simply bilateral CP, is a subtype of cerebral palsy. It is a lifelong condition characterized by limb muscles that are extremely tight (spastic) with the legs more affected than the arms (diplegia). However, spastic diplegia involves much more than tight leg muscles. This book provides a detailed explanation of spastic diplegia and shows how the condition develops over time. It describes the best management and treatment of the condition (at the time of writing) in childhood, adolescence, and adulthood.

My third son, Tommy, was born at term in Ireland in 1994. His older brothers, then aged four and six, had been easy babies, so by then my husband and I felt quite relaxed as parents. Tommy was born after an uneventful pregnancy and delivery, but from birth he cried incessantly. At three weeks our family physician insisted that I give up breastfeeding. She could see how frazzled I had become due to Tommy's constant crying, his difficulty with feeding (many feeds were being returned), and the fact that neither he nor I was getting much sleep.

At three months the incessant crying suddenly stopped; Tommy became a serene, happy, and placid child, and we all relaxed again. However, a few months later, at a routine developmental check, he was deemed "developmentally delayed." That started a long journey, beginning with the diagnosis of spastic diplegia when he was a year old and continuing with the management and treatment of his condition in our community as well as at the Central Remedial Clinic (CRC)[1] in Dublin. In the early years he also received conductive education,[2] and in adolescence he had a number of surgeries at Gillette Children's Specialty Healthcare (hereafter referred to as Gillette) in Minnesota. At the time of writing, Tommy, now 25 years old, is a college graduate, working full-time and living an independent life in the US.

Why a book on spastic diplegia is needed

CP is the most common cause of lifelong, childhood-onset physical disability in most countries, with an estimated prevalence of 17 million people worldwide [1]. Approximately one-third of those with CP have spastic diplegia [2]. Spastic diplegia is thus a common subtype of CP, affecting an estimated 6 million people worldwide—roughly the population of Ireland. If this book helps a tiny fraction of those affected by spastic diplegia, writing it will have been worthwhile.

A book on spastic diplegia that is accessible to laypeople does not exist. It did not exist when Tommy was diagnosed almost 25 years ago, and it still does not exist today. Many of the specialist centers that treat CP now have well-developed websites, but again, they do not offer much information specific to spastic diplegia.

Good texts on CP exist, but many cover all subtypes of CP together.[3] Explaining the different subtypes together is like having one book to explain all types of cancer and their treatments. Each subtype of CP is different, and each has a different prognosis for mobility and associated health challenges. Subtypes vary from generally mild to severe. Anyone with a condition is understandably rather selfish—they only want to learn about their specific condition. If my diagnosis is throat cancer, I only want to learn about throat cancer. If my diagnosis is spastic diplegia, I only want to learn about spastic diplegia. I do not need to know about health challenges that do not concern me.

---

1 The Central Remedial Clinic (CRC) in Dublin is a national treatment center for people with physical disabilities.

2 Conductive education is based on an educational rather than a medical model for treatment of children with CP. It combines educational and rehabilitation goals into a single program [3].

3 The subtypes of CP are spastic CP (monoplegia, hemiplegia, diplegia, triplegia, and quadriplegia), dyskinetic CP (dystonic and choreo-athetotic), ataxic CP, and mixed CP. These terms are fully explained in section 1.6.

Spastic diplegia is complex. How can a baby born with what appear to be typical bones, muscles, and joints grow into the young child who may walk with a gait[4] typical of a child with spastic diplegia? Although spastic diplegia is a complex condition, it becomes more understandable when logically explained.

Spastic diplegia is a lifelong condition, and we parents are key influencers of outcomes. My lack of understanding always held me back. My background is in science, and I was thirsty for knowledge that would further my understanding of the condition. In those early days, before the internet had become the resource it is today, I scoured bookshops in any city I visited, but all I could find were books on CP in general. The first book I found that offered specifics on spastic diplegia was one written by Dr. Jim Gage (1991), an orthopedic surgeon at Gillette who has since retired [4]. (This book was recommended to me by Tommy's community physical therapist, who had previously worked at Great Ormond Street Hospital in London and had visited Gillette.) Though I learned a lot from it, this book was not fully accessible to me because it was written for medical professionals. It took me many hours and much hard work to find the information I needed to understand the condition. That hard work culminated in my completing a master's degree over a decade ago—a case study providing a detailed picture of single-event multilevel surgery (SEMLS)[5] and rehabilitation, and evaluating outcome.

This book seeks to provide you, the reader, with an understanding of spastic diplegia without having to invest so much time and effort. Indeed, Bailes and colleagues (2018) pointed out that most of the time, health professionals underestimate the amount of information parents and caregivers want about their child's condition [5]. This problem extends to adulthood: lack of information about their condition was the highest area of unmet need reported by young adults with CP [6]. This included information on complications, consequences, and causes of CP.

The parent of a child with spastic diplegia does not have the full, long-term view of how spastic diplegia develops over time. Medical professionals have the benefit of their training and their clinical experience to put

---

4 Gait is a person's manner of walking.

5 Single-event multilevel surgery (SEMLS) involves multiple orthopedic surgical procedures performed on the lower limbs during a single operation.

things in context, but a parent does not. In the early days, I felt like I was trying to do a jigsaw puzzle without having the picture on the box as a reference. I had pieces but did not understand how they fit together. I wanted to help my child walk, but his physical therapist wanted me to help him roll.

A good explanation gives us parents a much better understanding of what we can and cannot change about our child's condition. Greater understanding should give us more confidence when helping our child. I so often had doubts: "am I doing this correctly?"[6] Greater understanding should lead to greater motivation to carry out the exercises we are given to do at home.

Parents also put in a huge effort to prevent future possible events—events of which we have no experience. Success is avoiding negatives. In some ways, that feels unsatisfactory. I'd never seen the problems resulting from excessive W-sitting;[7] they were as vague to me as being told as a young Catholic child, "Don't do this or you won't go to Heaven." Heaven was vague to the younger me. Hip subluxation[8] and contractures[9] were vague to the older me. I'd never seen them, nor the problems they caused. People who have plenty of money do not really understand the pain of poverty. People who have plenty to eat do not really understand the pain of hunger. People who already understand do not really feel the pain and frustration of just not understanding. Many prospective parents read books such as *What to Expect When You're Expecting* [7] to understand the different stages of pregnancy; this book could just as easily be called *What to Expect When You or Your Child Has Spastic Diplegia*.

Having a book just for spastic diplegia protects against unnecessary anxiety. Books and websites on CP frequently include a long list of other possible problems separate from the movement disorder, such as epilepsy or learning disabilities. However, the presence of other prob-

---

6 Regarding elements of the home program, for example.

7 "W-sitting" is the term used to describe the sitting position which the child with spastic diplegia (and other forms of spastic CP) adopts. The child's bottom is on the floor while their feet are out. Looking from the top, the legs form a "W" shape.

8 In a subluxated hip (hip subluxation), the ball is partially out of the socket but is still in contact with it—the ball is still partially covered by the socket.

9 A contracture is a limitation of the range of motion (ROM) of a joint.

lems largely depends on the CP subtype. Generic lists are not helpful and cause unnecessary anxiety for us parents, who already have enough to worry about. The opposite also holds true: if I have a child who is unlikely to ever walk independently, what use is it to read about gait analysis?

On the subject of anxiety, some may argue that if parents read this book—a book which details the issues associated with spastic diplegia in childhood, adolescence, and adulthood—they will not be able to handle the full story and will become even more anxious. I disagree. I would counter by noting that we parents find out quickly that our child's spastic diplegia is not going to go away. We see adolescents and adults with spastic diplegia in treatment centers and in the community, which gives us an idea of how the condition develops. Ignorance is not bliss. Fear of the unknown can be a bigger problem. Indeed, if we are given the long-term picture of how our child's particular condition will develop, it may be better than we fear. It may also mobilize us to early action. Outcomes in adulthood very much depend on management and treatment in childhood and adolescence (though spastic diplegia also presents its own challenges in adulthood). If you are a parent of a young child with spastic diplegia, I would advise you to read this book in full now, including the chapter on adulthood, to gain a full-life perspective on the condition.

Despite their best efforts, medical professionals use medical terms. This is a new language for us parents; we're not familiar with terms like "adduction" and "dorsiflexion." Professionals can either refrain from using such terms or continually explain them to parents. Alternatively, parents can gain an understanding of these commonly used terms. I think the latter is much easier all-around. This book includes an explanation of this "new" language for parents.

Treatment of CP does not involve just one discipline. It involves professionals from a number of disciplines, including physical therapy (PT, also termed physiotherapy), occupational therapy (OT), speech and language pathology/therapy (SLP/SLT), nursing, orthotics, pediatrics, neurology, neurosurgery, orthopedic surgery, and physical medicine and rehabilitation (PMR, also termed physiatry).[10] Within the multi-

---

10 These disciplines are explained in the glossary.

disciplinary team, no one professional is responsible for explaining the condition to parents; it is very ad hoc. At appointments, there is little time for explanation because the child is present and their treatment takes priority. (In addition, the child will get bored if the adults are talking too much.) Having medical professionals explain the condition to parent after parent is inefficient. It would be preferable, in my opinion, to have well-developed resources available to parents, and professionals can then answer specific questions.

Parents are co–decision makers with medical professionals. Unless we have a good understanding of the condition, how can we contribute in a meaningful way to this very important process? How can we be effective advocates for our child? A survey of 1,214 parents and caregivers of children with CP found that they judged available medical information to be inadequate to guide their decision-making [8]. Educating the parent is investing in a most vital member of the child's multidisciplinary team. Obviously, in time the role of the parent passes on to the adolescent—and then the adult—themselves.

How can we know if our child is getting the best management and treatment if we don't know what best management and treatment looks like? In an ideal world, management of spastic diplegia for all individuals would be at the current limits of medical science. This book details the best treatments available and the evidence base supporting each one. I regret that I did not know about selective dorsal rhizotomy (SDR)[11] back when it would have been a treatment of choice for Tommy. (For a number of reasons, the "ideal" candidate for SDR is aged four to seven years; reasons include that secondary contracture development is still minimal. By the time I learned of SDR, Tommy was nine and had already developed contractures.)

Parents are also bombarded with treatment ideas from well-meaning family and friends. In addition to describing evidence-based treatments, this book includes information on treatments that have been disproven or still lack an evidence base.

---

11   Selective dorsal rhizotomy (SDR) is an irreversible cutting of nerve rootlets in the spinal cord to reduce spasticity.

This book also explains the expert consensus on the best management plan for spastic diplegia. I would encourage readers to ask about their center's management plan, which may not exist—but if it doesn't, asking about it puts pressure on centers to develop one. I also hope that this book puts pressure on centers to provide the best evidence-based treatments—or, in their absence, to facilitate access to centers where such treatments are available. Treatment should not be limited by zip or postal code.

The world is changing. In all areas of medicine, patients now want good information. This book is motivated by that drive.

How this book was written

I was convinced of the need for this book but was not sufficiently knowledgeable or qualified to write it alone. I proposed the idea to Dr. Tom Novacheck at Gillette, and I am eternally grateful that he understood the need. Under his stewardship and with the great help of Jean Stout, Amy Schulz, and Candice Johnson, this book exists today. Indeed, this book bears testament to the fact that at Gillette, parents and professionals work well together.

The title of this book is *Spastic Diplegia—Bilateral Cerebral Palsy.* Throughout Tommy's life, the term "spastic diplegia" was used to describe his condition, and this term remains in use in the US today. Over the past 20 years, the term "bilateral[12] spastic CP" or simply "bilateral CP" has been adopted in Europe and Australia because it is thought to provide a more accurate description of the condition. If Tommy were diagnosed in Ireland today, his condition would be called "bilateral CP." Indeed, all three terms are used in the scientific literature.

The Gross Motor Function Classification System (GMFCS) is a five-level classification system that describes the functional mobilities of children and adolescents with CP [9]. Level I has the fewest limitations and level V has the greatest. The GMFCS offers an indication of the severity of the condition. This book is relevant to those at GMFCS levels I–III: people who are capable of walking independently or with a handheld mobility device. GMFCS levels I–III account for the majority

---

12 Both sides of the body are affected.

of children, adolescents, and adults with spastic diplegia. Because self-mobility is limited in spastic diplegia, GMFCS levels IV and V, these levels are best addressed in the book *Children and Youth with Complex Cerebral Palsy* [10].

At GMFCS levels I–III, the descriptors "spastic diplegia" and "bilateral spastic CP" are largely interchangeable. For simplicity, I use just one descriptor for the condition in the text. Because "spastic diplegia" is the descriptor with which I was familiar, and because of its continued use in the US, I have chosen to use it throughout this text. This book equally applies to people with bilateral spastic CP (or simply bilateral CP), GMFCS levels I–III. Indeed, while this book focuses on spastic diplegia, much of what is addressed also applies to other forms of spastic CP at GMFCS levels I–III (hemiplegia and spastic quadriplegia).[13]

Problems with bones, muscles, and joints (musculoskeletal problems) and with walking are generally the most significant issues one encounters in spastic diplegia, GMFCS levels I–III. Because of this, the development and management of musculoskeletal and mobility problems are the main focus of this book. However, children may have problems in other areas, such as with communication or with using their hands. These problems are beyond the scope of this book.

How to read this book

Though each chapter can be read independently, many build on information presented in previous chapters. It is best to first read the book in its entirety to get an overall sense of the condition; after that, you can ignore chapters that are not currently relevant and revisit them only if they become pertinent. Throughout the book, medical/scientific information is interspersed with personal experience. Orange-colored boxes are used to separate personal experience from the other information. In addition, Chapter 5 is devoted to the experiences of people who live with this condition. My son Tommy has written the epilogue. At the back of the book you'll find a glossary with definitions of key terms you will come across.

---

13 Terms explained in section 1.6.

A companion website for this book is available at www.Gillette ChildrensHealthcarePress.org/sdbook. This website contains several resources, including:

- All "Useful web links" throughout the book, collated on one page (helpful for those reading the hardcopy version of the book)[14]
- Appendix 7, which is available online only

For simplicity, throughout the book I refer to parents and children; I acknowledge, however, that family structures vary. The term "parent" is used as a generic that includes grandparents, relatives, and carers (caregivers) who are raising a child with spastic diplegia.

Who this book is for

This book is aimed at parents of young children with spastic diplegia as well as adolescents and adults who have the condition. It should also be useful for teachers, extended family members, and students taking under-graduate therapy and other courses (such as special education). It should be helpful for members of multidisciplinary teams because it provides a holistic view of spastic diplegia. A greater understanding of spastic diplegia should help answer many of the questions people have, keep pressure on treatment centers to provide the best evidence-based treatments, and improve quality of life for people who live with this condition.

From reading this book, you will learn that:

- Spastic diplegia arises from an injury to the brain of the developing fetus or infant before two or three years. The brain injury causes problems with movement, and as a consequence, over time, muscle growth and bone development are affected. Intelligence is typically not affected in spastic diplegia.
- There is currently no cure, nor is one imminent.
- People with spastic diplegia have a relatively normal life expectancy.
- The severity of spastic diplegia (i.e., GMFCS level) can be determined by age two. It is not possible to be certain of severity before this age because the baby's brain is still developing.

---

14 All web links were checked at the time of publication, but may change over time. These web links are checked regularly and any changes are noted on this companion website.

- Spastic diplegia is generally mild or moderate, not severe.
- Almost all children with spastic diplegia GMFCS levels I–III walk in childhood.
- A number of treatments are used individually or in combination (e.g., therapies, home program, orthoses,[15] and tone[16] reduction). These treatments are used to increase stretching (to stimulate muscle growth) and to facilitate the development of mobility. The aim is to prevent or delay the onset of muscle and bone abnormalities. The muscle and bone abnormalities that may develop may be addressed with orthopedic surgery.
- Disability can increase with age, and aging can occur earlier than normal in those with spastic diplegia. Good management in childhood and adolescence can optimize outcomes in adulthood.
- Though spastic diplegia affects muscle and bone development and mobility, people with spastic diplegia are able to compete in a variety of sports. Indeed, Paralympians are proof that spastic diplegia does not have to be a barrier to achieving great levels of fitness and skill.
- In the chapter on adulthood, you will read about studies which determined the percentage of adults with CP who, for example, had chronic pain, experienced a decline in walking, or were unemployed. There is much you can do to ensure that you or your child will be among those adults with CP who do not have chronic pain, do not experience a decline in walking, and who are employed.
- There is much that the parent, adolescent, or adult can do to control how much spastic diplegia affects their lives.

---

15 An orthosis (or brace) is a device designed to hold specific body parts in position in order to modify their structure and function. It is usually made of lightweight, custom-molded plastic or carbon fiber.

16 Muscle tone is the resting tension in a person's muscles. A range of "normal" muscle tone exists. Tone is considered "abnormal" when it falls outside the range of normal or typical. It can be too low (hypotonia) or too high (hypertonia).

CHAPTER 1

Cerebral Palsy (CP)

1.1

Introduction

So be sure when you step.
Step with care and great tact
and remember that Life's
a Great Balancing Act [...]
And will you succeed?
Yes! You will, indeed!
(98 and ¾ percent guaranteed.)
Kid, you'll move mountains!
Dr. Seuss, from *Oh, the Places You'll Go!*

To fully understand spastic diplegia, it is worth first having an understanding of the "umbrella term" cerebral palsy (CP). CP was first described in 1861 by an English doctor, William Little, and for many years it was known as "Little's disease." Over the years there has been much discussion of the definition of CP, and different definitions have been adopted and later discarded. The most recently adopted definition, published in 2007, is as follows:

Cerebral palsy (CP) describes a group of permanent disorders of the development of movement and posture, causing activity limitation, that are attributed to non-progressive disturbances that occurred in the developing fetal or infant brain. The motor disorders of cerebral palsy are often accompanied by disturbances of sensation, perception, cognition, communication, and behavior, by epilepsy, and by secondary musculoskeletal problems [1].

Table 1.1.1 explains the terms used in this definition.

Table 1.1.1 Explanation of terms in definition of CP

TERMS	EXPLANATION
Cerebral	Referring to the cerebrum, the front and upper part of the brain, one of the major areas responsible for the control of movement.
Palsy	*Palsy* means paralysis, though paralysis by pure definition is not a feature of CP.
Group	CP is not a single condition, unlike conditions such as type 1 diabetes. Rather, CP is a *group* of conditions. The location, timing, and type of brain injury vary, and the resulting effects of the brain injury are also varied. A simple blood test for glucose confirms a diagnosis of type 1 diabetes. A genetic test confirms Down syndrome. Unfortunately, there is no equivalent single test for CP.
Permanent	Refers to the fact that the brain injury remains for life: CP is a lifelong condition.
Disorders	A *disorder* is a disruption in the usual orderly process. To meet the definition of CP, the disorder must cause activity limitation.
Posture	The way a person holds their body when standing or sitting.
Activity limitation	*Activity* is the execution of a task or action by an individual. *Activity limitations* are difficulties an individual may have in executing activities. Walking with difficulty is an example of an activity limitation.
Non-progressive	The brain injury does not worsen, but its effects can develop/evolve over time.
Developing fetal or infant brain	The brain injury occurs in an immature, rather than a mature, brain. An injury to the *fetal or infant brain* happens before the brain is finished developing all of its neural connections.

Cont'd.

TERMS	EXPLANATION
Motor disorders	*Motor disorders* are conditions affecting the development of movement and posture. The term *motor impairment* can also be used.
Are often accompanied by	The motor problem is often associated with other problems.
Sensation, perception, cognition, communication, and behavior	*Sensation*: Refers to the senses; i.e., vision, hearing, and others. *Perception*: The ability to incorporate and interpret sensory and/or cognitive information. *Cognition*: The mental action or process of acquiring knowledge and understanding through thought, experience, and the senses. *Communication*: The imparting or exchanging of information. *Behavior*: The way one acts or conducts oneself.
Epilepsy	*Epilepsy* is a seizure disorder. A seizure is an abnormal electrical discharge in brain cells that disrupts normal activity, behavior, or movement. Seizures can vary in length and severity.
Secondary musculoskeletal problems	*Musculoskeletal* refers to both the muscles and the skeleton; i.e., the muscles, bones, and joints. *Musculoskeletal problems* appear with time and growth, hence they are termed *secondary problems* or *abnormalities*. They develop as a consequence of the brain injury. People with CP may develop a variety of musculoskeletal problems, such as muscle/tendon contracture or bone torsion (twist).

Adapted from Rosenbaum et al. (2007).

CP is a lifelong condition. There is currently no cure [2], nor is one imminent, but good management and treatment (addressed in Chapter 3) can help alleviate some or many of the effects of the brain injury.

When the brain injury occurs is important. The consequences of a brain injury to a fetus developing in the womb are generally different from those of a brain injury sustained at birth, which in turn are different from those of a brain injury acquired during infancy. It is generally accepted that only brain injuries occurring before the age of two or three fit the definition of CP [1]. A brain injury occurring after that age is called an acquired brain injury. This cutoff is due to the differences in brain maturity when the injury occurs.

This chapter contains background information on CP. It covers:

Section 1.2   Causes, risk factors, and prevalence
Section 1.3   Diagnosis
Section 1.4   The International Classification of Functioning, Disability and Health (ICF)
Section 1.5   Motor function, gross motor milestones
Section 1.6   Classification of CP

The term "cerebral palsy" first came into our lives when Tommy was about one year old. Until then it was a term I was vaguely familiar with but could not have explained.

Tommy missed developmental milestones and was initially described as "developmentally delayed." Months passed, but no diagnosis was forthcoming. By his first birthday he was unable to sit without support or even hold a bottle. I decided to seek a second opinion from a pediatrician known to be a straight talker. On the day of the appointment, I collected our two older children from school. They remained in the waiting room, happy with the promise of a visit to the McDonald's next door after the appointment.

After the usual brief introductory pleasantries, the pediatrician examined Tommy. The conversation that followed went something like this:

Pediatrician: Do you not know what's wrong with this child?

Me: (*Politely*) No. (*Thinking:* If I did, I wouldn't be here.)

Pediatrician: (*Matter-of-fact*) He has cerebral palsy. And what's more, if I want to know how this child will turn out, I don't look at the child, I look at the mother.

Though this was certainly not what I had expected, nor what I wanted to hear, I felt a strange sense of relief after the months of uncertainty and worry. I appreciated knowing, and I appreciated the doctor's straight-talking manner.

That day, three lively children and one dazed mother visited McDonald's. That day, I had no opinion on the matter, but 25 years later I definitely agree with the pediatrician: we parents are key influencers of outcome. That day, having received Tommy's diagnosis, I wish I could have been given this book.

Useful web links

- Cerebral Palsy Alliance (2014) *What Is Cerebral Palsy?* [video] youtube.com/watch?v=Rsk3VQ-gr34

- Cerebral Palsy Foundation (2016) *What Is Cerebral Palsy?* [video] youtube.com/watch?v=8XH0WPasBzQ

- Ontario Brain Institute (2017) *Meet Jessica. This Is What She Wants You to Know about Cerebral Palsy.* [video] youtu.be/ MSd3LwwJksU

- CP Now (2015) *The Cerebral Palsy Toolkit: From Diagnosis to Understanding.* [pdf] cpnowfoundation.org/wp/wp-content/ uploads/2015/11/CP-ToolKit.pdf

- UK National Institute for Health and Care Excellence (NICE) (2017) *Cerebral Palsy in Under 25s: Assessment and Management.* [online] nice.org.uk/guidance/ng62

- Gillette Children's Specialty Healthcare (2016) *Cerebral Palsy Road Map: What to Expect as Your Child Grows.* [pdf] gillettechildrens.org/assets/uploads/care-and-conditions/ CP_Roadmap.pdf (The road map covers all types of CP and all GMFCS levels. It is organized into four age groups from birth to age 18. It covers 10 areas of interest including mobility, musculoskeletal, and interventions.)

1.2

Causes, risk factors, and prevalence

The little reed, bending to the force of the wind,
soon stood upright again when the storm had passed over.

Aesop

Causes and risk factors

The term "cause" is self-explanatory. The term "risk factor" can be defined as "any attribute, characteristic, or exposure of an individual that increases the likelihood of developing a disease or injury" [1]. Causes thus have a stronger relationship with CP than risk factors. Significant deprivation of oxygen to the infant's brain, for example, is a cause of CP. Preterm birth is a risk factor but not a cause of CP—in other words, not every preterm baby is found to have CP. There are many possible causes of brain injury, including events before and during pregnancy, during birth, or in early infant life. Much is known about the causes and risk factors for CP, but much remains unknown as well. Depending on what you read, you may come across different lists of causes and risk factors for CP. The following are from the Gillette website [2].

a) Causes of CP

Developing fetuses and infants (up to age two to three) can develop CP if they experience brain injury or disruptions in brain development caused by:

- Bleeding in the brain before, during, or after birth
- Infections of the brain, including meningitis or encephalitis[17]
- Shock—a state in which organs and tissues do not receive adequate blood flow
- Traumatic brain injuries, such as from a serious car accident
- Seizures at birth or in the first month following birth
- Certain genetic conditions

b) Risk factors for CP

Risk factors for CP include:

- Preterm birth and low birth weight. A typical pregnancy lasts 40 weeks. Babies born before 37 weeks have a greater risk of having CP. The risk increases the earlier a baby is born and the lower the baby's birth weight. Twins and other multiple-birth siblings are at particular risk because they tend to be born earlier and at lower birth weights.
- Serious illness, stroke, or infection in the mother. CP is more common in children whose mothers:
  - Experience certain viral and bacterial infections and/or high fevers during pregnancy.
  - Have coagulation (clotting) disorders or experience blood clots during pregnancy.
  - Receive excessive exposure to harmful substances during pregnancy.
  - Have thyroid problems, seizure disorders, or other serious health concerns.
- Serious illness, stroke, or infection in the baby. Infants who experience serious illnesses, strokes, or seizures around the time of birth are at greater risk of having CP. Such illnesses might include:
  - Severe jaundice. (Kernicterus is a rare kind of preventable brain damage that can happen in newborns with jaundice.)
  - Seizures during the first 48 hours after birth.

---

17 Encephalitis is an acute inflammation (swelling) of the brain, normally resulting from a viral infection or the immune system mistakenly attacking the brain tissue.

- ○ Infections of the brain, such as meningitis or encephalitis.
- ○ Strokes caused by broken or clogged blood vessels or abnormal blood cells.
- Pregnancy and birth complications. For example, not enough nutrition through the placenta or a lack of oxygen during labor and birth. Incompatible blood types between mother and baby.
- Genetic issues.

c) What the literature tells us

- Although any one risk factor, if severe, may be sufficient to cause CP, more often it is the presence of multiple risk factors that leads to CP. One factor may interact with another to cause the brain injury, such as an event (or events) during pregnancy combined with the stress of birth combined with a genetic vulnerability [3].
- The literature suggests that events during pregnancy are more likely to cause CP than events during labor or delivery. More specifically:
  - ○ A major US study, called the Collaborative Perinatal Project, conducted between 1959 and 1974 followed approximately 50,000 women and their children from the first prenatal visit until the children were seven years old. It found that events during labor and delivery were not major contributors to the occurrence of CP; most cases had their origins before labor began. A second finding was that intrauterine inflammation[18] was a major cause of adverse pregnancy outcome [4].
  - ○ At least 70 percent of cases of CP have antecedents[19] during pregnancy, and only 10 to 20 percent of cases are related to the child's birth [5]. Neither the routine use of fetal monitoring during labor nor the increased incidence of caesarean births (factors which reduce risk during labor and delivery) have reduced the number of cases of CP [5].
  - ○ Most brain injuries which cause CP occur in the second half of pregnancy, a period when the rate of brain development is fastest [6].

---

18 Inflammation occurs when part of the body becomes reddened, swollen, hot, and often painful, especially as a reaction to injury or infection.

19 Things that existed before or that logically preceded another event.

- Some risk factors are on the decline, but others are increasing [5,7]. Advances in neonatal care have reduced the risk of birth injury. However, with these advances more preterm infants and infants with low birth weight are surviving, some of whom may develop CP. In vitro fertilization has led to more multiple births, and multiple births, as noted above, is a risk factor for CP. The fact that some risk factors are decreasing while others are increasing is leading to a change in the type of CP that develops. For example, an injury to a brain at 24 weeks can have a different effect than one at 28 weeks or 36 weeks. Until recently, babies born at 24 weeks would not have survived. Now, thankfully, many of these babies survive; however, some may develop CP. The most common types of CP differ in different parts of the world, depending on risk factors.
- In approximately 90 percent of cases, CP results from healthy brain tissue becoming damaged rather than from abnormalities in brain development [7].
- Confirmation of the presence of a brain injury by magnetic resonance imaging (MRI) occurs in many but not all cases. Up to 17 percent of people with CP have normal MRI brain scans [7]. Imaging may also help determine when the brain injury occurred [7].
- The cause of CP in an individual child is very often unknown [8].

> We don't know what caused Tommy's CP, but that is not unusual. Like many other parents, I would like to have known.

Prevalence

The prevalence of a condition is how many people in a defined population have the condition at a specific point in time. Prevalence rates can vary geographically. A 2013 worldwide review found that the overall prevalence of CP was 2.11 per 1,000 live births [9].[20] It also found that the prevalence of CP has remained constant despite increased survival of at-risk preterm infants. A recent (2019) study, however, reported that the birth prevalence[21] of CP declined across Australian states between

---

20 Births up to 2004.

21 This was formerly referred to as "incidence," but the term "birth prevalence" is now felt to be more accurate [10].

1995 and 2009 [10]. The percentage of children with CP whose disability was moderate to severe also decreased. This is encouraging.

Some further points:
- CP is the most common cause of physical disability in children [7].
- Males are at higher risk of CP than females. Recent data from Australia found that 57 percent of those with CP were male, while males represented 51 percent of all births [11]. This may be because males have certain nerve cell vulnerabilities that may result in CP [5]. It is noteworthy that there are frequently more male than female participants in CP studies.
- Relative to its prevalence and its impact on the life span of those with the condition, funding for CP research is very low. The National Institutes of Health (NIH) is the primary US body responsible for health research; it reports research funding by condition. Although the reported prevalence of CP was three times higher than that of Down syndrome (0.3 percent versus 0.1 percent), funding allocated to CP research in 2018 ($26 million) was significantly lower than that allocated to Down syndrome research ($60 million) [12]. Funding estimates for 2019 and 2020 are $28 and $24 million, respectively, for CP and $72 and $65 million for Down syndrome.

I believe it would be beneficial if, once a child is diagnosed with CP (up to three years after birth), there were some way of conveying this diagnosis to the obstetrician who provided care to the mother and infant during pregnancy and birth. This information may inform future practice. Or parents could consider giving consent to have their child added to a properly governed regional or national CP register and allowing appropriate access to medical records from pregnancy and birth.

Though I did not know what caused Tommy's CP, in the early days I wasted a lot of time feeling guilty. I had worked very hard and was stressed during his pregnancy, and I felt responsible. Today I no longer feel that sense of guilt. I didn't knowingly do anything wrong: my life circumstances were such that I was very busy, and besides, there are multiple possible causes of brain injury. I encourage parents to waste no time on guilt—we are where we are and we must move forward.

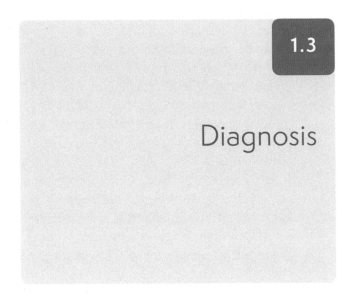

1.3

Diagnosis

Acceptance is knowing that grief is a raging river.
And you have to get into it.
Because when you do, it carries you to the next place.
It eventually takes you to open land,
somewhere where it will turn out OK in the end.
Simone George

Sometimes it is obvious from birth that a new baby has CP, but in many cases it is not. The possibility may be anticipated because of problems in pregnancy or a preterm or difficult birth, or the suspicion may only arise when developmental milestones are missed. Even if a professional is suspicious of CP, that suspicion may not be communicated to parents. Unfortunately, unlike with other conditions, such as Down syndrome, there is no definitive test for CP.

The difficulty of diagnosing CP arises more in the mild and moderate forms of the condition since the severe forms are generally apparent early on. The majority of spastic diplegia is mild or moderate, thus the difficulty of diagnosis is a very real issue. However, there seems to be a recent shift toward earlier diagnosis:

- McIntyre and colleagues (2011) proposed a change from referring an infant for intervention following a formal—most often late—diagnosis of CP to doing so as soon as the infant is considered "at risk" of CP. (Their paper was titled "Cerebral Palsy—Don't Delay." [1])
- Graham and colleagues (2016) noted that any infant with known risk factors should be considered at risk and enhanced screening should be offered [2].
- A number of assessments can be used for diagnosis before five months corrected age,[22] including MRI, Prechtl's General Movements Assessment, Test of Infant Motor Performance (TIMP),[23] and a standardized neurological examination [3,4].

Novak and colleagues (2017) noted that clinicians[24] should understand the importance of prompt referral to diagnostic-specific early intervention in order to [4]:

- Optimize infant motor and cognitive plasticity[25]
- Prevent secondary musculoskeletal problems
- Support the parents after they have received the diagnosis

Parents' chief criticisms of medical professionals responsible for diagnosis relate to unclear information and communication of a pessimistic outlook [5].

Diagnosis has been described as a process, not an event [6]. There's only so much parents can absorb in the first meeting, so subsequent follow-up is needed.

---

22 With preterm babies, it takes time to determine whether the delays are related to being preterm or are true delays. The term "corrected age" refers to how old a baby would be if they had been born on their due date rather than preterm. "Chronological age" refers to how old a baby is from their date of birth. Corrected age is often used when assessing growth and developmental skills.

23 Prechtl's General Movements Assessment and Test of Infant Motor Performance (TIMP) are assessments of infant movement.

24 Clinicians are medical professionals who have direct contact with patients rather than being involved with, for example, research or laboratory work.

25 "Cognition" may be defined as the process of acquiring knowledge and understanding. Motor and cognitive plasticity are types of neuroplasticity. "Plasticity" refers to the ability of the human brain to recover after an injury through the ability of nerve cells to alter their structure and function in response to a variety of external and internal pressures, including behavioral training [7].

Receiving the news that your beautiful child has CP is very tough for parents, who may then go through a grieving process. Looking back, I found that the diagnosis was almost a help after all the months of uncertainty. It galvanized me into immediate action to find out how I could best help my child. This was probably my way of coping with the news. Every parent will deal with the diagnosis in their own way, but I would encourage all parents to try to get as good an understanding of the condition as they can, as soon as they can. To that end this book may be helpful.

One of the early readers of this book, a nurse and psychotherapist who has a son with spastic diplegia, wrote a piece about the different stages of dealing with a diagnosis. I've included it in Appendix 1.

Looking back at photographs from Tommy's first year, I can now see that the signs of his CP were obvious from very early on. In retrospect, I feel his diagnosis could have been made much earlier. Because he wasn't diagnosed until he was a year old, intervention only started in earnest then. If a clinician suspects a child of having CP, I believe they should communicate this to the parents immediately. The possible harm done by delaying diagnosis, and therefore intervention, is to my mind greater than the possible harm done by raising a suspicion that later proves unwarranted. The only intervention the child is likely to receive during that period is physical therapy, which won't do them any harm.

You may ask, why would a diagnosis be delayed? One reason is that a physician might not want to give parents this significant diagnosis until they are very sure that it is accurate.

What should a medical professional who is not responsible for diagnosis do if they strongly suspects a child in their care has CP? In my view, such a professional has a responsibility to communicate, without delay, with the person responsible for diagnosis. Likewise, if parents have any suspicion that their child may have a problem, they should communicate it to their physician as soon as possible.

I remember discussing diagnosis with a friend who made an interesting point: sometimes the parent would rather not hear bad news; having one foot out the door, so to speak, may be easiest for both the physician and the parent. But this doesn't make sense—it just prolongs the anxiety and delays intervention while the clock is ticking.

I was happy to read in the literature about the recent shift toward earlier diagnosis. I was also heartened to read a paper by Graham and colleagues (2016) noting that mothers of children with CP who have previously had a typically developing child often sense that something is wrong at a very early stage [8]. This paper advised professionals to take the concerns of an experienced parent seriously. I sensed that something was wrong when Tommy was just a day old. He cried so incessantly that by evening I asked if he could be checked by a pediatrician. I did not feel all was fine; his prolonged crying had an unusual pitch. The on-duty pediatrician came to see him and reassured me that all was well, and I accepted her reassurance. Years later, I remember gently suggesting to a close friend that she have her baby assessed because I felt he had a very unusual cry. My friend's baby turned out to have a significant developmental problem.

When Tommy was very young, I read a short essay titled "Welcome to Holland." It was written in 1987 by Emily Perl Kingsley, a writer on the TV series *Sesame Street*, about parenting her son, who was born with Down syndrome. She described it as going on vacation, but not to the expected destination. Though some people may find it overly sentimental, the essay resonates with me to this day. I've included a web link to it at the end of this section.

Useful web links

- Cerebral Palsy Alliance (2018) *Prechtl's General Movements Assessment.* [pdf] cerebralpalsy.org.au/wp-content/uploads/2018/03/Parental-Fact-Sheets.pdf

- National Down Syndrome Society (1987) "A Parent's Perspective: Welcome to Holland by Emily Perl Kingsley." [online] ndss.org/resources/a-parents-perspective/

- CP-NET (2015) *Creating Possibilities for Cerebral Palsy.* [video] vimeo.com/141592022

1.4

The International Classification of Functioning, Disability and Health (ICF)

The individual is rarely going to be altered very much,
whereas the environment slowly but surely can.

Tom Shakespeare

The World Health Organization (WHO)[26] developed a framework for considering any health condition called the International Classification of Functioning, Disability and Health [1]. The framework[27] helps show the impact of a health condition at different levels and how those levels are interconnected. It reminds us to look at the full picture—to look at the person with a disability in the context of their world. The framework's long title is abbreviated to ICF; the F stands for Functioning, which shows where its emphasis lies.

The framework gives us a way of looking at the concepts of health and disability. It acknowledges that every human being can experience

---

26 The World Health Organization (WHO) is the agency of the United Nations concerned with public health. In 1948, the year it was established, the WHO adopted the following definition of health: "Health is a state of complete physical, mental, and social well-being and not merely the absence of disease or infirmity." This is a very interesting and broad definition. It is also interesting that this 1948 definition has not been amended—it has stood the test of time.

27 A framework is a structure to explain a particular concept.

a decrease in health and thereby experience some disability. It is not something that happens only to a minority of people. The ICF thus "mainstreams" disability and recognizes it as a widespread human experience. By shifting the focus from the *cause* to the *impact* of a health condition, the ICF places all health conditions on an equal footing, allowing them to be compared [2].

You might wonder why we need a framework to understand a health condition. As I became more familiar with the ICF, I could really see its usefulness. The idea that every human being can experience a decrease in health and therefore experience some disability is useful because it illustrates that people don't fit neatly into one of two boxes (metaphorically speaking), healthy or disabled. There is, rather, a continuum between health and disability. The framework is helpful because it focuses on how a person with CP functions in their life.

See Figure 1.4.1.

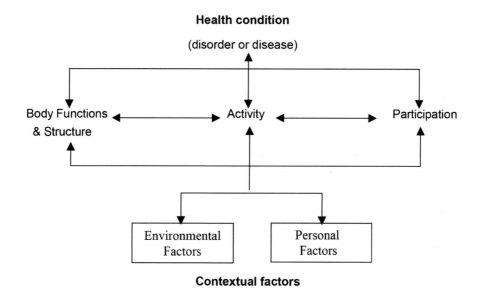

Figure 1.4.1 International Classification of Functioning, Disability and Health (ICF). Reproduced with kind permission from WHO.

The framework describes three levels of human functioning and characterizes disability as difficulty functioning at one or more of these three levels [1,2]:

- **Body functions and structure** refers to functioning at the level of the body or a body part.[28] Spasticity is at this level. **Impairments** are problems in body function or structure, such as a significant deviation or loss.
- **Activity** is the execution of a task or action by an individual. Is the person able to walk or kick a ball? **Activity limitations** are difficulties an individual may have in executing activities. To meet the latest (2007) definition of CP, a permanent motor disorder has to cause activity limitation [3].
- **Participation** is involvement in a life situation. Being able to play sports with friends or having a job are examples of participating in society. **Participation restrictions** are problems an individual may experience with their involvement in life situations.

The framework also includes factors that influence any of the three levels of functioning (termed contextual factors):

- **Environmental factors** make up the physical, social, and attitudinal environment in which people live and conduct their lives [2]. Examples of physical environment include structural barriers at home and in the community, such as steps or stairs without handrails in the house, or a school building with stairs but no elevator.
- **Personal factors** include gender, age, coping style, social background, education, profession, past and present experiences, and other factors that influence how disability is experienced by the person [2]. Examples of personal factors include a person's attitude, determination, motivation, and perseverance.

The three levels of human functioning, plus environmental and personal factors, are all interconnected with the health condition.

With regard to activity, the ICF distinguishes between **motor capacity**—what a person can do in a standardized, controlled environment, and **motor performance**—what a person actually does in their daily

---

28 The WHO formally defines "body functions" as physiological functions of body systems (including psychological functions). "Body structures" are defined as anatomical parts of the body such as organs, limbs, and their components [2].

environment. For example: is the child walking at an appointment on a smooth surface with the medical professional and parent watching and encouraging them the same as their walking in a crowded playground on possibly uneven surfaces?

There is a third concept to keep in mind when considering activity: **motor capability**—what a person can do in their daily environment [4]. For example, a child may be able to ride a bike to school—they have the capability—but they may choose not to. Their performance is influenced by their choice. Holsbeeke and colleagues (2009) noted that physical and social environment and personal factors such as motivation influence the relationship between capacity, capability, and performance.

A series of "F-words" have been developed and inserted into the different areas of the ICF, providing a useful adaptation of the framework [5]. See Figure 1.4.2. The authors highlighted **fitness, function, friends, family, fun,** and **future** as areas of focus for the child with a health condition. Indeed, these also apply to adults. Web links to a number of useful videos on the F-words are included at the end of this section.

I've observed how becoming familiar with the ICF has influenced my thinking over the years. In the early days, I was very focused on issues at the level of body functions and structure. Later I came to understand the relationship between the three levels. For example, orthopedic surgery leads to improvements at the level of body functions and structure by addressing muscle and bone problems. As a result, the child may walk more easily and their walking might consume less energy. This is an improvement at the activity level. If walking is less tiring, the child might be able to keep up and do more with their peers—an improvement at the participation level. I also came to understand that treatments need to benefit a child at the level of activity and/or participation rather than purely at the level of body functions and structure. It is important to keep in mind that one cannot assume that a treatment at one level will necessarily help the child at another [6].

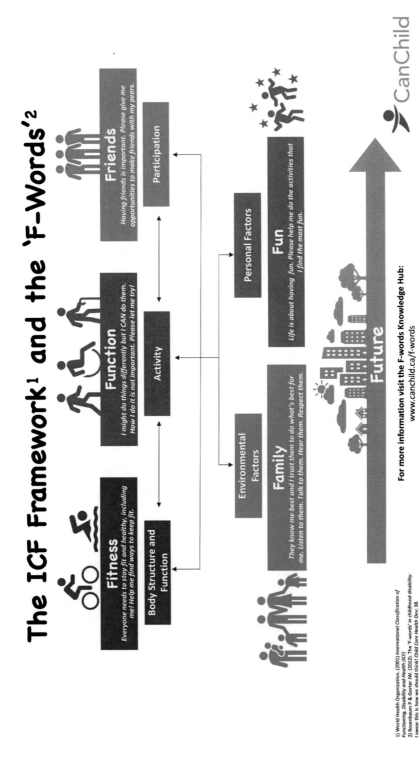

The ICF Framework[1] and the 'F-Words'[2]

Fitness
Everyone needs to stay fit and healthy, including me! Help me find ways to keep fit.

Body Structure and Function

Function
I might do things differently but I CAN do them. How I do it is not important. Please let me try!

Activity

Friends
Having friends is important. Please give me opportunities to make friends with my peers.

Participation

Environmental Factors

Family
They know me best and I trust them to do what's best for me. Listen to them. Talk to them. Hear them. Respect them.

Personal Factors

Fun
Life is about having fun. Please help me do the activities that I find the most fun.

Future

CanChild

1) World Health Organization. (2001) *International Classification of Functioning, Disability and Health (ICF)*
2) Rosenbaum P & Gorter JW. (2012). The 'F-words' in childhood disability: I swear this is how we should think! *Child Care Health Dev*; 38.

For more information visit the F-words Knowledge Hub:
www.canchild.ca/f-words

Figure 1.4.2 The ICF framework (WHO 2001) and the F-words (Rosenbaum and Gorter 2012). Reproduced with kind permission from CanChild.

Useful web links

- CanChild (2019) *The ICF for Parents (P-ICF)*. [online] canchild.ca/en/the-icf-for-parents-p-icf (Scroll down the page for a very useful video series on the ICF.)

- Cerebral Palsy Foundation (2016) *The F Words of Disability*. [video] youtu.be/tFeV166kuUY

- CP-NET (2018) *My Favourite Words*. [video] vimeo.com/252166407

- CP-NET (2015) *These Six F-Words Won't Fill up Your Swear Jar: What Do the F-Words Mean to Youth with Impairments?* [video] vimeo.com/236235559

1.5

Motor function, gross motor milestones

That's one small step for man,
one giant leap for mankind.

Neil Armstrong

Motor function

Motor function is divided into two types: gross motor function and fine motor function.

- **Gross motor function** (or **gross motor skills** or **gross motor activities**) refers to the movement of the arms, legs, and other large body parts. It involves the use of large muscles. Examples include sitting, crawling, standing, running, jumping, swimming, throwing, catching, and kicking. These movements involve maintaining balance and changing position.

- **Fine motor function** (or **fine motor skills** or **fine motor activities**) refers to smaller movements that occur in the wrists, hands, fingers, feet, and toes. It involves the control of small muscles. Examples include picking up objects between the thumb and forefinger, and writing. These movements typically involve hand-eye coordination and require a high degree of precision of hand and finger movement.

The development of gross and fine motor skills is under neurological control (i.e., under the control of the nervous system) and is affected to varying degrees in CP. Gross and fine motor function may improve somewhat without treatment, but treatment is essential to maximize the individual's motor function as early as possible, which is why early intervention is so important.

Gross motor milestones

There is a usual sequence and timing to the achievement of gross motor milestones in the typically developing child. A large study conducted by the WHO found that, with some variation, almost all typically developing children have achieved independent sitting by nine months and independent walking by 18 months [1].[29] The average age and age range for achieving each of the six gross motor milestones are as follows:
- Sitting without support ···························· 6.0 (3.8–9.2) months
- Standing with assistance ···················· 7.6 (4.8–11.4) months
- Hands and knees crawling ················· 8.5 (5.2–13.5) months
- Walking with assistance ···················· 9.2 (5.9–13.7) months
- Standing alone ······························ 11.0 (6.9–16.9) months
- Walking alone ······························· 12.1 (8.2–17.6) months

These milestones are an important reference when a child appears to be late in development compared with typically developing children. One of the hallmarks of CP is that the child may be late achieving gross motor milestones. In fact, that may be what first alerts parents and/or professionals to a problem. It is also worth noting that not all children crawl (even typically developing children).

The earlier motor development stages—sitting, standing, crawling—are important for the development of walking. Earlier developmental stages include the precursors of later ones. To the extent possible, following (going through) these motor development stages is important for the child with CP. However, there is a balance to be achieved. For example, research has shown that providing powered mobility to children as young as 2.5 years of age who have more severe motor disabilities is beneficial in terms of function and development [2,3]. With powered

29 The study collected data from 816 healthy children over multiple years in different regions and is representative of children worldwide. The study found no difference between boys and girls.

mobility the children's language, exploration, social function, and efforts at self-initiated movement showed improvement. Even for children with less severe motor disability, there may be a balance between following normal motor development stages and promoting the child's activity and participation.

A web link to the WHO gross motor milestones is included at the end of this section. A web link to the developmental milestones published by the US Centers for Disease Control and Prevention (CDC)[30] is also included. In addition to movement and physical development, the CDC's information sheet includes social/emotional, language/communication, and cognitive (learning, thinking, and problem-solving) development for children up to five years of age.

Measuring gross motor function

One commonly used method for measuring gross motor function in CP is the Gross Motor Function Measure (GMFM) [4]. The GMFM-88 consists of 88 items (skills) that measure a child's abilities in five areas of increasing gross motor function:

- Lying and rolling
- Sitting
- Crawling and kneeling
- Standing
- Walking, running, and jumping

The 88 items are skills that are well established in typically developing children by the age of five. A web link to the full 88 GMFM items is included at the end of this section. It is worth consulting because it gives you an idea of the skills that exist beyond independent walking (item 69 on the GMFM). They include stepping over obstacles, kicking a ball, running, jumping, and stair climbing. These skills involve balance. The assessment is completed (usually by a physical therapist) with the child in bare feet—that is, without walking aids, orthoses, or shoes. (The assistance these supports provide can be checked by repeating the assessment with them. A child may be able to walk with orthoses, shoes,

---

30 The Centers for Disease Control and Prevention (CDC) is the leading national public health institute in the US.

and crutches for support, for example, but not without them.) Most children with even mild CP fail to complete all items.[31]

The results for each item are then totaled and expressed as a percentage of the maximum possible score. The higher a child's gross motor function, the higher their GMFM-88 score. There is also a shorter, 66-item version called the GMFM-66 [5]. The GMFM-66 requires software to compute the result.[32] It is scored 0–100.

In relation to the ICF, the GMFM measures skills at the activity level. GMFM is a measure of what the child can do, not how well they do it. For example, item 69 tests whether the child can walk forward 10 steps, not how well they walk that distance. (In addition, as noted above, the child may not be able to walk the distance in bare feet but may be able to walk it with an aid, such as crutches.)

Further information on gross motor function is included in Appendix 2.

As a parent, I never thought too much about walking. My two older children walked before their first birthdays and developed running and jumping skills without my ever having to notice or think about them. It is only when there is a problem that we begin to think about what walking actually involves.

The reason I include so much information on gross motor function in this section is to ensure that readers understand what it means to improve gross motor function. It's about more than merely achieving the gross motor milestones: a small increase in gross motor function, as measured by the GMFM, can have a big effect on the child's life.

---

31 Gross motor function is not exclusively measured by the GMFM. There are a number of tools that are used to screen for developmental motor delays in addition to motor function depending on the age of the child. They include Test of Infant Motor Performance, Bayley Scales of Infant and Toddler Development, Peabody Development Motor Scales, and Bruininks Oseretsky Test of Motor Proficiency.

32 In the GMFM-66 items are graded by difficulty, whereas in the GMFM-88 all items contribute equally to the overall result regardless of difficulty.

Useful web links

- CanChild (2013) *GMFM Score Sheet*. [pdf] canchild.ca/system/
tenon/assets/attachments/000/000/218/original/gmfm-88_and_66_
scoresheet.pdf

- WHO (2019) *Motor Development Milestones*. [online]
who.int/childgrowth/standards/motor_milestones/en/

- CDC (2019) *CDC's Developmental Milestones*. [online]
cdc.gov/ncbddd/actearly/milestones/index.html

- Healthy Children (2019) *Does My Child Have Physical
Developmental Delays?* [online] healthychildren.org/English/
MotorDelay/Pages/default.aspx#/ (Healthy Children is a website
of the American Academy of Pediatrics.)

1.6

Classification
of CP

*Order and simplification are the first
steps toward the mastery of a subject.
The actual enemy is the unknown.*
Thomas Mann, from *The Magic Mountain*

Classification of CP

Over the years, there has been much discussion of the classification of CP. Classification, or dividing into groups, is useful for a number of reasons. First, it provides information about the nature of the condition and its severity (its level or magnitude). Second, it allows us to learn from people who have the condition at a similar level.

A good measurement or classification system must be:
- **Valid:** It actually measures what it claims to measure.
- **Reliable:** It provides the same answer when used by different people or by the same person at different times.
- **Accurate:** It measures how close a value is to its true value. (An example would be how close an arrow gets to the target.)
- **Precise:** It measures how repeatable a measurement is. (An example

would be how close the second arrow is to the first one, regardless of whether either is near the target.)

A kitchen scale (weighing scales) can be used to illustrate the different concepts:
- If the scale claims to measure weight and does so, then the scale is valid.
- If it provides the same reading regardless of who uses it or when they use it, then the scale is reliable.
- If the reading is correct when a known standard weight is weighed, then the scale is accurate.
- If repeated weighings of the same item give the same reading (whether accurate or not), then the scale is precise.

In this section we cover three main methods of classifying CP. These are based on:
a) **Topography:** The area of the body affected
b) **Motor impairment:** The type of motor disorder (a motor disorder affects the development of movement and posture)
c) **Gross motor function:** The level of functional mobility

a) Classification of CP on the basis of topography

The historical method of classifying CP is on the basis of topography—the area of the body affected [1,2]. The suffix "-plegia" is derived from the Greek word for stroke. The prefixes "mono-," "hemi-," "di-," "tri-," and "quad-," again derived from the Greek or Latin words, indicate the area of the body affected. See Table 1.6.1.

One of the disadvantages of this classification system is a lack of precision. However, this method of classifying CP has been and continues to be used extensively, particularly the terms "hemiplegia," "diplegia," and "quadriplegia" in the US.

A recently adopted classification system, again based on topography, was adopted by the Surveillance of Cerebral Palsy in Europe (SCPE) group [3]. The SCPE's classification system is thought to be reasonably reliable with room for improvement [4]. It is now generally used in Europe and Australia. It identifies two main types of CP: unilateral and bilateral. See Table 1.6.2.

Table 1.6.1 Classification of CP on the basis of topography—historically [1,2]

CP SUBTYPE	AREA OF BODY AFFECTED	
Monoplegia	*Mono* = One Affecting one limb, usually the lower limb.	
Hemiplegia	*Hemi* = Half Affecting the upper and lower limbs on one side of the body. The upper limb is usually more affected than the lower limb.	
Diplegia	*Di* = Two Affecting all limbs, but the lower limbs are much more affected than the upper limbs, which frequently only show fine motor impairment.	
Triplegia	*Tri* = Three Affecting three limbs, usually the two lower limbs and one upper limb. The lower limb is usually more affected on the side of the upper-limb involvement.	
Quadriplegia	*Quad* = Four Affecting all four limbs and the trunk. This is also known as tetraplegia.	

Table 1.6.2 Classification of CP on the basis of topography—SCPE [3]

CP SUBTYPE	AREA OF BODY AFFECTED	
Unilateral	One side of the body is affected.	
Bilateral	Both sides of the body are affected.	

b) Classification of CP on the basis of motor impairment

Another method classifies CP into subtypes based on the predominant features of the motor impairment.[33] CP is characterized by abnormal muscle tone and problems with motor control which may or may not include involuntary movements. A brief explanation of the subtypes is included in Table 1.6.3.

Most studies report that spasticity is the most common type of motor impairment, though the exact percentage varies. The general consensus is that 60 to 85 percent of those with CP have the spastic form [5]. Only spastic CP is subdivided into bilateral or unilateral [3]. This is because dyskinetic and ataxic CP generally affect the whole body.

A web link to a useful video titled *Types of CP* is included at the end of this section.

---

33 A motor impairment or motor disorder is a condition affecting the development of movement and posture.

Table 1.6.3 Classification of CP on the basis of motor impairment

CP SUBTYPE	EXPLANATION
Spastic (spasticity)	*Spasticity* is a condition in which there is an abnormal increase in muscle tone or stiffness of muscle which might interfere with movement, speech, or be associated with discomfort or pain [6]. Lance (1980) included "a velocity-dependent increase in the stretch reflex" in his definition of spasticity [7]. Spastic CP can be subdivided into *unilateral* or *bilateral* based on whether one or two sides of the body are involved [3].
Dyskinetic (dyskinesia)	*Dyskinetic* CP is defined as "abnormal patterns of posture and/or movement associated with involuntary, uncontrolled, recurring, occasionally stereotyped movement patterns" [1]. (*Stereotyped movement patterns* means the movements are in a particular pattern, specific to that person, which is repeated.) Dyskinetic CP can be subdivided into either *dystonic* or *choreo-athetotic* CP [3]. • **Dystonic (dystonia):** The dystonias are movement disorders in which sustained muscle contractions cause twisting and repetitive movements or abnormal postures. The movements, which are involuntary and sometimes painful, may affect a single muscle; a group of muscles such as those in the arms, legs, or neck; or the entire body [8]. • **Choreo-athetotic (choreo-athetosis):** *Chorea* is characterized by brief, irregular contractions that are not repetitive or rhythmic but appear to flow from one muscle to the next. Chorea often occurs with *athetosis*, which adds twisting and writhing movements [9].
Ataxic (ataxia)	People with *ataxia* experience a failure of muscle control in their arms and legs, resulting in a lack of balance and coordination or a disturbance of gait [10].
Mixed	Some people have a mixture of both abnormal muscle tone and/or involuntary movements. For example, some people with spastic diplegia may have both spasticity and dystonia. CP is classified by the predominant feature: if spasticity is the predominant feature, then the person is said to have spastic CP; if dystonia is the predominant feature, then the person is said to have dystonic CP. However, some people can be classed as having *mixed* CP where there is no clear predominant feature.

c) Classification of CP on the basis of gross motor function

The final method of classifying CP is on the basis of gross motor function using the Gross Motor Function Classification System (GMFCS). As noted in the previous section, gross motor function involves the movement of the arms, legs, and other large body parts.

The GMFCS is a five-level classification system that describes the functional mobility of children and adolescents with CP [11]. It is based on how children and adolescents move on their own, with emphasis on sitting, transfers (moving from one position to another), and mobility. The GMFCS includes descriptions for five age groups: less than two years, two to four years, four to six years, six to 12 years, and 12 to 18 years. The emphasis is on the child/adolescent's usual performance in their daily environment (i.e, their home and community).[34] By choosing which description best matches the child at their current age, a child can be assigned a GMFCS level.

The following are descriptions of the five levels; these correspond to the method that best describes the child's functional mobility after age six. Level I has the fewest movement limitations and level V has the greatest, thus the severity of the movement limitations increases with each increasing level. It is important to note, however, that the differences between the levels are not even.
- **Level I** ······ Walks without limitations
- **Level II** ······ Walks with limitations
- **Level III** ····· Walks using a handheld mobility device
- **Level IV** ····· Self-mobility with limitations; may use powered mobility
- **Level V** ······ Transported in a manual wheelchair

Although the levels are based on the method of functional mobility that best describes the child's performance after age six, a child can be classified much earlier using these descriptions.

---

34 In this context, "community" may be interpreted as "away from home." Moving about at home is generally easier since home is likely well suited or adapted to the person's needs. The community may be more challenging. It is important to keep in mind the impact of environmental and personal factors on what children and adolescents are able to do in their daily environment (home or community). This was addressed in Section 1.4, The International Classification of Functioning, Disability and Health (ICF).

The following summarizes the commencement of walking for children with CP at GMFCS levels I–III [12]:

- At GMFCS level I, children walk between 18 months and two years without the need for any assistive mobility device.[35] (Note that even at GMFCS level I, this is later than for typically developing children, as noted in the gross motor milestones in section 1.5.)
- At GMFCS level II, children aged two to four walk using an assistive mobility device as their preferred method of mobility. At ages four to six, they walk without the need for a handheld mobility device indoors and for short distances on level surfaces outdoors.
- At GMFCS level III, children aged two to four may walk short distances indoors using a handheld mobility device (walker) and adult assistance for steering and turning. At ages four to six, they walk with a handheld mobility device on level surfaces.

The full version of the GMFCS is a short document that contains very useful information. A web link to it is included at the end of this section. The document contains further detail on mobility for each age and GMFCS level. It also includes a summary of the distinctions between each level to help determine the level that most closely resembles a particular child/adolescent's current gross motor function. Web links to videos explaining the GMFCS are also included at the end of this section.

The GMFCS has been proven to be relatively stable over time after age 2 [11]. A recent Swedish study provided further evidence of the stability of the GMFCS [13]. Because the GMFCS level is stable, once a child's GMFCS level is known, it offers insight into what the future may hold in terms of the child's mobility. It helps answer some of the many questions we parents have in the early days, such as, "Will our child walk?" or, "How serious is their CP?"

It is important to note that just as a child's diagnosis of spastic diplegia is generally stable throughout their life, their GMFCS level is generally stable. In other words, the area of the body affected and the severity of the condition (the GMFCS level) generally do not change.

---

35 Assistive mobility devices (also termed assistive devices, walking aids, mobility aids, and gait aids) include walking sticks (canes), crutches, reverse walker, gait trainer (a device which is more supportive than a walker but less supportive than a wheelchair), and wheelchair.

Traditionally, medical professionals made the assessment, but the *GMFCS Family Report Questionnaire* (web link also included) now allows parents or the young person themselves to do so. Professional and family reports have been shown to be consistent [14]. Useful illustrations have been developed based on the GMFCS for the two upper age bands (six to 12 years and 12 to 18 years) by staff at the Royal Children's Hospital in Melbourne. See Figures 1.6.1 and 1.6.2.

The SCPE classified walking ability into three levels according to the GMFCS [15]:
- **Mild** ⋯⋯⋯⋯⋯⋯⋯ Independent walker; GMFCS levels I–II
- **Moderate** ⋯⋯⋯⋯⋯ Walker with aid; GMFCS level III
- **Severe** ⋯⋯⋯⋯⋯⋯ Wheelchair; GMFCS levels IV–V

The GMFCS has been translated into many languages and is used all over the world. One of its many advantages is its simplicity. Though the GMFCS is now used in adulthood, particularly in research studies, it has not yet been validated for adults. Hopefully it will be. One study compared the GMFCS level of adults with CP with their GMFCS level at age 12 and found that GMFCS level observed around age 12 was highly predictive of motor function in adulthood [16].

Let us now look at how individuals with spastic diplegia are distributed across the different GMFCS levels. Figure 1.6.3 shows the proportion of children with CP by topography (area of the body affected) and gross motor function (GMFCS level) using data collated from five studies [17–21].

Figure 1.6.3 shows that:
- 36 percent of people with CP had hemiplegia, 36 percent had diplegia, and 28 percent had quadriplegia.[36]
- Of those with hemiplegia, 96 percent were at GMFCS levels I–III.
- Of those with diplegia, 85 percent were at GMFCS levels I–III.
- Of those with quadriplegia, 27 percent were at GMFCS levels I–III.

Thus this data shows that the majority of individuals with spastic diplegia were at GMFCS levels I–III.

---

36   In one study [21], the number of people with hemiplegia also included those with monoplegia.

GMFCS E & R between 6th and 12th birthday: Descriptors and illustrations

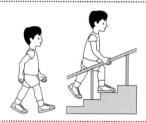

GMFCS Level I

Children walk at home, school, outdoors and in the community. They can climb stairs without the use of a railing. Children perform gross motor skills such as running and jumping, but speed, balance and coordination are limited.

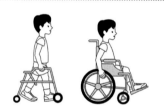

GMFCS Level II

Children walk in most settings and climb stairs holding onto a railing. They may experience difficulty walking long distances and balancing on uneven terrain, inclines, in crowded areas or confined spaces. Children may walk with physical assistance, a hand-held mobility device or used wheeled mobility over long distances. Children have only minimal ability to perform gross motor skills such as running and jumping.

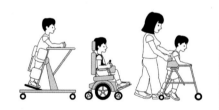

GMFCS Level III

Children walk using a hand-held mobility device in most indoor settings. They may climb stairs holding onto a railing with supervision or assistance. Children use wheeled mobility when traveling long distances and may self-propel for shorter distances.

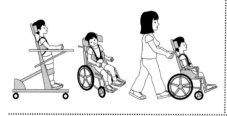

GMFCS Level IV

Children use methods of mobility that require physical assistance or powered mobility in most settings. They may walk for short distances at home with physical assistance or use powered mobility or a body support walker when positioned. At school, outdoors and in the community children are transported in a manual wheelchair or use powered mobility.

GMFCS Level V

Children are transported in a manual wheelchair in all settings. Children are limited in their ability to maintain antigravity head and trunk postures and control leg and arm movements.

GMFCS descriptors: Palisano et al. (1997) Dev Med Child Neurol 39:214-23
CanChild: www.canchild.ca

Illustrations Version 2 © Bill Reid, Kate Willoughby, Adrienne Harvey and Kerr Graham, The Royal Children's Hospital Melbourne   ERC151050

Figure 1.6.1 GMFCS E & R between 6th and 12th birthday: descriptors and illustrations. Reproduced with kind permission from K. Graham and K. Willoughby, Royal Children's Hospital Melbourne, Australia.

GMFCS E & R between 12th and 18th birthday: Descriptors and illustrations

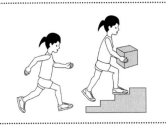

GMFCS Level I

Youth walk at home, school, outdoors and in the community. Youth are able to climb curbs and stairs without physical assistance or a railing. They perform gross motor skills such as running and jumping but speed, balance and coordination are limited.

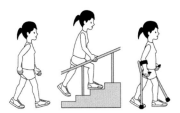

GMFCS Level II

Youth walk in most settings but environmental factors and personal choice influence mobility choices. At school or work they may require a hand held mobility device for safety and climb stairs holding onto a railing. Outdoors and in the community youth may use wheeled mobility when traveling long distances.

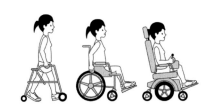

GMFCS Level III

Youth are capable of walking using a hand-held mobility device. Youth may climb stairs holding onto a railing with supervision or assistance. At school they may self-propel a manual wheelchair or use powered mobility. Outdoors and in the community youth are transported in a wheelchair or use powered mobility.

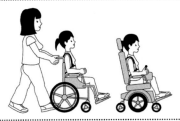

GMFCS Level IV

Youth use wheeled mobility in most settings. Physical assistance of 1-2 people is required for transfers. Indoors, youth may walk short distances with physical assistance, use wheeled mobility or a body support walker when positioned. They may operate a powered chair, otherwise are transported in a manual wheelchair.

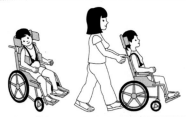

GMFCS Level V

Youth are transported in a manual wheelchair in all settings. Youth are limited in their ability to maintain antigravity head and trunk postures and control leg and arm movements. Self-mobility is severely limited, even with the use of assistive technology.

GMFCS descriptors: Palisano et al. (1997) Dev Med Child Neurol 39:214-23
CanChild: www.canchild.ca

Illustrations Version 2 © Bill Reid, Kate Willoughby, Adrienne Harvey and Kerr Graham,
The Royal Children's Hospital Melbourne   ERC151050

Figure 1.6.2 GMFCS E & R between 12th and 18th birthday: descriptors and illustrations. Reproduced with kind permission from K. Graham and K. Willoughby, Royal Children's Hospital Melbourne, Australia.

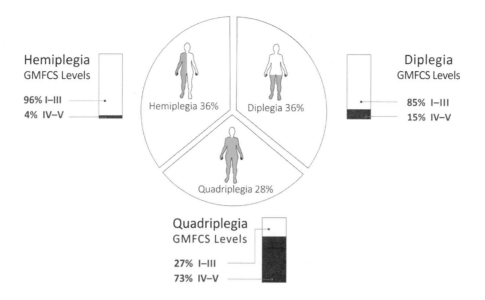

Figure 1.6.3 Proportion of CP by topography (area of the body affected) and severity (GMFCS level). Data collated from five studies [17–21].

As noted earlier, the SCPE subdivided spastic CP into unilateral or bilateral based on whether one or two sides of the body were involved. From the data above, one can broadly assume that:

- At GMFCS levels I–III, the majority of children with bilateral spastic CP have spastic diplegia.
- At GMFCS levels IV and V, the majority of children with bilateral spastic CP have spastic quadriplegia.

This explains why at GMFCS levels I–III the descriptors "spastic diplegia" and "bilateral spastic CP" (or simply "bilateral CP") can largely be used interchangeably.

Classification systems similar to the GMFCS have since been developed for function in other areas:

- The **Manual Ability Classification System (MACS)** is a five-level classification system that describes how children with CP aged four to 18 years use their hands to handle objects in daily activities [22]. There is a separate **Mini-MACS** for children aged one to four [23].

- The **Communication Function Classification System (CFCS)** is a five-level classification system that describes everyday communication performance [24].[37]

Web links to the MACS, Mini-MACS, and CFCS are included at the end of this section. Table 1.6.4 summarizes the five levels of the three classification systems (GMFCS, MACS, and CFCS).

Table 1.6.4 Description of the five levels of the GMFCS, MACS, and CFCS [11,12,22,24]

LEVEL	GROSS MOTOR FUNCTION CLASSIFICATION SYSTEM (GMFCS)	MANUAL ABILITY CLASSIFICATION SYSTEM (MACS)	COMMUNICATION FUNCTION CLASSIFICATION SYSTEM (CFCS)
I	Walks without limitations.	Handles objects easily and successfully.	Effective Sender and Receiver with unfamiliar and familiar partners.
II	Walks with limitations.	Handles most objects but with somewhat reduced quality and/or speed of achievement.	Effective but slower paced Sender and/or Receiver with unfamiliar and/or familiar partners.
III	Walks using a hand-held mobility device.	Handles objects with difficulty; needs help to prepare and/or modify activities.	Effective Sender and Receiver with familiar partners.
IV	Self-mobility with limitations; may use powered mobility.	Handles a limited selection of easily managed objects in adapted situations.	Inconsistent Sender and/or Receiver with familiar partners.

Cont'd.

37 Communication occurs when a "Sender" transmits a message and a "Receiver" understands the message. In conversation, for example, the Sender is the speaker and the Receiver is the listener. Unfamiliar conversation partners are strangers or acquaintances who only occasionally communicate with the person. Familiar conversation partners such as relatives, caregivers, and friends may be able to communicate more effectively with the person because of previous knowledge and personal experience [24].

LEVEL	GROSS MOTOR FUNCTION CLASSIFICATION SYSTEM (GMFCS)	MANUAL ABILITY CLASSIFICATION SYSTEM (MACS)	COMMUNICATION FUNCTION CLASSIFICATION SYSTEM (CFCS)
V	Transported in a manual wheelchair.	Does not handle objects and has severely limited ability to perform even simple actions.	Seldom-effective Sender and Receiver even with familiar partners.

A study looked at the correlation between distribution of gross motor function, manual ability, and communication function [20]. Table 1.6.5 shows the distribution for children and adolescents with spastic diplegia across the five levels of each classification (GMFCS, MACS, and CFCS).

Table 1.6.5 Distribution of GMFCS, MACS, and CFCS levels for children and adolescents with spastic diplegia

	GMFCS (GROSS MOTOR FUNCTION)	MACS (MANUAL ABILITY)	CFCS (COMMUNICATION)
Level I	38%	44%	55%
Level II	38%	44%	17%
Level III	15%	11%	18%
Level IV	8%	0%	9%
Level V	2%	2%	2%

Data from reference [20].

Table 1.6.5 shows that in this study:
- 91 percent of children and adolescents with spastic diplegia were at GMFCS levels I–III.[38]
- 99 percent of children and adolescents with spastic diplegia were at MACS levels I–III.

---

38 Variation is to be expected between studies carried out at different times and in different geographical regions.

- 90 percent of children and adolescents with spastic diplegia were at CFCS levels I–II.
- The distribution across the three classification systems does not precisely correlate. For example, 38 percent of children and adolescents with spastic diplegia were at GMFCS level I, but 55 percent were at CFCS level I. This underscores the important point that the GMFCS does not predict functionality in domains other than mobility. (The same point applies to the MACS and the CFCS.)

Most children with spastic diplegia can be considered to have a mild or moderate (not severe) level of disability with regard to gross motor function (walking ability). Likewise, they can be considered to have a mild or moderate level of disability with regard to manual ability and communication.

We have now looked at the three main classification systems for CP. Of the three, only the GMFCS (and its offshoots, the MACS, Mini-MACS, and CFCS) has been proven to be valid and reliable.

Finally, it should be obvious from the information above that although CP is a single diagnosis, it is far from a uniform condition. Similar to autism, a name change from "cerebral palsy" to "cerebral palsy spectrum disorder" has recently been suggested [25].

Gross motor development curves

The GMFCS led to the development of the gross motor development curves [26,27]. The curves show the change in gross motor function over time as measured by the GMFM-66. There are five curves, one for each GMFCS level. See Figure 1.6.4.

What do the curves show us?
- The curves represent the average GMFM-66 score (y-axis) at each GMFCS level by age (x-axis).
- For each GMFCS level there is an initial rapid rise in GMFM-66 score to a peak level, then the score plateaus (GMFCS levels I–II) or decreases (levels III–V).
- The GMFM-66 score (y-axis) is highest for level I and lowest for level V.

- The dotted lines show the timing of the peak in GMFM-66 score and the decrease from the peak to age 21 years for levels III–V.
- Even a child/adolescent at GMFCS level I does not reach 100, the maximum, on the GMFM-66 scale.

Why are the curves useful? They help answer some of the many questions we parents have in the early days. Knowing our child's GMFCS level at age two, the curves allow us to see how our child's gross motor function, as measured by the GMFM-66, is likely to develop over time.

The curves are based on averages, and while they are very useful, it is important to remember that some children were above and some below the line at each level. While remaining very realistic in our expectations, we should focus on helping our child reach their maximum possible gross motor function, not just hitting the average. The curves should guide, but not limit, our child's potential.

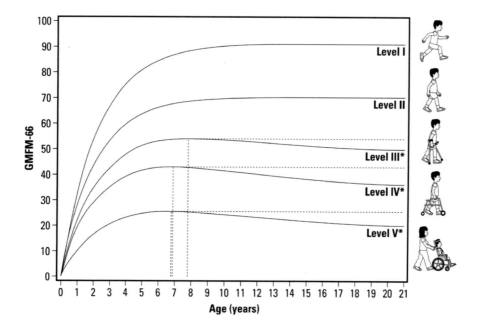

Figure 1.6.4 Gross motor curves in children with CP and the five levels of the GMFCS, modified from Hanna et al. (2008). Reproduced with kind permission from *Cerebral Palsy: Science and Clinical Practice*, edited by Bernard Dan, Margaret Mayston, Nigel Paneth, and Lewis Rosenbloom, published by Mac Keith Press (mackeith.co.uk) in its Clinics in Developmental Medicine Series, 2014, 978-1-909962-38-5.

Tommy was born in 1994. The first GMFCS to age 12 was published in 1997, and the curves were published in 2002. Looking back, I can see how useful they could have been earlier in Tommy's life. Before these tools emerged, questions like, "Will our child walk?" were difficult for professionals to answer; they likely did not want to overpromise.

When I asked whether Tommy would walk, I was told he would walk before age seven but would likely need to use a wheelchair in college. As it turned out, Tommy began to walk independently just after his third birthday and continued to walk independently right through college. (In fact, my favorite photograph from his college graduation is one I took of the family and a friend walking to dinner that evening. It was special because not only was Tommy graduating, he was also walking unaided beside his dad and brothers. I sent a copy of that photograph, with great gratitude, to the many professionals who had treated him over the years.)

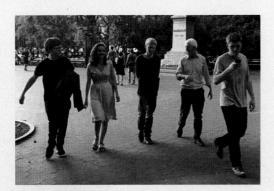

Tommy (far left), with a friend and his dad and brothers

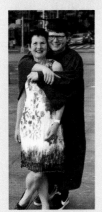

Tommy and me

While I do not have a record of his earlier GMFM-66 scores, Tommy's GMFM-66 score just before his 10th birthday was 78. Plotting that score on the curves put him between levels I and II, and at that time he was classed as level II (walks with limitations). This accurately describes how Tommy, now 25, walks today.

Useful web links

- Cerebral Palsy Alliance (2015) *Types of Cerebral Palsy.* [video] youtube.com/watch?v=cOfUGUNxEqU

- CanChild (2007) *Gross Motor Function Classification System Expanded and Revised.* [pdf] canchild.ca/system/tenon/assets/ attachments/000/000/058/original/GMFCS-ER_English.pdf

- CanChild (2018) *GMFCS Video.* [video] vimeo.com/293380093

- Cerebral Palsy Foundation (n.d.) *Insights from Experts: Motor Classification.* [video] yourcpf.org/expert-videos/gmfcs/

- CanChild (2011) *GMFCS Family Report Questionnaire.* [pdf] canchild.ca/system/tenon/assets/attachments/000/000/481/ original/GMFCS_Family.pdf (Scroll down to find separate sheets for each of the four age groups: 2–4, 4–6, 6–12, and 12–18.)

- MACS (2010) *Manual Ability Classification System for Children with Cerebral Palsy 4–18 Years.* [pdf] macs.nu/files/MACS_ English_2010.pdf

- MACS (2013) *Mini-Manual Ability Classification System for Children with Cerebral Palsy 1–4 Years of Age.* [pdf] macs.nu/files/ Mini-MACS_English_2016.pdf

- CFCS (2011) *Communication Function Classification System (CFCS).* [pdf] cfcs.us/wp-content/uploads/2014/02/CFCS_ universal_2012_06_06.pdf

Key points Chapter 1

- There are many possible causes of the brain injury that results in CP, including events before and during pregnancy, during birth, or in early infant life.
- Confirmation of the presence of a brain injury by MRI occurs in many but not all cases of CP. Up to 17 percent of people with CP have normal MRI brain scans.
- There seems to be a recent shift toward earlier diagnosis of CP.
- CP is a lifelong condition. There is currently no cure for CP, nor is one imminent.
- A 2013 worldwide review found that the overall prevalence of CP was 2.11 per 1,000 live births.
- Relative to its prevalence and its impact on the life span of those with the condition, funding for CP research is very low.
- The International Classification of Functioning, Disability and Health (ICF) is a very useful framework for CP. It describes human functioning at three levels: body functions and structure, activity, and participation. Environmental and personal factors may influence any of these three levels.
- The World Health Organization (WHO) identified the age at which typically developing children achieve each of the six gross motor milestones. Delay in reaching these milestones is one of the hallmarks of CP.
- One commonly used method for measuring gross motor function in CP is the Gross Motor Function Measure (GMFM). The GMFM can measure and detect changes over time in gross motor function.
- CP may be classified on the basis of topography (the area of the body affected) as monoplegia, hemiplegia, diplegia, triplegia, or quadriplegia. An alternative classification system, also based on topography, classifies CP as unilateral or bilateral.
- CP may be classified on the basis of the predominant feature of the motor impairment. Most studies report that spasticity is the most common type of motor impairment.
- Spastic diplegia is a common subtype of CP, accounting for roughly one-third of cases.
- The GMFCS is a five-level classification system that describes the functional mobility of children and adolescents with CP. The

GMFCS and the gross motor development curves can help predict functional mobility and gross motor function over time.

- The majority of children with spastic diplegia are classified as GMFCS levels I–III: mild or moderate CP.
- At GMFCS levels I–III, the descriptors "spastic diplegia" and "bilateral spastic CP" or simply "bilateral CP" can largely be used interchangeably.
- The GMFCS does not predict function in domains other than mobility.

CHAPTER 2

Spastic Diplegia—
Bilateral CP

2.1

Introduction

Nothing in life is to be feared, it is only to be understood.
Now is the time to understand more, so that we may fear less.
Marie Curie

I remember a TV advertisement for a particular brand of cider that showed an orchard of trees laden with apples. Its catchphrase was "just add time." Children with spastic diplegia are born with what appear to be typical bones, muscles, and joints. The problems of spastic diplegia emerge when we "just add time."

Spastic diplegia is a complex and lifelong condition. There is currently no cure. However, good management and treatment can help reduce its effects. This chapter focuses on the musculoskeletal and mobility issues associated with spastic diplegia from birth through adolescence. A separate chapter is devoted to spastic diplegia in adulthood.

This chapter should contribute to your understanding of how the condition arises and develops over time. It provides much of the information I wish I'd had when Tommy was diagnosed all those years ago.

In his 1991 book, Gage described spastic diplegia as follows [1]:

The involvement is primarily in the lower extremities with relatively normal upper extremity function. The "classic" diplegic child has normal intelligence, absence of seizures, near-normal upper extremity function, and virtually pure spastic involvement. [...] Most diplegic children will walk, although balance, particularly posterior balance, is a much greater problem for these children than for those with hemiplegia. [...] The "typical" gait of a child with diplegia [...] is one of flexion, adduction, and internal rotation at the hips and flexion at the knees. The feet usually have a valgus hindfoot and [...] abducted forefoot.

In their 2007 book, Horstmann and Bleck described it as follows [2]:

When we observe the posture and gait of a child with spastic diplegia anywhere in the world it is as though each child came from the same mold. The common pattern [...] is flexed, adducted, and internally rotated hips [...] We see an increased anterior pelvic tilt, lumbar lordosis, either flexed or hyperextended knees, and equinus.

Table 2.1.1 explains each of the terms used in these descriptions. Together, they paint a picture of spastic diplegia: of a child who walks with flexed knees and hips and whose bones are twisted.

Table 2.1.1 Features of spastic diplegia

TERM USED IN DESCRIPTIONS	EXPLANATION	ILLUSTRATION
Posterior balance	Balance in the backward direction is affected. The person often falls backward.	N/A
Lumbar lordosis	An exaggerated inward curve in the lumbar region of the spine, often called a swayback.	
Anterior pelvic tilt	A tipping forward of the pelvis to the front. (The triangle indicates the pelvis.)	

Cont'd.

TERM USED IN DESCRIPTIONS	EXPLANATION	ILLUSTRATION
Adduction and internal rotation at the hips	*Adduction* is movement toward the middle of the body. *Internal rotation* is a twisting movement around the long axis of a bone toward the middle of the body. With *adduction and internal rotation at the hips*, the thigh turns inward and toward the middle of the body.	
Flexion at the hips and knees	The hips and knees are bent.	
Hyperextended knees	*Hyperextended* means beyond straight or over-straightened. This is also termed *genu recurvatum*. The knee on the left is hyperextended; the knee on the right is normal.	
Abducted forefoot	The front part of the foot moves away (outward) from the back part of the foot. The foot on the left is abducted; the foot on the right is normal.	
Valgus hindfoot	The heels of both feet are turned away from the middle of the body to an abnormal degree; i.e., the heels are turned outward.	
Equinus	The person is walking on their toes.	

This chapter explains how a baby born with what appear to be typical bones, muscles, and joints can grow into a child who fits the descriptions above. I say "appear to be typical" because research is ongoing; there may be slight differences between the bones, muscles, and joints of a baby with spastic diplegia and those of a typically developing baby. Our understanding may change over time.

This chapter addresses:

Section 2.2   The brain injury
Section 2.3   Growth
Section 2.4   Bones, muscles, joints, and movements
Section 2.5   Normal walking
Section 2.6   Primary abnormalities
Section 2.7   Secondary abnormalities
Section 2.8   Tertiary abnormalities
Section 2.9   Walking in individuals with spastic diplegia

Section 2.4 may seem like an anatomy lesson, but because spastic diplegia affects the bones, muscles, joints, and movements, particularly of the lower limbs, a basic understanding helps enormously in understanding both the condition and its treatment. Spastic diplegia also affects mobility, and therefore a basic understanding of normal walking, addressed in section 2.5, is beneficial.

I read the description of spastic diplegia in Dr. Gage's book when Tommy was about five years old. It was a lightbulb moment for me. His assertion that the "classic" diplegic child has normal intelligence was the first positive statement on intelligence in spastic diplegia I had read or heard.

Tommy had a CT scan when he was approximately one year old; phrases like "significant brain damage," "not much active brain," and "go home and mind the other children" conveyed the consultant's concern about what he saw on the scan. I was perplexed: how could this consultant say these things when he had never actually met our very alert and engaging child? It turned out Tommy had normal intelligence.

In the early days we had also been advised to watch out for seizures. Reading Dr. Gage's book, I learned that seizures were not typical in spastic diplegia. Tommy never had a seizure.

Those two descriptions by Drs. Gage, Horstmann, and Bleck described Tommy pretty accurately as a young child. In the early days I thought the way Tommy walked was particular to him. Later, as I observed other people with spastic diplegia, I realized Tommy's manner of walking was characteristic of the condition. The concept that each child with spastic diplegia "came from the same mold" really resonated with me.

In hindsight, the only differences between Tommy and his two older brothers (who do not have spastic diplegia) as a baby were that he cried incessantly for the first three months, he was difficult to feed, and his legs felt strong and stiff from birth. That early stiffness was probably spasticity, though I would only become familiar with the term much later. The photograph below shows our eldest son holding a very rigid Tommy.

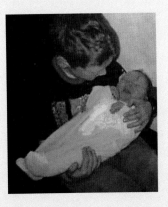

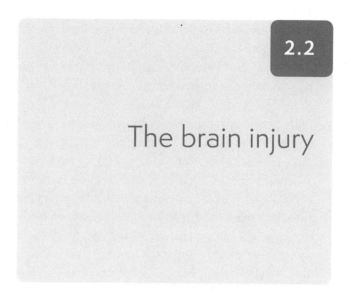

2.2

The brain injury

*The greater danger for most of us lies not in
setting our aim too high and falling short;
but in setting our aim too low, and achieving our mark.*

Michelangelo

When and where an injury occurs in the brain determines the effect of that injury. Different subtypes of CP result from damage at different times in development and to different areas of the brain. Spastic diplegia is most commonly associated with preterm birth or an injury in the late second or early third trimester [1,2]. In this section we briefly address the brain injury that causes spastic diplegia.

The classic brain injury of spastic diplegia is called periventricular leukomalacia (PVL). The following is an explanation of the terms:

- **Periventricular:** The ventricles are the black, kidney-shaped areas shown in Figure 2.2.1. The injury (yellow area) occurs near these ventricles, hence the term "periventricular," which means "around the ventricles."
- **Leukomalacia:** "Leuko" means "white" and "malacia" means "abnormal softening of tissue." The term "leukomalacia" therefore means "softening of the white tissue." The white tissue in that area

includes the communication tracts (pyramidal tracts) that connect the brain (cerebral cortex) and spinal cord, shown as lines in Figure 2.2.1.The communication tracts in the region around the ventricles are involved in the control of movement and posture.

The full term "periventricular leukomalacia" thus means "softening of the white tissue around the ventricles."

PVL results in the motor problems we see in spastic diplegia. The communication tracts closest to the ventricles relate to the ankle, those next closest relate to the knee, and those next closest relate to the hip. We will see later that this mirrors the pattern of problems in spastic diplegia: the ankle is more involved than the knee, which in turn is more involved than the hip. There is less upper limb involvement in spastic diplegia, and as we can see in the diagram, those tracts are even further from the site of the injury. The injury is usually bilateral (affecting both sides of the brain), but it can be uneven. The severity of spastic diplegia depends on the severity of the brain injury.

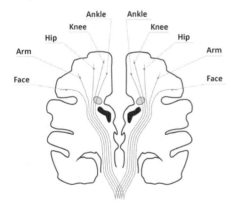

Figure 2.2.1 Drawing of the pyramidal tracts as they descend from their origin in the cerebral cortex to the spinal cord. The ventricles are the black, kidney-shaped areas. The injury (yellow area) occurs near these ventricles, hence the term "periventricular," which means "around the ventricles." Adapted from Gage (1991) [1].

Knowledge of the brain injury can sometimes confirm symptoms seen in a child. If a child is suspected of having CP, and an MRI scan reveals damage in the periventricular area, this helps confirm the diagnosis of CP and specifically of spastic diplegia. MRI scans are becoming more routine in CP. However, up to 17 percent of people with CP have normal MRI brain scans [3].

The brain injury is unchanging (i.e., the size and location do not change and it is permanent). However, the effects of the brain injury emerge with time. To some extent the word "unchanging" may be a bit misleading. "Unchanging" might describe the brain injury, but it does not describe its effects. With time, growth, and maturation of the brain and other structures, the effects of the brain injury result in altered musculoskeletal anatomy and motor delays.

A growing body of evidence demonstrates that the brain is capable of recovery after an injury. This is due to the ability of nerve cells to adapt their structure and function in response to a variety of external and internal stimuli, such as behavioral training. This is known as neuroplasticity[39] [4]. This is why early therapy is so important.

Therapy approaches that induce neuroplasticity have become more common in CP [5]. Constraint-induced movement therapy (CIMT) is a therapy used mostly in hemiplegia. It involves restricting the unaffected "good" hand (in a mitt or cast) to allow intensive training of the affected hand.

We address the therapies used to treat spastic diplegia (physical therapy, occupational therapy, and speech and language pathology/therapy) in the next chapter. These therapies recognize that the brain has the ability to change, though change takes a lot of practice. A review of interventions for children with CP by Novak and colleagues (2013) found that the majority of effective therapy evidence generated in the last 10 years arose from two main therapy approaches, one of which involved inducing neuroplasticity [5]. The other was aimed at improving the performance of activities. Children appear to have more neuroplasticity than adults, again underscoring the importance of early therapy.

Useful web link

- Cerebral Palsy Foundation (2016) The Brain. [video] youtu.bc/vFrdANVTYGk

---

39 Also known as brain plasticity, neural plasticity, neuronal plasticity, and neuroelasticity.

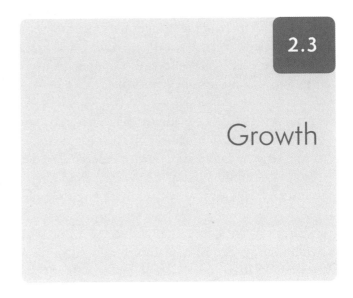

2.3

Growth

You have to do your own growing no matter how tall your grandfather was.

Abraham Lincoln

An understanding of normal growth is helpful for understanding how the problems of spastic diplegia develop. This section addresses growth in typically developing children and adolescents as well as those with CP.

The Centers for Disease Control and Prevention (CDC) publishes separate growth charts for typically developing boys and girls. For both sexes, the growth charts are divided into two age groups: birth to 36 months and two to 20 years, 20 years being the age at which growth in height is generally complete. Web links to all four growth charts are included at the end of this section. Figure 2.3.1 shows the chart for boys aged birth to 36 months [1].

Many parents may be familiar with these charts. The graphs show percentiles—or 100 equal parts that illustrate how tall your child is in relation to all other children of the same age. The 50th percentile is always the midpoint.

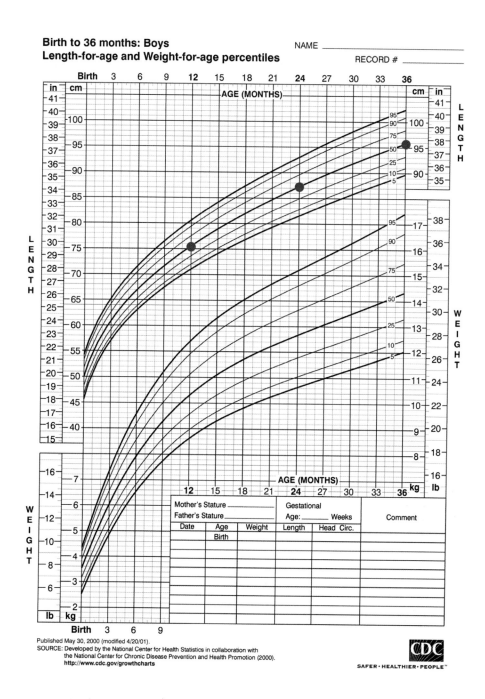

Figure 2.3.1 Height (referred to as "length") and weight chart for boys aged 0–36 months [1]. The seven curves are for the 5th, 10th, 25th, 50th, 75th, 90th, and 95th percentiles. Reproduced with kind permission from the Centers for Disease Control and Prevention (CDC). Length at 12, 24, and 36 months is marked.

When height is measured and plotted on the relevant height graph, the plotted value will lie close to one of the percentile curves. Referring to Figure 2.3.1:

- If a boy's height is close to the 75th percentile curve, they are the same height or taller than 75 percent of boys.
- If a boy's height is close to the 50th percentile curve, they are the same height or taller than 50 percent of boys.

The taller the boy, the higher the percentile curve their height will match.

What is of interest when it comes to spastic diplegia is not so much growth as growth velocity; i.e., the rate (or speed) of growth. See Figure 2.3.1 again. Using the 50th percentile height to represent the average boy, we see that they are:

- 50 cm long at birth
- 75 cm at one year old: a 50 percent increase over the previous year
- 87 cm at two years old: a 16 percent increase over the previous year
- 96 cm at three years old: a 10 percent increase over the previous year

Thus, in the first three years of life, growth is vigorous. It is most vigorous in the first year and then gradually decreases. By age three, the average child has almost doubled in height from 50 cm to 96 cm. We can continue to follow the growth of a typical boy on the two to 20 years growth chart.

Keogh and Sugden (1985) noted that growth occurs in three major phases during a child's life, as shown in Table 2.3.1 [2].

Of the three major phases of growth, there are two phases of rapid growth: from birth to three years and during puberty.[40] If the problems of spastic diplegia emerge with growth, then these periods of rapid growth are especially significant. By the time the child with spastic diplegia is three years old and has almost doubled in height, some of the typical features of spastic diplegia, such as contractures, may already have appeared. Bone growth stops at maturity (around age 20); thus the

---

40 According to the CDC, puberty starts and ends at different times for everyone. Girls develop and change more between the ages of nine and 13. For boys, puberty typically starts a little later, when they are between 10 and 15 years old [3].

challenge of keeping muscle growth at pace with bone growth ceases at this age.

Table 2.3.1 Growth velocity [2]

AGE	CHANGE IN HEIGHT	COMMENT
Birth to age three	Very rapid	From birth to age three the speed of growth is great, but is steadily decreasing.
Three years to puberty	Slow, consistent	From three years to puberty growth occurs at a slowly decreasing linear rate.
Puberty to maturity	Rapid	At puberty the speed of growth increases for 18–24 months, achieves a peak, then decreases until the skeleton is mature.
Maturity onward	No change	

It is important to note certain differences between the sexes in relation to growth:
- Until puberty, there is only a small difference in height between the sexes.
- At puberty, boys grow rapidly taller. By age 20, typically developing boys are on average 14 cm taller than girls.

This has relevance in spastic diplegia. Since the problems of spastic diplegia emerge with growth, and since boys are taller than girls, the problems of spastic diplegia can be somewhat more challenging for boys.

A large US study of growth in children with CP led to the development of growth charts for boys and girls with CP aged two to 20. These were developed for each GMFCS level [4,5]. Web links are included at the end of this section.

Table 2.3.2 was compiled by taking the 50th percentile height at four age points from the growth charts of children and adolescents with CP and typically developing peers.

Table 2.3.2 Growth patterns of boys and girls with CP compared with typically developing peers

GMFCS LEVEL	HEIGHT AT AGE 3 IN CM	HEIGHT AT AGE 8 IN CM	HEIGHT AT AGE 14 IN CM	HEIGHT AT AGE 20 IN CM
Typically developing boys	95	128	164	177
Boys with CP level I	90	121	155	170
Boys with CP level II	88	118	150	165
Boys with CP level III	87	114	142	159
Typically developing girls	94	127	160	163
Girls with CP level I	88	120	152	158
Girls with CP level II	87	117	147	155
Girls with CP level III	84	113	142	151

Data collated from references [4–7].

Table 2.3.2 shows that:
- Across all GMFCS levels, the average height of boys and girls with CP at each age was lower than that of typically developing peers.
- The difference in height between boys and girls with CP and typically developing peers increased with GMFCS level.

Similar trends in height difference among children and adolescents with CP have been observed in other parts of the world [8].

Since growth is such an important factor in spastic diplegia, I would advise parents to keep a growth chart for their child in order to keep a focus on growth (and, as we will see, the need for stretching). I suggest you print the appropriate chart (boy or girl with CP and relevant GMFCS level) from the web links included at the end of this section.

Though any growth chart shows how much a typical child grows each year, an experienced parent knows that a child does not grow evenly throughout the year. Sometimes it felt like our sons shot up overnight. (I found this often followed a period of them eating more than usual.)

The difference in height between people with CP and typically developing peers was borne out at home: Tommy is not as tall as his two brothers.

The fact that the first three years are a period of very rapid growth is to some extent unfortunate timing in spastic diplegia. This period of very rapid growth coincides with the time before diagnosis or when we parents are only just learning about and coming to terms with the diagnosis. Yet this is a period when intervention is needed because the problems of spastic diplegia emerge with growth. The fact that the first year of life is the period of most rapid growth again emphasizes the importance of early diagnosis and intervention.

Useful web links

Note: Depending on age, height is referred to as either "length" or "stature" in these resources.

- CDC (2001) *Birth to 36 Months: Boys.* [pdf] cdc.gov/growthcharts/data/set1clinical/cj41l017.pdf

- CDC (2000) *2 to 20 Years: Boys.* [pdf] cdc.gov/growthcharts/data/set1clinical/cj41l021.pdf

- CDC (2001) *Birth to 36 Months: Girls.* [pdf] cdc.gov/growthcharts/data/set1clinical/cj41l018.pdf

- CDC (2000) *2 to 20 Years: Girls.* [pdf] cdc.gov/growthcharts/data/set2clinical/cj41c072.pdf

- Life Expectancy Project (2011) *New Growth Charts.* [online] lifeexpectancy.org/articles/NewGrowthCharts.shtml

2.4

Bones, muscles, joints, and movements

It is not by muscle, speed, or physical dexterity that great things are achieved, but by reflection, force of character, and judgment.

Marcus Tullius Cicero

This section contains an introduction to bones, muscles, joints, and movements.

Bones form the framework of the body. Joints are the points, or pivots, around which the bones move. There are three types of muscle:

- **Cardiac:** Muscle which forms the bulk of the wall of the heart
- **Smooth:** Muscle located in the walls of hollow internal structures such as the blood vessels, stomach, and intestines
- **Skeletal:** Muscle attached (mostly) to bones

Spastic diplegia primarily affects skeletal muscle.[41] In this book, when I refer to muscle, I am referring to skeletal muscle only. Skeletal muscles exert force on the bones to produce movement and maintain posture.

---

41   There are some reports of bladder muscle being affected.

In a sense, the bones are like the limbs of a marionette (or puppet, see Figure 2.4.1). The marionette cannot stand up on its own. Similarly, the bones cannot stand up on their own; gravity would pull them down. When muscles contract, in addition to causing movement, they exert force, which keeps the body erect. Without these forces opposing gravity, the bones would collapse in a heap on the ground.

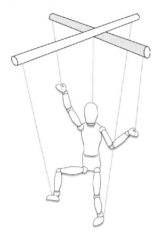

Figure 2.4.1 A marionette (puppet)

My father lived to a very old age. Just before he died, his trunk muscles became so weak that they were no longer able to keep him erect. He needed support even when sitting. His trunk muscles were no longer strong enough to oppose the force of gravity.

When it comes to movement, the muscles are the "action men" and the bones just follow. Bones act as levers. In physics, a lever is a rigid bar resting on a pivot, which moves a load on one end when pressure is applied to the other (see Figure 2.4.2).

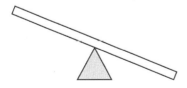

Figure 2.4.2 A lever

A seesaw (or teeter-totter) is a type of lever. A child on one end generates a force, acting on a lever (the horizontal beam of the seesaw) about a joint (the pivot of the seesaw) to cause the child at the other end to move (go up).

Bones—the levers—move in relation to each other when muscles exert their force. In biomechanics, a "moment" is a turning effect produced by a force (e.g., a muscle contraction) acting on a lever (the bone) about a pivot (the joint). An example is when the knee bends: the hamstring muscles behind the knee contract (exerting force), which causes the lower leg (the lever) to move toward the upper leg (generating movement). The knee joint is the pivot.

A muscle has to contract to produce a force. The force it produces can be very small (e.g., to pick up a feather) or very large (e.g., to pick up a bucket of water). There are three types of muscle contraction:

- **Concentric contraction:** The muscle shortens. For example, going up a flight of stairs, the quadriceps (the muscles in front of the knee joint) contract concentrically—they shorten so that the knee extends.
- **Eccentric contraction:** The muscle lengthens. Eccentric contraction allows controlled movement against gravity. For example, going down a flight of stairs, the quadriceps contract eccentrically—they lengthen so that the knee bends. The lengthening contraction controls the bending of the knee against gravity.
- **Isometric contraction:** No change in muscle length. If there is no movement—for example, when maintaining posture (i.e., opposing the force of gravity)—the muscle is contracting isometrically, without getting longer or shorter.

Every muscle has its own length when it is at rest. Muscles produce optimal force in the middle of that resting length.

The details of the different types of contractions are not important as such, but it is helpful to keep in mind that during walking our lower limb muscles move in fractions of a second between these different types of contractions to produce the gait cycle.

In addition to having contractile elements, muscles also contain non-contractile elements. The latter form the tendon and various sheaths. The tendon is the cord-like structure that attaches the muscle to the bone: the Achilles tendon, for example, attaches the gastrocnemius and soleus muscles—both calf muscles—at the ankle joint. The combination of the muscle, tendon, and other structures is collectively known as the muscle-tendon unit (MTU).

There is a difference between muscle strength and muscle power. Muscle strength is the amount of force that a muscle can generate during a specific movement—for example, the weight you can lift at the gym in a single repetition. Muscle power is the rate of force production (i.e, how fast the force is being produced). There is a strength aspect to power, but it is also about the speed of the movement. Jumping is an example of a power-based activity. In the gym example, the weight would have to be much lower so that you could move it quickly. Both muscle strength and muscle power are important for everyday activities like walking and running.

The range of motion (ROM), also called range of movement, of a joint is a measure of the joint's flexibility. The actual ROM through which a joint moves is measured in degrees. An instrument called a goniometer[42] is used to measure the ROM of a joint. A web link to a video about measuring ROM is included at the end of this section.

Table 2.4.1 explains the key movements and lower limb muscles affected in spastic diplegia.

I compiled a version of this table many years ago, and it greatly helped my understanding of the condition. It came in handy when medical professionals referred to various movements or muscles or to a joint being tight (having a decreased ROM). I also found it helpful to be aware of the normal ROM for each joint. When surgery was planned, it helped me understand why procedures such as psoas, adductor, and gastrocnemius lengthening were needed. For these reasons, it is worth taking some time to study this table. It will also be useful as a reference when reading later sections of this book.

---

42 A goniometer is like a movable protractor. A protractor is an instrument used for measuring angles; it is typically a piece of semicircular plastic marked with degrees along the curved edge.

Table 2.4.1 Movements, joint ROMs [1,2], and key muscles

MOVEMENT AFFECTED BY SPASTIC MUSCLES	MOVEMENT	KEY MUSCLES RESPONSIBLE FOR MOVEMENT	STICK DRAWING OF MUSCLES
Hip flexion Movement of the thigh up toward the pelvis. **ROM 0–125°**		**Hip flexors** • Psoas (2J [spine & hip] major) • Iliacus (1J [hip] major) • Rectus femoris (2J [hip & knee] minor)	
Hip adduction Movement of the thigh toward the midline. **ROM 0–20°**		**Hip adductors** • A longus (1J [hip] major) • A magnus (1J [hip] major) • A brevis (1J [hip] minor) • Gracilis (2J [hip & knee] minor)	
Hip internal rotation Rotary movement of the thigh toward the midline. Also known as inward or medial rotation. **ROM 0–45°**		*(Note: Internal rotation is included to show the movement, but unlike the other four movements on this side of the table, the major internal rotator muscles are single-joint muscles that are unlikely to be affected by spasticity. The minor internal rotator muscles [medial hamstrings and adductors] are affected by spasticity.)*	
Knee flexion Increasing the angle between the thigh and lower leg. **ROM 0–140°** *(Note: reference point is the straight leg. The angle increases the nearer the lower leg moves to the thigh.)*		**Knee flexors** • Hamstrings (2J [hip & knee] major) • Gastrocnemius (2J [knee & ankle] minor)	
Ankle plantar flexion Movement of the foot away from the lower leg. **ROM 0–45°**		**Ankle plantar flexors** • Gastrocnemius (2J [knee & ankle] major) • Soleus (1J [ankle] major)	

Cont'd.

CORRESPONDING MOVEMENT	MOVEMENT	KEY MUSCLES RESPONSIBLE FOR MOVEMENT	STICK DRAWING OF MUSCLES
Hip extension Movement of the thigh away from the pelvis. **ROM 0–10°**		**Hip extensors** • Gluteus maximus (1J [hip] major) • Hamstrings (2J [hip & knee] minor)	
Hip abduction Movement of the thigh away from the midline. **ROM 0–45°**		**Hip abductors** • Gluteus medius (1J [hip] major)	
Hip external rotation Rotary movement of the thigh away from the midline. Also known as outward or lateral rotation. **ROM 0–45°**			
Knee extension Decreasing the angle between the thigh and lower leg. **ROM 140–0°** *(Note: reference point is the straight leg. The angle decreases the further the lower leg moves away from the thigh.)*		**Knee extensors** The quadriceps (quads) consist of four muscles: • Rectus femoris (2J [hip & knee] major) • Vastus intermedius (1J [knee] major) • Vastus lateralis (1J [knee] major) • Vastus medialis (1J [knee] major)	
Ankle dorsiflexion Movement of the foot toward the lower leg. **ROM 0–20°**		**Ankle dorsiflexors** • Tibialis anterior (1J [ankle] major) • Toe extensors (Minor) *Not shown in diagram*	

Some points with reference to Table 2.4.1:

- Muscles are arranged in pairs around a joint. The muscles of one pair move the joint in one direction, while the muscles of the other pair move the joint in the opposite direction.
- Lower limb movements include hip flexion and extension, hip adduction and abduction, hip internal and external rotation, knee flexion and extension, and ankle plantar flexion and dorsiflexion.
- Movements caused by muscles affected by spasticity are shown on the left side of the table. The only exception to this is hip internal rotation. As far as is known, the hip internal rotators are not affected by spasticity.
- The main muscles affected by spasticity are the rectus femoris, psoas, adductor longus, gracilis, hamstrings, and gastrocnemius [3–5]. Each of these muscles, except the adductor longus, cross two joints. They are called two-joint muscles.
- Two-joint muscles play a role in movement at two joints. For example, the gastrocnemius (which crosses both the ankle and knee joints) is a major ankle plantar flexor but also a minor knee flexor.
- Abbreviations used in table: 1J or 2J = Muscles that cross one joint (1J) or two joints (2J); Major or Minor = Muscles that make a big (major) or small (minor) contribution to the movement. Note: Although key muscles have been identified at each joint, further minor muscles have not been included.

To stretch a muscle, one does the opposite of that muscle's action. To stretch a flexor muscle, for example, one must extend the joint. To stretch an extensor muscle, one must flex the joint. To fully stretch a muscle, one must move the joint through its full ROM. Because some muscles cross two joints rather than one, both joints are involved in the stretching of two-jointed muscles. To stretch the two-jointed hamstrings, for example, one has to extend the knee while flexing the hip. Long sitting (sitting with the legs extended) is a good method of stretching the hamstrings because the knees are extended while the hips are flexed.

Useful web link

- CDC (2016) ROM Measurement Procedures: Knee Flexion and Extension. [video] youtube.com/watch?v=lpeFU7yzcY0

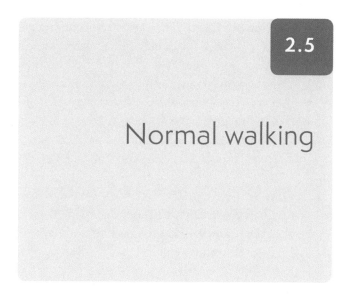

2.5

Normal walking

A journey of a thousand miles begins with a single step.
Lao Tzu

In general, we take walking for granted. It is only when we encounter a problem that we stop to think about what walking entails. The term "gait" refers to a person's manner of walking. "Normal" gait refers to the typically developing person's manner of walking, which has been studied extensively. Because problems with walking are one of the hallmarks of spastic diplegia, this section briefly looks at the features of normal walking.

Walking is a phenomenal achievement. It involves generating forces, managing gravity, speed, balance, and more. In evolutionary terms, walking on two limbs was advantageous because it freed our upper limbs for other tasks. It is no surprise that crawling comes before walking in human gross motor development: a crawling baby has four limbs on the floor, and is therefore more stable. Walking, which involves balancing on two limbs, is a more advanced and more demanding form of movement. A young foal is able to walk very soon after birth, whereas a human only starts walking around the one-year mark: one reason is that walking on two limbs as opposed to four is more challenging. (Another reason is that the human brain matures and grows after birth.)

The requirements of walking

Walking has four requirements [1]:
- **A control system:** The central nervous system (the brain and spinal cord) provides the control system for walking.
- **An energy source:** Energy is required for walking, and that energy is supplied by oxygen and the breakdown of food.
- **Levers:** The levers are the bones.
- **Forces to move the levers:** Muscle contraction provides the forces for walking. As we saw in the previous section, movement is generated by muscle forces acting on the levers (the bones).

Imagine getting a marionette to "walk" across a space. The control system is the person who pulls the strings; the energy comes from that person; the levers are the marionette's limbs; and the forces are provided by the person pulling the strings.

The gait cycle

One complete walking (or gait) cycle refers to the time between two successive occurrences of the same event in walking—for example, the time between when one foot strikes the ground and when that same foot strikes the ground again. See Figure 2.5.1, which shows a complete gait cycle for the right leg.

The gait cycle is divided into two major phases:
- **Stance phase:** The period of time when the foot is on the ground
- **Swing phase:** The period of time when the foot is in the air

Stance phase occupies approximately 60 percent of the gait cycle and swing phase occupies approximately 40 percent. There are two periods in the gait cycle when both limbs are on the ground; this is termed "double stance" (or "double support"). Single stance (or single support) is when just one limb is on the ground. Walking involves alternately balancing on each single limb as we move forward.

You don't need to know the terminology, but you can get an appreciation for what happens as the limb proceeds through the gait cycle in Figure 2.5.1. I recommend you observe what is happening at each of the different stages in the diagram.

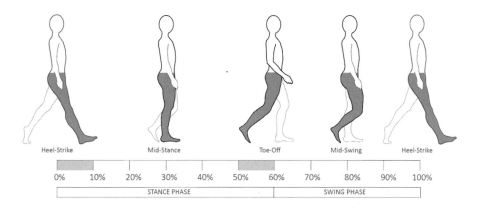

Figure 2.5.1 The gait cycle for the right leg. Stance phase, the period of time when the foot is on the ground, occupies 60 percent of the gait cycle. Swing phase, the period of time when the foot is in the air, occupies 40 percent. The two periods of double stance (each 10 percent), when both limbs are on the ground, are shaded.

Attributes of normal walking

The following are attributes of normal walking which are frequently lost in individuals with spastic diplegic gait [1]:

- **Stability in stance:** This is a reflection of good balance.
- **Foot clearance in swing:** To cleanly move the foot forward (e.g., without dragging the toe).
- **Pre-positioning of the foot for initial contact:** This prepares the foot to strike the ground with the heel (heel strike). See Figure 2.5.1.
- **Adequate step length:** A sufficiently long step is taken during each gait cycle.
- **Energy conservation:** Walking is energy-efficient.

Problems with the first four attributes contribute to problems with the fifth, the energy cost of walking.

When a typically developing child begins to walk, they do so without these attributes. The knees are relatively stiff and they walk with a wide base of support (i.e., the legs are far apart). As the child develops balance and their motor system becomes more mature, their gait evolves toward the adult pattern; this happens by about 3.5 years of age. It appears that walking is innate rather than learned, and it depends on the progressive maturing of the central nervous system.

2.6

Primary abnormalities

Divide each difficulty into as many parts as is feasible and necessary to resolve it.

Descartes

We saw that the child with spastic diplegia is born with what appear to be typical bones, muscles, and joints, and that the problems of spastic diplegia develop as they grow. We now address the abnormalities (impairments) of spastic diplegia and how their combination results in the typical gait observed in individuals with spastic diplegia.

Based on clinical expertise, Gage (1991) proposed a useful framework for classifying the abnormalities that occur in spastic CP [1]. Gage and Novacheck (2001) further refined this framework [2]. They divided the problems into primary, secondary, and tertiary abnormalities.

Primary abnormalities are caused by the brain injury and are therefore present from when the brain injury occurred: they are known as "neurological problems." Secondary abnormalities develop over time in the growing child: they are problems of abnormal muscle growth and bone shape development, and are referred to as "growth problems."

The tertiary abnormalities are the "coping responses" which arise to compensate for or counteract the primary and secondary abnormalities.

Understanding the primary (this section), secondary (next section, 2.7), and tertiary (section 2.8) abnormalities and how they combine to affect gait (section 2.9) is key to understanding spastic diplegia. These sections are long, but they are worth reading in order to gain a full understanding of the condition. Your physical therapist or physician may be able to answer any questions you may have. It may also help to use Table 2.4.1 as a reference.

Understanding this classification really helped me understand what was going on in spastic diplegia. It was one of the lightbulb moments I referred to earlier. I found the problems difficult to understand in the first place, but I also had trouble grasping how the condition would change over time. This classification was first published in 1991, almost 30 years ago, and it has stood the test of time.

We saw in section 2.2 that the typical brain injury in people with spastic diplegia is PVL, which involves damage to the white matter—the pyramidal tracts. (The pyramidal tracts are the communication tracts between the cerebral cortex and the spinal cord.) Graham and colleagues (2016) explained that the brain injury results in two types of effect [3]. One is loss of pyramidal tract connections from specific nerve cells in the brain to nerve cells in the spinal cord, and hence to certain muscles. The other is loss of the dampening input to nerve cells in the spinal cord (and again to certain muscles) across those same connections. (The latter results in something that should be dampened down not being dampened down.)

The primary abnormalities include the following, and we examine each in turn:
- **Loss of selective motor control**
- **Poor balance**
- **Abnormal tone**
- **Muscle weakness**
- **Sensory and other problems**

Loss of selective motor control

Loss of selective motor control results from the brain damage and the disruption of messages usually delivered by the pyramidal tract, including messages from the cerebrum and other areas of the brain.

In simple terms, "selective motor control" refers to the ability to isolate a muscle or combination of muscles to produce a particular movement. I cannot wink my right eye, no matter how hard I try—I do not have good selective motor control over the muscles responsible for winking my right eye. A child with spastic diplegia has problems with selective motor control and therefore has difficulty performing some movements.

Selective motor control can be checked by asking the child to perform certain movements, such as ankle dorsiflexion/plantar flexion (moving the foot up and down). Each limb and joint is tested separately. This evaluates whether the child:

- Can do the full movement in both directions
- Can do the movement without involving other body movements
- Can do the movement without doing a mirror movement, or other movement, in the same or the other lower limb

The degree to which loss of selective motor control occurs in spastic diplegia depends on the extent of the brain injury.

People with spastic diplegia typically demonstrate fairly good selective motor control at the hip, less control at the knee, and the least control at the ankle and foot [4]. As we saw in section 2.2, the brain injury associated with spastic diplegia occurs in the pyramidal tracts near the ventricles of the brain. Figure 2.2.1 shows that the tracts to the ankle are closer to the site of the injury than those to the knee, which in turn are closer than those to the hip. Thus the distal muscles (those further from the trunk) are more involved than the proximal muscles (those nearer the trunk).

Selective motor control is tested as part of a clinical assessment. It involves isolating movements upon request, with appropriate timing and without any overflow movement.

Tommy has difficulty dorsiflexing his right foot (bringing his right foot up). When he tries to dorsiflex his right foot, a mirror movement automatically occurs in his left foot.

Poor balance

Good balance is important in normal walking, and the task of maintaining balance while walking is quite complex. We saw in the previous section that walking involves alternately balancing on each single limb as we move forward. Balance is one of the areas affected in spastic diplegia as a result of the brain injury and loss of communication between brain centers and the spinal cord. It is particularly affected in the anterior-posterior plane ("anterior" refers to what is in front of the person, "posterior" to what is behind them).

Balance reactions can be tested by pushing the child forward and backward and side to side. A child with normal balance will easily maintain their balance and, if necessary, take a compensatory step to regain their balance. A child with balance problems may fall over or take longer to regain their balance (more than one step). In spastic diplegia the child often falls backward due to poor posterior balance. These balance problems can be seen when balance is challenged (even in children with mild spastic diplegia), such as when the person tries to avoid an object or quickly changes direction.

Balance can also be tested by getting a child (from about age four) to hop on one foot. If they can hop on one foot, their balance reactions are OK. If they are unable to hop, they can try another test: standing on one foot for 10 seconds. Many children with spastic diplegia who walk independently still fail this single-foot standing test.

There seem to be conflicting views in the literature as to whether poor balance reactions can be improved by training and/or therapy [5].

Tommy also has some balance problems; he is prone to falling backward. Though he walks independently, he does not pass these balance tests.

Abnormal tone

Muscle tone is the resting tension in a person's muscles. A range of "normal" muscle tone exists. Tone is considered "abnormal" when it falls outside the range of normal or typical. It can be too low (hypotonia) or too high (hypertonia). Abnormal muscle tone occurs in all types of CP. In children with spastic diplegia tone is typically too high in the legs and arms due to spasticity, but it can be low in the trunk.

Spasticity is one type of hypertonia (high tone). There are a number of definitions of spasticity. One definition is "a condition in which there is an abnormal increase in muscle tone or stiffness of muscle, which might interfere with movement, speech, or be associated with discomfort or pain" [6]. Another highlights the velocity-dependent nature of spasticity [7]. Spasticity results from a loss of the dampening input from specific nerve cells in the brain across the pyramidal tract connections to nerve cells in the spinal cord, and hence to certain muscles.

Since spasticity is such an important contributor to the gait problems seen in spastic diplegia, it is worth having a good understanding of it. The following is an explanation of spasticity:

- A muscle with spasticity reacts to rapid stretching by contracting (i.e., the muscle tightens rather than continuing to stretch or lengthen). This is a type of hyperactive stretch reflex: it is an overreactive response to the stretch because of the loss of inhibition—the dampening effect. (The muscle contraction can be felt as resistance by the person doing a quick passive stretch of the muscle.)[43] The muscle stretching that occurs during walking is quick (an entire gait cycle occurs in about one second), thus the spastic response happens in people with spastic diplegia while walking.
- Clonus is the purest form of spasticity and is related to the hyperactive stretch reflex. It involves a series of involuntary, rhythmic muscular contractions and relaxations. It can be seen in the gastrocnemius muscle, for example: if an examiner forcibly dorsiflexes the foot (moves the foot up), the foot may then plantar flex (move down) and continue to move up and down uncontrollably for a number of seconds. A web link to a video depicting clonus is included at the end of this section.

---

43   Passive stretching is when another person stretches an individual's muscle.

- The speed of the stretch is important because the spastic reaction only happens with a *quick* stretch. If the stretch is slow, it does not elicit a spastic reaction. (The effect of speed can be noted by comparing a muscle's response to slow and quick passive stretching.)
- In spastic diplegia, some muscles exhibit spasticity while others do not. Spasticity generally affects the two-joint muscles rather than the one-joint muscles. Spasticity particularly affects the rectus femoris, psoas, adductor longus, gracilis, hamstrings, and gastrocnemius [8–10]. All of these, except for the adductor longus, are two-joint muscles. The level of spasticity can vary from mild to severe.
- Although spasticity typically affects the muscles of the lower limbs in spastic diplegia, some upper limb muscles may also exhibit spasticity.
- Spasticity involves both the nervous and muscular systems, thus it is a neuromuscular problem [3,6,7].

Dystonia is another type of hypertonia (high tone) that may occur in spastic diplegia. In contrast to spasticity, dystonia does not occur as a result of rapid stretch. In a person with dystonia, sustained muscle contractions cause twisting and repetitive movements or abnormal postures [11]. Examples of dystonia include the leg muscles tightening when talking or playing a video game (where there is excitement or tension), or uncontrolled, writhing/posturing movements of the fingers or toes.

Spasticity and dystonia occur as a result of damage in different parts of the brain.

Tommy has spasticity in the muscles listed above. The mirror movement that occurs when Tommy tries to dorsiflex his right foot may be a sign of some level of dystonia.

Muscle weakness

Weakness, in general terms, is the inability to generate muscle force. Table 2.4.1 shows the main lower limb muscles arranged in pairs around each joint. A study found that the strength of the major muscle groups of both legs of children with spastic diplegia was lower than that of those of age-matched, typically developing peers [12]. The authors concluded that reduced muscle strength could be observed even in children with mild CP.

Muscle strength can be measured by manual muscle testing (MMT) or with a handheld machine called a dynamometer. It is sometimes challenging to measure muscle strength in spastic diplegia, however, because of the loss of selective motor control.

> Muscle weakness in the major muscle groups of both legs is a problem for Tommy.

Sensory and other problems

The brain damage may also result in sensory and other problems. Sensory problems can include decreased sensation, inability to sense where a limb is in space (proprioception), and inability to identify an object by feeling it (stereognosis). It may be more difficult for the child with spastic diplegia to identify sensory deficits because of their bilateral involvement (affecting both sides of the body) compared to a child with hemiplegia (unilateral involvement, or one side of the body affected). In other words, the child with hemiplegia may notice a difference between the two sides of their body, whereas the child with spastic diplegia may not sense any difference because both sides are affected. Other problems may include visual impairments and difficulties with visual perception[44] [13,14].

The prevalence of problems with vision, communication, feeding, and seizures was generally found to be lower among those with spastic diplegia and at GMFCS levels I–III compared with other CP subtypes and GMFCS levels [15–17].

---

44 Visual perception is the process of extracting and organizing information, giving meaning to what is seen. It is required to perform everyday tasks such as reading, copying information from a board, and understanding symbols. For those who have visual perception problems, assessment by a neuropsychologist, occupational therapist, or other expert is crucial, as is early intervention and learning adaptations from a young age. For those affected, learning strategies and/or accommodations can be very beneficial.

Tommy had visual perception difficulties such as trouble doing jigsaw puzzles and copying information from the board or from a textbook in class. The latter was initially thought to be carelessness, but it wasn't. Though these difficulties sound small, they can have big implications in education and, later, in the workplace. This underscores the importance of understanding the condition and finding appropriate supports and accommodations.

The primary abnormalities are neurological problems, present from when the brain injury occurred. In general they are difficult to change or improve.

Useful web link

- Med School Made Easy (2013) *Clonus*. [video] youtube.com/watch?v=UX75k8s5QUE

2.7

Secondary abnormalities

The human foot is a masterpiece of engineering and a work of art.
Leonardo da Vinci

Just as the twig is bent the tree's inclined.
Alexander Pope

The secondary abnormalities in spastic diplegia develop slowly over time and in direct proportion to the rate of bone growth. They also depend on the amount and type of usage of the muscles. We saw earlier that the periods of most rapid growth are from birth to age three and during puberty. These are therefore periods of great change in the child with spastic diplegia.

Now that we have an understanding of the primary abnormalities present from birth, we can look at what happens when we "just add time." With time, secondary abnormalities arise as a result of the abnormal forces imposed on the growing skeleton by the effects of the primary brain injury. In other words, the primary abnormalities drive the secondary abnormalities. The good news is that the secondary abnormalities can be treated.

This section covers:
- **Abnormal muscle growth**
- **Abnormal bone development**
- **Common bone abnormalities in spastic diplegia and the concept of lever-arm dysfunction**

Abnormal muscle growth

The following is a simplified explanation of abnormal muscle growth in spastic diplegia. This is a very complex subject, and more is still being learned about the differences between muscles in typically developing individuals and in people with spastic CP.

Children born preterm have impaired muscle growth, which is due in part to decreased pyramidal input [1,2]. This impaired muscle growth may also contribute to alterations in the ability of the muscle to grow and develop in the typical manner.

When a typically developing child is born, they have hip flexion and possibly dorsiflexion (foot up) contractures as a result of the folded position of their limbs in the womb. In the typically developing child, normal tone and normal movement resolve these contractures over time. Because of the lack of both normal tone and normal movement in the child with spastic diplegia, these infantile contractures may persist.

A muscle grows in length when it is stretched, and stretching can occur both passively and actively. It has been shown that for normal muscle growth to occur, two to four hours of stretch per day is required [3]. Bones grow during sleep. In a typically developing child whose bones have grown during sleep, this amount of stretch occurs when the child gets up and starts to move about, to run, and to play. Normal movement moves the joints through their full ROM and fully stretches the muscles of the typically developing child. This stretch provides the stimulus for laying down new muscle cells, which is how a muscle grows in length. Thus, bone growth leads to stretching of the muscle, which leads to the muscle growing in length.

A child with spastic diplegia, however, has spastic muscles and does not have the same ability to move about and exercise as the typically developing child. Even with movement, the child with spastic diplegia may not fully stretch out their muscles (i.e., they may not stretch their muscles through the full ROM of the joints). Thus the reduced stretching range may become the norm.

The reasons why the child with spastic diplegia does not have the same ability to move about and exercise as the typically developing child include:

- **Muscle spasticity:** When spastic muscles are quickly stretched, they contract, and this interferes with movement.
- **Muscle weakness:** If muscles are weak, it is more difficult to generate the effective muscle force required for normal movement.
- **Poor balance:** Movement may be restricted due to balance challenges.
- **Loss of selective motor control:** The child with spastic diplegia may not be able to produce certain movements.
- **Sensory and other problems:** The child may not be able to sense where a limb is in space, for example.
- **Difficulty transitioning between positions:** In addition to and because of the above, the child may find it difficult to transition between positions and may stay in certain positions for prolonged periods of time.

As a result of the above, the muscles fail to grow adequately in length and width[45] and contractures develop, which result in joints having reduced ROM.[46] Indeed, in the past CP was called "short muscle disease." It is worth noting that despite this title, the problem arises from muscles failing to grow in length and width rather than becoming shortened. With lack of movement, the muscles also become stiff.

Contractures are dynamic at first, in that the full ROM of the joint can be achieved when the muscle is relaxed; for example, during sleep. Over time, however, the contractures may become fixed, meaning that the full joint ROM cannot be achieved at any time. Even though a contracture may be dynamic at first and full ROM of the joint may be possible when the muscle is relaxed, full ROM may not be achievable during movement—a dynamic contracture may therefore behave as a fixed contracture and reduced ROM becomes the norm. A study

---

45 Muscles also grow in width. Growth in width has been shown to be decreased as well [2].

46 To be more precise, the contracture occurs in the muscle-tendon unit (MTU) and/or capsule of the joint, not just the muscle.

found decreasing ROM in children with CP from age two to 14 as fixed contractures developed [4].

Contractures particularly affect the two-joint muscles [5]. They interfere with positioning and movement. For example, the young child may not be able to long sit comfortably because of hamstring contractures. Contractures may also interfere with the normal movements that lead up to achieving gross motor milestones. Hamstring contractures may result in walking with flexed knees. Decreased mobility at any age may lead to activity limitation and reduced participation. Nordmark and colleagues (2009) described the circular nature of the problem: a decrease in ROM with age may result in decreased mobility and a further decrease in muscle excursion (loss of extensibility of the muscle). Loss of extensibility of the muscle may in turn result in a further decrease in ROM— a vicious circle [4].

In addition to the factors outlined above which cause contractures to develop over time, there may be differences at a tissue level between muscle contractures and typically developing muscles, including [5]:
- The muscles contain fibers of reduced diameter, which may partially explain muscle weakness.
- Increased stiffness of muscle fibers.
- Lengthened and fewer sarcomeres (the functional unit of contraction of a muscle), though the muscle itself is shortened. This could also contribute to muscle weakness.
- Enlargement of the extracellular matrix (the network surrounding the muscle cells, consisting of collagen, proteins, and more), which leads to increased muscle stiffness.
- Decrease in the number of early muscle cells. These are responsible for the majority of muscle growth.

Thus, in addition to the muscles becoming shortened, the actual composition of the spastic muscles may become altered. They may become smaller (less muscle bulk), stiffer, and less elastic compared with those of typically developing children. Smaller muscle size has been reported in children with spastic CP compared to typically developing children and in children as young as 15 months [6–8].

Thus it is to be expected that the muscles of a 14-year-old with spastic CP are very different from those of a one-year-old with spastic CP. We have more to learn about altered muscle composition in spastic CP.

To compensate for the fact that the muscles of a child with CP may not get enough stretching, a big part of what we parents have to ensure is that our child gets adequate opportunity to stretch and move their spastic muscles. Traditionally, this included the parent doing daily slow stretches of the child's spastic muscles through their full ROM. (This is called passive stretching; the slow stretching does not elicit the spastic response). However, because of the high number of hours of stretching needed to achieve muscle growth, the current thinking places a greater emphasis on other methods of stretching, including positioning, orthoses, casting,[47] and active movement. Because of its importance, a detailed section on stretching is included in the next chapter. The aim is to keep full ROM for as long as possible to prevent contractures from developing to the greatest possible extent. Working on ROM is not something that can begin when the child is older. It has to start right at the time of diagnosis. However, despite our best efforts, it is inevitable that some contractures may develop.

Not surprisingly, the rate of development of contractures often mirrors the rate of growth of the child—i.e., contractures tend to develop during periods of rapid growth (which is why keeping a growth chart is useful). While great attention needs to be paid to stretching during periods of active growth, stretching is needed throughout childhood and adolescence. Even in the "quieter" growth years, the child will still gain a few centimeters in height. See Table 2.4.1 for the normal ROMs of joints.

Graham and Selber (2003) succinctly summed up normal muscle growth as follows [9]:

> *The conditions for normal muscle growth are regular stretching of relaxed muscle, under physiologic[48] loading conditions and normal levels of activity.*

---

47 Casting consists of putting a joint in a plaster of Paris or fiberglass cast (e.g., a below-knee cast) for sustained passive stretching of the joint.

48 "Physiologic" means the right forces acting on bones, muscles, and joints in the correct position at the correct stage of development. If, for example, the joint has decreased ROM, this can be problematic.

> When Tommy was a small child, passive stretching was given more prominence than it is today (though still in combination with positioning, orthoses, casting, and active movement). My husband and I did the daily passive stretching, and organizing a typical day often included deciding which of us would "do Tommy's stretches."
>
> Over the years, Tommy developed contractures in a number of muscles.

Abnormal bone development

Abnormal muscle and abnormal bone growth in spastic diplegia are interlinked. The long bones of the body grow in a particular area of the bone called the growth plates, but it is the forces acting on the bones that determine their ultimate shape. Growing bone is "plastic" and models (takes shape) as a result of the forces exerted on it. The expressions "If you put a twist on a growing bone, it will take the twist" and "Just as the twig is bent the tree's inclined" illustrate this concept.

The bones are levers on which the muscles exert their force (pull). Bones form in response to the forces that act on them. If the forces are correct and occur at the correct time in development, then the final shape of the bone will be correct as well. We covered the six main gross motor milestones in Chapter 1; the movements that achieve the milestones[49] and the timing at which they occur are part of the normal forces acting on the bones.

One of the hallmarks of spastic diplegia is that the child is late achieving gross motor milestones. If the child is late meeting their gross motor milestones, they may have missed the opportunity for the correct forces to act on their bones. For example, a two-year-old's bones are not as malleable as a one-year-old's. In a child with spastic diplegia, the forces acting on the bones are not always normal, nor do they occur at the correct time in development. I compare it to providing opportunities for our children: we have to provide them at the right time. Peekaboo will delight your six-month-old baby, but your six-year-old child will likely

---

49   The milestones are significant, but so are the movements leading up to the milestones. For example, when a child is able to stand holding on to furniture, they may also be able to hold on with one hand and turn their body to bend down and pick up an object. All of these movements, not just the main movements, contribute to the normal forces that act on the bones.

roll their eyes if you try to play Peekaboo with them. In the presence of spastic diplegia, normal bone modeling (shaping) may not occur as the bone grows.

In addition to bone modeling, a certain amount of bone remodeling (reshaping) occurs in development. We saw that a newborn may have persistent infantile contractures that resolve over time. A certain amount of bone remodeling therefore occurs after birth: as contractures resolve, that resolution also helps reshape the bone. An example is femoral anteversion, which remodels over the course of early development (this will be addressed in the next section). In the presence of spastic diplegia, however, due to the abnormal forces, there may also be problems with bone remodeling.

Common bone abnormalities in spastic diplegia and the concept of lever-arm dysfunction

As noted earlier, a moment is a turning effect produced by a force (e.g., a muscle contraction) acting on a lever (the bone) about a pivot (the joint). The magnitude of the turning effect—the moment—is a combination of the force applied and the length of the "arm," or lever. Imagine a wrench tightening a bolt. The lever is the handle of the wrench, and the force is the pull on the handle. The moment is the turning effect produced to rotate the bolt.

The effectiveness of the muscle action to produce movement depends not only on the muscles but also on the shape and length of the bones and the position of the joints. We have already reviewed the muscle problems that develop with growth in children with CP. If the position or shape of the bone and joint are not correct, then the bone is less effective as a lever. This interferes with muscle action and movement. For example, if the femur is twisted, the hip abductors cannot work effectively because the pulling force of the muscle will now be in an incorrect direction. Gage (1991) coined the term "lever-arm dysfunction" to describe the influence of bone problems on movement [10]. These problems include lever-arms (bones) that are short, flexible, twisted, and/or in the wrong position.

The following are examples of common bone abnormalities that lead to lever-arm dysfunction in spastic diplegia. These result from disruption of bone remodeling and/or modeling and may greatly interfere with movement. They include:
a) **Hip displacement (subluxation/dislocation)**
b) **Excessive femoral anteversion and femoral torsion**
c) **Tibial torsion**
d) **Pes valgus**

Each is explained below.

a) Hip displacement (subluxation/dislocation)

The hip joint is a ball-and-socket joint that is formed by the head of the femur (ball) and the acetabulum (socket) of the hip bone. Under the influence of bone growth and spastic muscles, a child's hip may become displaced: the ball moves partially or fully out of the socket.

- In a **subluxated hip (hip subluxation)**, the ball is partially out of the socket but is still in contact with it—the ball is still partially covered by the socket.
- In a **dislocated hip (hip dislocation)**, the ball moves completely out of the socket.

The development of hip displacement is a slow process. It can lead to pain and reduced function. See Figure 2.7.1.

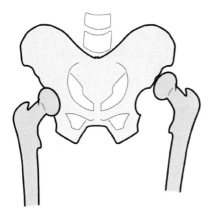

Figure 2.7.1 A dislocated hip. The subject's right hip is normal. The subject's left hip is dislocated: the head of the femur (ball) has moved completely out of the acetabulum (socket) of the hip bone.

The American Academy for Cerebral Palsy and Developmental Medicine (AACPDM) has developed a program to monitor hip development in children and adolescents with CP [11] (a web link is included at the end of this section). The program includes clinical examination and X-rays. Formal hip surveillance (monitoring) programs for children and adolescents with CP have been implemented in Australia and Sweden and are in development in other countries [5,12]. Surveillance frequency increases with increasing GMFCS level.

The measure used in X-rays for hip surveillance is called the migration percentage (MP), also known as the migration index (MI). Both terms refer to the percentage of the ball that has moved out of the socket. Hip displacement is defined as an MP greater than 30 percent. "Normal" is less than 10 percent [5]. Once the MP is greater than 30 percent, the likelihood of further displacement is almost certain (if there is growth remaining).

Research has shown that the risk of hip displacement increases with GMFCS level [13,14]. The risk of hip displacement for children with CP has been found to be:
- 0 percent (the same as typically developing children) for GMFCS level I
- 15 percent for GMFCS level II
- 41 percent for GMFCS level III

You may also come across the term "hip dysplasia." Though closely related to hip displacement, it is not the same thing. Hip dysplasia is the medical term for a hip socket that doesn't develop correctly and becomes shallow.

b) Excessive femoral anteversion and femoral torsion

"Femoral" refers to the femur (thigh bone). Though the terms "femoral anteversion" and "femoral torsion" are sometimes used interchangeably, they describe two different concepts. This section explains both.

The important parts of the femur for the purposes of this discussion are the head (ball), neck, and shaft. The neck connects the head with the shaft. See Figure 2.7.2.

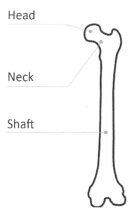

Head

Neck

Shaft

Figure 2.7.2 A femur

"Version" refers to the angle of the neck of the femur relative to the shaft. "Ante" means "forward." "Femoral anteversion" therefore refers to the fact that the neck of the femur is rotated forward relative to the shaft. See Figure 2.7.3, which provides a view of a normal hip and leg from the top down. The range of "normal" values for femoral anteversion varies depending on the reference one uses, but typically it is around 0–30 degrees in adults [15,16].

At birth, an infant has approximately 40 degrees of femoral anteversion [17]. In typically developing children with normal movement, it slowly corrects itself. It models and reshapes, and the angle reduces rapidly in the first three to four years, and further reduces until puberty to the normal value for adults. However, children with spastic diplegia do not have normal muscle forces. They also have delays in the timing of their early motor milestones. In children with spastic diplegia, therefore, femoral anteversion may not be corrected with growth. In fact, the femoral anteversion present at birth not only fails to reduce with growth but may increase. As a result, children with spastic diplegia not only retain femoral anteversion, they may also develop greater anteversion than originally present at birth. This is termed "excessive femoral anteversion." See Figure 2.7.3.

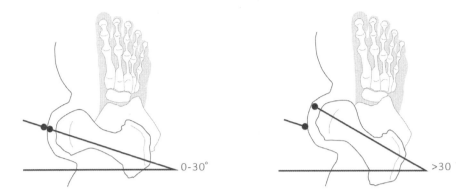

Figure 2.7.3 Femoral anteversion. Left: Normal femoral anteversion. The neck of the femur is correctly aligned with the acetabulum (socket) of the hip bone. Right: Excessive femoral anteversion. The neck of the femur is not correctly aligned with the acetabulum: it is rotated excessively forward relative to the shaft.

Mean femoral anteversion for children with CP increases with GMFCS level [14]:
- 30 degrees for GMFCS level I
- 36 degrees for GMFCS level II
- 40 degrees for GMFCS level III

People with excessive femoral anteversion often compensate by walking with the knee and foot turned in. This helps the hip abductors be in a better position to act more effectively. However, this turning in of the knee and foot exerts an abnormal inward pull on the femur, and over time it can lead to femoral torsion, a twisted femur. Femoral anteversion is present at birth, but femoral torsion develops over time. Excessive femoral anteversion and femoral torsion are examples of rotational malalignment of bones.

c) Tibial torsion

Tibial torsion is another example of rotational malalignment. Tibial torsion is a twist in the tibia (shinbone). At birth, the typically developing child has internal tibial torsion (i.e., an inward twist on the tibia). As with the femur, with the right forces acting at the right time and in the right sequence, the internal tibial torsion present in the infant turns into the 10–15 degrees of external tibial torsion in the adult [18]. However, in the child with spastic diplegia, the internal tibial torsion may overcorrect over time and become "excessive external" tibial torsion, with the foot now turning out too much. See Figure 2.7.4.

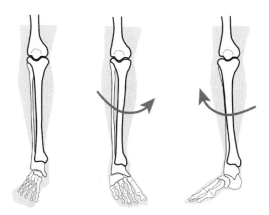

Figure 2.7.4 Tibial torsion of the right leg. Left: The leg exhibits 10–15 degrees of external tibial torsion, which is normal for an adult. The foot is slightly turned out. Middle: The leg exhibits internal tibial torsion—the foot is turned in. Right: The leg exhibits excessive external tibial torsion—the foot is excessively turned out.

The internal tibial torsion present at birth sometimes persists in children with spastic diplegia, but, as noted above, it often develops into an excessive external twist. Persistent internal tibial torsion may be seen in the younger child with spastic diplegia, while excessive external tibial torsion may be seen in the older child with spastic diplegia.

It is worth noting that in a child with femoral torsion *and* external tibial torsion, the femur (upper leg) is turned inward but the tibia (lower leg) is turned outward.

d) Pes valgus

Pes valgus is a series of complex segmental malalignments of the hindfoot, midfoot, and forefoot [14].[50] The malalignments consist of:
i)   **Valgus hindfoot**
ii) **Pronation of the midfoot**
iii) **Abduction of the forefoot**

---

50 The hindfoot is the heel. The midfoot is the middle of the foot around the arch. The forefoot comprises the toes and the long bones leading up to the toes.

i) Valgus hindfoot

In a valgus hindfoot, the heel is turned outward, away from the midline of the body, to an abnormal degree. See Figure 2.7.5.

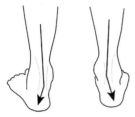

Figure 2.7.5 Valgus hindfoot. Both feet have a valgus hindfoot.

ii) Pronation of the midfoot

Pronation consists of a rotation of the bones on the inside of the arch so that in walking, the arch falls to the floor. (Some runners have pronated feet.) See Figure 2.7.6.

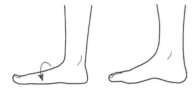

Figure 2.7.6 Pronation of the midfoot. The foot on the left is pronated; the foot on the right is normal.

iii) Abduction of the forefoot

In an abducted forefoot, the forefoot is turned outward. See Figure 2.7.7.

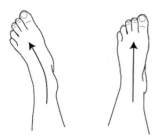

Figure 2.7.7 Abduction of the forefoot. The forefoot on the left is abducted; the forefoot on the right is normal.

These three different foot problems develop over time in response to the abnormal forces exerted on the bones, and they are commonly seen together. These problems reduce the effectiveness of the bones as lever-arms and thus interfere with movement. For example, think of a person whose foot is turned outward as they attempt to walk forward. The foot needs to be stiff in the last part of the stance phase of the gait cycle to propel the body forward. If the foot is too flexible, it becomes ineffective at doing its job. This is an example of a lever-arm that is too flexible.

Conclusion

The secondary abnormalities develop slowly over time as a result of the abnormal forces imposed on the growing skeleton by the effects of the primary brain injury. Though secondary abnormalities can be corrected with orthopedic surgery, it is important to note that they may redevelop over time as their underlying cause (the primary abnormalities) remains.

As a snapshot in time, Tommy's secondary problems at age nine included:
- Reduced ROM in many joints (both sides)
- Excessive femoral anteversion and femoral torsion (right side)
- Excessive external tibial torsion (right side)
- Pronation of the midfoot (both sides)

Useful web link

- American Academy for Cerebral Palsy and Developmental Medicine (AACPDM) (2017) *Hip Surveillance in Cerebral Palsy.* [online] aacpdm.org/publications/care-pathways/hip-surveillance

2.8

Tertiary abnormalities

Our greatest glory is not in never falling,
but in rising every time we fall.

Confucius

The tertiary abnormalities in spastic diplegia are the coping responses or compensations which arise in response to the individual's need to deal with or get around the primary and secondary abnormalities [1]. The following are some examples of tertiary abnormalities in spastic diplegia:

- **Pelvic obliquity:** One hip is higher than the other when viewed from the front. This may be the result of the child being up on the toes of one foot but not the other (asymmetric equinus). The asymmetry at the feet causes the hips to be at different levels.
- **Truncal sway:** A side-to-side sway in walking, generally a compensation for abductor weakness.
- **Retracted pelvis:** A person may walk with the pelvis tilted back on one side (retracted) and forward on the other side (protracted). This may help position the lower limb.
- **Vaulting:** Vaulting is a mechanism by which an individual compensates to clear an extremity during swing by plantar flexing or springing up on the stance side. It's a common compensation used by amputees, but it is also common in children with CP.

To correct the tertiary abnormalities, the root cause, not the compensation, has to be corrected. In the case of truncal sway, for example, addressing abductor weakness may reduce the sway. Too often vaulting is treated with lengthening, which makes gait worse. While compensations are often the most visually apparent features of CP, they do not require treatment: these compensations—the tertiary abnormalities—generally disappear when the underlying cause is treated and they are no longer required.[51]

Tommy's tertiary problems at age nine included both pelvic obliquity and truncal sway.

Conclusion

Other than spasticity, and to some extent weakness, the primary abnormalities (the neurological problems) are difficult to treat. The secondary abnormalities (the growth problems) can be treated, and treatment for the tertiary abnormalities (coping responses or compensations) is not necessary. Gait analysis, which provides an objective measurement of walking, is a very useful tool for classifying the abnormalities, which are sometimes difficult to separate.

Classifying the abnormalities of spastic diplegia into primary, secondary, and tertiary abnormalities is helpful because:

- For parents, it aids our understanding of the many problems we may encounter in spastic diplegia. The classification helps explain how the problems develop and the sequence in which they develop. It also explains how and why the condition changes over time.
- For the medical professional, it is important to separate out the different abnormalities to decide what can, cannot, and should not be treated. This separation provides a road map for treatment. Just as there is sequence in which problems develop, there is a logical sequence to treatment.

We now look at how the combination of the primary, secondary, and tertiary abnormalities affect gait in spastic diplegia.

---

51 It is worth noting that these compensations are general gait compensations that may be found in other disabilities, not just CP.

2.9

Walking in individuals with spastic diplegia

I get up. I walk. I fall down. Meanwhile I keep dancing.

Daniel Hillel

Gait is a person's manner of walking. The manner in which a person with spastic diplegia walks results from a combination of the neurological problems present from birth (the primary abnormalities), the muscle and bone problems that develop with growth (the secondary abnormalities), and any coping responses that they develop as a result (the tertiary abnormalities).

In a typically developing child, once mature walking has developed by around 3.5 years of age [1], their manner of walking changes little. This is not true of children with spastic diplegia. Delayed walking is one of the hallmarks of spastic diplegia. We saw in section 1.6 that [2]:

- At GMFCS level I, children walk between 18 months and two years without the need for any assistive mobility device.
- At GMFCS level II, children aged two to four walk using an assistive mobility device as their preferred method of mobility. At ages four to six, they walk without the need for a handheld mobility device indoors and for short distances on level surfaces outdoors.

- At GMFCS level III, children aged two to four may walk short distances indoors using a handheld mobility device (walker) and adult assistance for steering and turning. At ages four to six, they walk with a handheld mobility device on level surfaces.

Though commencement of walking is delayed, the gait of a person with spastic diplegia may also change over time as growth occurs and more abnormal muscle and growth problems accumulate.

Rodda and colleagues (2004) classified the gait patterns seen in spastic diplegia, identifying four groups with increasing severity, from Group I, true equinus, in which the child walks on their toes but with extended hips and knees, to Group IV, in which the child walks in crouch gait (persistent flexed-knee gait) [3].[52] This classification shows a progression (deterioration) in gait over time. It is important to remember, however, that not all children with spastic diplegia develop crouch gait. We address crouch gait in detail in this section.

We saw in section 2.5 that energy conservation is one of the five attributes of normal walking. Walking with spastic diplegia is less energy-efficient than normal walking (however, for that person, their walking is the most energy-efficient they can manage). For a child with spastic diplegia, walking is roughly as demanding as climbing stairs would be for a typically developing child. This is why fatigue is common in people with spastic diplegia. A study of 573 individuals with bilateral CP found that oxygen consumption during gait, a measure of energy consumption, was 2.9 times that of speed-matched typically developing peers [4]. All of the factors that cause the reduced energy efficiency of walking in spastic diplegia are not yet fully understood.

---

52 The Rodda et al. (2004) classification is as follows [3]:
- Group I: True equinus. The child is walking on their toes but with extended hips and knees. It is commonly seen in younger children when they first learn to walk.
- Group II: Jump gait. Characterized by toe-walking (equinus) and some degree of flexion at the knee and hip. It is the most common pattern in the preadolescent.
- Group III: Apparent equinus. The child walks on their toes, though they still have full ROM in their ankle joints, hence the term "apparent." This is often a transitional stage, as the majority of children go on to develop crouch gait.
- Group IV: Crouch gait (explained in this section). Some people might regard Groups II and III as forms of crouch gait.

Think of energy expenditure during walking like the fuel efficiency of a car. A more efficient car will consume less fuel while traveling a set distance. Children can generate energy at a finite rate. A person with spastic diplegia, and thus an energy-inefficient gait, travels a shorter distance for a given amount of energy or gets tired more easily when they have to walk a set distance.[53] This obviously has important consequences for activity and participation. Can the child or adolescent keep up with their peers in terms of speed or the distance they cover? Do they frequently feel fatigued and need to rest?

Navigating high school and college campuses can involve a lot of walking, and there is a balance to be struck between independent walking and using walking/mobility aids (such as sticks, crutches, a walker, or a wheelchair). The latter may reduce fatigue and/or pain to allow the child or adolescent to participate more in everyday life.

Three-dimensional (3D) computerized motion analysis is a very important tool for understanding the gait deviations that arise in spastic diplegia and planning treatment. Gait is analyzed simultaneously in three planes (hence "3D"). The three planes are:
- From back or front: coronal plane
- From the side: sagittal plane
- From top or bottom: transverse plane

Two children with spastic diplegia may walk the same, but the mechanisms behind their walking may differ. 3D computerized motion analysis helps explain each child's gait and the problems contributing to it.

Gait problems generally increase with increasing GMFCS level. Studies have shown a higher prevalence [5] and greater severity [6] of gait problems with increasing GMFCS level. However, the authors of one of these studies [6] also found there was a wide variation in gait problems within GMFCS level; thus GMFCS level is not a useful guide to gait problems. Two children at GMFCS level II, for example, could have very different gaits: one could be walking relatively erect but the other could be walking in crouch.

---

53   On a related note, if any treatment improves the energy efficiency of walking, the amount of food the child consumes may need to be adjusted so that the improved energy efficiency does not inadvertently lead to weight gain.

Three longitudinal studies of gait in children and adolescents showed deterioration in gait over time in untreated spastic diplegia [7–9] (the outcome of an untreated condition is known as the natural history of the condition). The time interval for deterioration was as low as 1.5 years. These studies underscore the importance of treating gait problems.

Crouch gait

Because crouch gait is one of the most prevalent and functional gait problems seen in spastic diplegia, we address it in detail here. Crouch gait is the typical spastic diplegic gait, described by Drs. Gage, Horstmann, and Bleck at the beginning of this chapter. As noted earlier, not all children with spastic diplegia progress to crouch gait.

Crouch gait can be defined as persistent flexed-knee gait. The exact degree of knee flexion that constitutes crouch gait varies in the literature but is typically greater than or equal to 20 degrees. This knee flexion is normally also accompanied by persistent hip flexion. The foot position can be variable; it can either be in plantar flexion (the child is on their toes) or dorsiflexion (the child has flat feet and flexed knees). Crouch gait may progress as the child grows. It should be thought of as a continuum of deformity from mild to severe.

Stout and colleagues [10] classified crouch gait as:
- **Mild crouch:** Typically seen in the younger child. This may be associated with internal hip rotation and the child being in equinus (up on their toes).
- **Moderate crouch:** Typically seen in adolescence in the person who has been walking in this posture for longer, and hamstring contracture may have developed.
- **Severe crouch:** Typically seen in older children.

This classification is similar to other classification systems [3,11]. See Figure 2.9.1.

Crouch gait looks like a person placed their hand on the child and pushed them downward. The child flexes at both the hips and the knees. The child stands and walks with this posture.

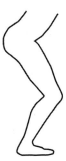

Figure 2.9.1 Crouch gait

There are many problems associated with crouch gait, particularly when it becomes severe:
- It can worsen with time and lead to decreasing walking ability or loss of walking ability.
- Knee pain, caused by pressure on the kneecap, may be a problem. Chondromalacia[54] and fracture of the patella (kneecap) may be present.
- Back pain may be a problem.
- Crouch gait may affect the child/adolescent's self-image and confidence.

Crouch may be caused by a number (and any combination) of factors, including:
- Hip flexion contractures or tightness (secondary abnormality)
- Knee flexion contractures or tightness (secondary abnormality)
- Weak antigravity muscles (primary and secondary abnormalities)
- Any treatment that weakens the ankle plantar flexors (soleus/ gastrocnemius)
- Lever-arm deformities; i.e., bone abnormalities (secondary abnormality)
- Problems with balance and selective motor control (primary abnormality)

Although crouch gait is common in spastic diplegia, professionals are still learning about it and may not yet fully understand all the factors that contribute to it.

---

54 Chondromalacia is a condition in which the cartilage on the undersurface of the patella deteriorates and softens. It can be painful.

The antigravity muscles that contribute to our extension posture are the hip extensors, knee extensors, and ankle plantar flexors (see Table 2.4.1). In crouch gait, it is mainly the hip extensors and ankle plantar flexors that are weak. Keeping adequate strength in these muscle groups is important. Keeping the ankle plantar flexors strong is particularly important because they make a significant contribution to our extension posture. The plantar flexors (particularly the soleus) control the tibia (shinbone); they pull the tibia back to straighten (extend) the knee.

The mechanics of crouch gait are complicated. When standing, gravity acts on the body to exert a downward force, while an opposite upward force is produced by the ground. The latter is called the ground reaction force (GRF).[55] The position and shape of the body/body parts determine where the GRF acts on the joints and the muscles or positions that are required to counteract it:

- When standing with extended knees (i.e., with knees straight), the GRF acts in front of the knees and helps keep them extended (straight). This is useful because less muscle action is required to keep the knees extended.
- When standing with knees excessively flexed, the GRF moves behind the knees and causes a flexion force. This results in the antigravity muscles having to work much harder to resist the GRF, which is acting to collapse the knees. See Figure 2.9.2.

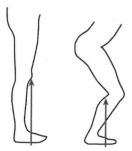

Figure 2.9.2 Position of ground reaction force (GRF) in relation to the knee.
Left: The GRF acts in front of the knees and helps keep them extended (straight).
Right: The GRF is behind the knees and causes a flexion force.

---

55 Consider a box on the floor. The GRF from the floor is sufficient to oppose the pull of gravity on the box. Now, imagine a paper bag with handles, and put a heavy object in it. The reaction force of the bag is not sufficient (does not have enough resistance) against the heavy object, which bursts through the bottom of the bag and falls out. The pull of gravity on the object is stronger than the reaction force from the bag; thus the bag cannot support the object.

If the plantar flexors have been weakened, they cannot function effectively to straighten the knee (by pulling the tibia back) in standing or walking, thus the knee extensors and hip extensors have to work hard to keep the body erect. Because of the flexed knees in crouch gait, this "free" extension force is lost. Gage (1991) coined the term "plantar flexor/knee extension couple," referring to the concept that plantar flexion action can extend the knee [12].

Once crouch starts to develop, it can become self-perpetuating. Walking continuously in a flexed pattern means that:
- Certain muscles may be continuously in a shortened state, causing contractures.
- Other muscle-tendon units are continuously in a lengthened state, becoming over-lengthened. This particularly affects the patellar tendon (the tendon that connects the kneecap [patella] to the tibia).

In section 2.4, we saw that muscles generate optimal force when operating in the middle of the ROM of the joint (i.e., when the muscle is neither too short nor too long). Muscles that are over-shortened (with contractures) or over-lengthened are not as effective at generating force. It's like trying to get a child to operate a seesaw but placing them closer to the center of the apparatus. No matter how hard they try, they will not be able to generate sufficient force to make their side of the seesaw go down. The same occurs in spastic diplegia, except here the muscles may have multiple disadvantages (they may be excessively short, excessively long, spastic, and/or weak) and may be trying to exert that force on a bone that may itself not be normal (in shape and/or position).

As a child grows, the rate of increase in muscle mass is far higher than the rate of increase in muscle strength. This is because muscle mass, which is related to muscle volume, increases as a function of the cube law, but strength, which is related to the cross-sectional area of the muscles, only increases as a function of the square.[56,57]

---

56 Here is a very simple example to illustrate the point. A young child has a muscle mass of 2 units and muscle strength of 2 units. If muscle mass increases as a function of the cube but muscle strength increases as a function of the square, then after a number of years, the older child's muscle mass will be 8 units (2 x 2 x 2) whereas their muscle strength will be 4 units (2 x 2). The older child has much less muscle strength for their muscle mass than the younger child.

57 There is a subtle difference between mass and weight. Mass is the actual amount of material in an object, measured in kilograms or pounds. Weight is the force exerted by gravity on that object. Weight is different on the Earth and the Moon (where gravity is one-sixth of that on Earth), whereas mass is the same on both.

The unfavorable strength-to-mass ratio that develops as a child grows may exacerbate an already developing crouch gait. Young children are relatively strong for their mass, but as they grow, their muscle strength may not keep pace. Thus crouch often gets worse as the child gains mass. (This strength-to-mass ratio change applies to all children and adolescents, not just those with spastic diplegia. It just goes unnoticed in typically developing children because their muscles are sufficiently strong). It is therefore very important for the child with spastic diplegia to have maximal muscle strength as they grow. Preserving plantar flexor strength and maintaining an effective plantar flexor/knee extension couple is important for preventing crouch gait.

As a snapshot in time, Tommy at nine years old walked with moderate crouch gait. His oxygen consumption while walking was 2.5 times normal, meaning his walking was two and a half times more energy-demanding than normal.

Gait analysis helped identify his particular problems at that point in time and develop a tailored treatment plan. The logical classification of his abnormalities and the ensuing treatment plan to address his particular problems gave us confidence that this was the correct path to follow.

Key points Chapter 2

- Children with spastic diplegia are born with seemingly typical bones, muscles, and joints. The problems of spastic diplegia emerge when we "just add time."
- Spastic diplegia is most commonly associated with preterm birth or an injury in the late second or early third trimester.
- The classic brain injury of spastic diplegia is called periventricular leukomalacia (PVL). It disrupts communication tracts (pyramidal tracts) that connect the brain and spinal cord and the ability to receive input from other areas of the brain. Because of the relative positions of the tracts, the ankle is more involved than the knee, and the knee is more involved than the hip.
- Growth is a very important factor in spastic diplegia. There are two periods of rapid growth: from birth to age three and during puberty. Bone growth typically ceases around age 20.
- Studies have shown that the average height of both boys and girls with CP at all ages and all GMFCS levels was lower than that of typically developing peers.
- The abnormalities that occur in spastic CP can be divided into primary, secondary, and tertiary abnormalities.
- The primary abnormalities are caused by the brain injury and are therefore present from when the brain injury occurred: they are neurological problems. They include loss of selective motor control, poor balance, abnormal tone, muscle weakness, and sensory and other problems.
- The secondary abnormalities develop over time in the growing child. They are problems of abnormal muscle growth and bone development, and are therefore referred to as growth problems.
- The tertiary abnormalities are coping responses or compensations which arise to compensate for or counteract the primary and secondary abnormalities.
- The development of contractures is a complex process that results from a number of factors, including failure of the muscles to grow adequately in length or width. Contractures arise in the muscle-tendon unit, not just the muscle.
- Common bone abnormalities that lead to lever-arm dysfunction in spastic diplegia include hip displacement (subluxation/dislocation),

excessive femoral anteversion and femoral torsion, tibial torsion, and pes valgus. These result from bone modeling and/or remodeling problems.

- In biomechanics, a "moment" is a turning effect produced by a force (e.g., a muscle contraction) acting on a lever (the bone) about a pivot (the joint). The effectiveness of a muscle action to produce movement depends not only on the muscle but also on the position and shape of the bone and joint. If the position or shape of the bone and joint are not correct, then the bone is less effective as lever, which interferes with mobility and walking.

- Formal hip surveillance programs throughout childhood and adolescence are in place in several countries. Surveillance frequency increases with increasing GMFCS level.

- The manner in which a child with spastic diplegia walks (their gait) results from a combination of the primary, secondary, and tertiary abnormalities. Gait may change over time as the child with spastic diplegia grows.

- Gait patterns in spastic diplegia can be divided into four groups with increasing severity, from Group I, true equinus, in which the child walks on their toes but with extended hips and knees, to Group IV, in which the child walks in crouch gait.

- Crouch gait can be defined as persistent flexed-knee gait. This knee flexion is also normally accompanied by persistent hip flexion. Crouch gait can vary from mild to severe.

- Walking with spastic diplegia is less energy-efficient than normal walking. This is one reason why people with spastic diplegia often experience fatigue. This may have consequences for activity and participation.

CHAPTER 3

Management and Treatment of Spastic Diplegia—Bilateral CP to Age 20

3.1

Introduction

Knowing is not enough; we must apply.
Willing is not enough; we must do.
Johann Wolfgang von Goethe

The difference between management and treatment is subtle. "Management" is the broader term which takes into account all aspects of the child's life, whereas "treatment" may be regarded as the use of a specific intervention, for example physical therapy, orthoses, or orthopedic surgery. The terms "treatment" and "intervention" are largely interchangeable.

Rosenbaum, Rosenbloom, and Mayston (2012) summed up the distinction as follows [1]:

Management implies looking at the child's day from a 24-hour perspective and ensuring that all aspects of their life are being given appropriate attention and intervention, hence the need to integrate therapy into the total management package and to appreciate the contribution of the many team members. We provide treatment to achieve management in order to enhance function and life quality.

The overall goal of management is to help the child with spastic diplegia reach their true potential—to promote their self-confidence and independence to the greatest possible extent. This is no different from the goal we have for any of our children. However, when it comes to the child with spastic diplegia, we, the family and professionals, have to work hard to ensure the condition does not hold them back from achieving their potential. Reflecting the ICF model addressed in section 1.4, the aim of management is to promote optimal participation in daily life by enhancing activities and minimizing problems with body functions and structure.

Treatment depends on the person's age and GMFCS level. Age is important because the secondary abnormalities develop with growth and thus with time. GMFCS level is important because in general the higher the GMFCS level, the greater the extent of the problems. We will see that a number of treatments are used to increase stretching and thus to stimulate muscle growth. These treatments are often accompanied by treatments to reduce muscle tone. The goal is to prevent or delay the onset of muscle contractures and bone deformities and allow the child the typical experience of activity and participation at every stage of life. The muscle and bone abnormalities that still develop may be addressed with orthopedic surgery.

Treatments in spastic diplegia are not isolated but integrated. A person may receive multiple treatments at the same time. In some cases, one type of treatment enhances the effectiveness of another. This is one element of the integrated management approach to spastic diplegia, and it underscores the importance of the multidisciplinary team.

This chapter examines what good management and treatment looks like. It addresses management and treatment to age 20. The following chapter addresses spastic diplegia in adulthood. This age cutoff is appropriate for a number of reasons:

- Growth is an important factor in spastic diplegia. As we saw in the growth charts in Chapter 2, growth is generally complete by age 20.
- Around age 18 to 20, health services in most countries transition from pediatric to adult. Sadly, health services for adults with CP are much less developed than those for children.

This chapter is organized as follows:

Section 3.2   What does best practice look like?
Section 3.3   Therapies
Section 3.4   The home program
Section 3.5   Orthoses
Section 3.6   Tone reduction
Section 3.7   Orthopedic surgery
Section 3.8   The overall musculoskeletal management plan to age 20
Section 3.9   Alternative and complementary treatments
Section 3.10   What the parent can do to help the child, what the adolescent can do to help themselves

3.2

What does best practice look like?

"Would you tell me, please, which way I ought to go from here?"
"That depends a good deal on where you want to get to," said the Cat.
"I don't much care where—" said Alice.
"Then it doesn't matter which way you go," said the Cat.
Lewis Carroll, from *Alice's Adventures in Wonderland*

It is important to understand best practice and know what it looks like. This section provides an overview of the generally accepted principles underpinning best practice in the management and treatment of spastic diplegia at the time of writing. Best practice is likely to continue to evolve over time.

Best practice currently includes:
- **Family-centered care and patient-centered care**
- **Evidence-based medicine**
- **Data-driven decision-making**
- **A multidisciplinary team approach**
- **Specialist centers**
- **Early intervention**
- **Setting goals**
- **Measuring outcome**

Family-centered care and patient-centered care

When a child is diagnosed with spastic diplegia, the whole family is affected: parents, siblings, and extended family members. Family-centered care is a way of ensuring that care is planned around the whole family, not just the child with the condition.[58] Family-centered care can be thought of as a meeting of experts, who pool their knowledge to jointly develop the most appropriate plan of care for the child. The parent is the expert on their child, while the professional is the expert on the condition and its treatment. Professionals who practice family-centered care see themselves not as the sole authority but as a partner with the parent in the provision of care for the child [1].

Family-centered care and patient-centered care are closely related. The latter evolves from the former as the child grows. In patient-centered care, the patient is an active participant in their own medical care and decision-making. A few points on patient-centered care:

- Patient-centered care involves the professional engaging the child from an early stage in conversations. A study of factors that predict whether a child will answer questions during primary care pediatric visits found that if a doctor simply looks at a very young child when they ask a question, that child is more likely to engage in the medical process [2].
- Patient-centered care promotes the opposite of the concept of "learned helplessness," the belief that nothing one chooses to do can affect what is happening [3]. Learned helplessness can be regarded as a secondary disability [1].
- A study found that having learned how to take personal responsibility for personal health during childhood was significantly associated with regular physical activity in adults with CP [4].

---

58 Family-centered care is also termed "family-centered service." CanChild defined family-centered care as follows (web link included at the end of this section) [5]:

Family-centred service is made up of a set of values, attitudes, and approaches to services for children with special needs and their families. Family-centred service recognizes that each family is unique; that the family is the constant in the child's life; and that they are the experts on the child's abilities and needs. The family works together with service providers to make informed decisions about the services and supports the child and family receive. In family-centred service, the strengths and needs of all family members are considered.

The change from family-centered care to patient-centered care is a gradual one that parents and providers can help facilitate over time.

In the early days, the child cannot speak for themselves, so the parent has to be their advocate and decision-maker. A friend of mine signed all official paperwork for her young son as "Deirdre [Surname], voice of John [Surname]." This clearly summed up how she viewed her role.

As experts on our children, we parents must not forget to speak up on their behalf. Our child is depending on us. Here's an example. Once, a well-meaning occupational therapist suggested Tommy get a special adjustable table and chair at school to promote good posture while sitting. He was about eight or nine years old at the time. The downside was that instead of sitting at a table for two like all of his peers and having the company of a friend, he was now sitting alone at a very different-looking table. He did not like it at all. Whatever the marginal gain in posture, the loss in terms of participation was simply not worth it. He stopped using it after about a year.

I advise parents to be mindful of the cost-benefit ratio of treatments. (I'm not talking about financial cost.) Remember, you are the expert on your child, and you should feel empowered to weigh the pros and cons of medical professionals' recommendations to make sure they are truly what's best for your child. Don't be afraid to offer another perspective (even if you only realize it after the fact, as I did in the example above). Trust your judgement.

Evidence-based medicine

Evidence-based medicine (or evidence-based practice) is "the conscientious, explicit, and judicious use of current best evidence in making decisions about the care of individual patients." It combines the best available external clinical evidence from research with the clinical expertise of the professional [6].

Unfortunately, though evidence-based practice is the goal, a number of authors in the field of CP have noted that there is a long way to go to achieve it [7,8]. The transfer of research into clinical practice can be slow: this applies to all medical fields, not just CP. It was found that it takes an average of 17 years for research evidence to reach clinical practice [9]. For example, the GMFCS was first published in 1997; a survey of 283 pediatric physical therapists in 2015 found that fewer than half used the GMFCS consistently [10]. A recent study found that fewer than half of 303 caregivers knew their child's GMFCS level [11]. This demonstrates how long it takes for medical advances to be implemented in practice.

While evidence is essential in medicine, absence of evidence does not necessarily mean absence of effectiveness. Evidence-based medicine combines the best available evidence from research with the clinical expertise of the professional. The professional's clinical expertise is usually what gives rise to the development of new treatments, and research proving a treatment's efficacy generally follows. For example, single-event multilevel surgery (SEMLS) was first developed in the 1980s based on the clinical expertise of leading surgeons in the field, but the research followed later. Though SEMLS was first performed in the 1980s, the first randomized controlled trial (RCT)[59] to evaluate its effectiveness as a treatment for CP was only conducted in 2011 [12]. Many children would have missed out on the benefits of SEMLS if they'd had to wait for the evidence to prove its effectiveness. Indeed, given that new research (and hopefully new treatments) is continually emerging, this book will need to be updated in time.

In addition:
- Sometimes scientific evidence is conflicting. Some authors may support a treatment, yet others may raise concerns. Evidence-based medicine involves evaluating the quality and quantity of the research and paying attention when concerns are raised. A treatment may be well researched but problems may become evident only after the treatment has been used over a long period of time. New research may emerge which causes the field to question and/

---

59   The randomized controlled trial (RCT) is the gold standard in research. An RCT is a scientific experiment that has very strict guidelines to ensure that the only aspect that makes the two groups different is that one receives the treatment and the other does not. In an RCT, people are randomly assigned to either the group receiving the treatment or the non-treatment group (also known as the control group). Comparing the outcome of the two groups allows the researcher to determine whether the treatment was effective.

or change widely held opinions. Scientific research is not static—it is continually evolving.

- Not all CP treatments have adequate evidence supporting their efficacy.
- In addition to short-term effects, it is important to track the long-term effects of any treatment. There are few long-term studies in CP, but thankfully these are growing in number.
- Tools like the GMFCS allow researchers to better describe participants in research studies. This greatly improves our ability to evaluate the relevance of a study to a particular situation. Research studies that included participants with spastic diplegia, GMFCS levels I–III were most relevant for this book.
- Studies report the average results for a group of participants. Results may be good for some participants and less good for others. Many factors contribute to outcome; though there may be strong evidence supporting a treatment, this does not guarantee the treatment will work for every person. It is important to keep this in mind when applying the findings of studies to a particular situation. For example, studies report positive outcomes following SEMLS for groups of children. However, the outcome following SEMLS for each individual child is unique, based on factors including their level of disability, the original treatment plan, and the plan of care following surgery. This point applies to all treatments.
- The budget allocated to CP research is very small, which makes the choice of research actually conducted very important. A recent US initiative to set a patient-centered research agenda for CP involved a collaboration between all stakeholders—including caregivers and people with CP [13]—based on the belief that a research agenda developed collaboratively would be more useful to the entire community than one developed by professionals alone. It was built around the concept of "nothing about us without us."[60]

Data-driven decision-making

Best practice demands decision-making be data-driven. (This can also be called data-informed decision-making.) For example, in orthopedic

---

60 Sixteen top research priorities were identified. Leading themes included the comparative effectiveness of interventions, physical activity, and understanding aging. It also highlighted the need to focus on longitudinal research that includes outcomes related to participation and quality of life.

surgical decision-making in CP (e.g., for SEMLS), data is drawn from multiple sources:

- Medical history
- Physical examination
- Imaging
- Gait analysis
- Examination under anesthesia

The skilled evaluation of multiple sources of data is essential for good decision-making.

A multidisciplinary team approach

Treatment of CP does not involve just one discipline. It involves medical professionals from a number of disciplines, including physical therapy (PT), occupational therapy (OT), speech and language pathology (SLP, also termed speech and language therapy, SLT),[61] nursing, orthotics,[62] pediatrics,[63] neurology,[64] neurosurgery,[65] orthopedic surgery,[66] physical medicine and rehabilitation (PMR, also termed physiatry),[67] and more.

The multidisciplinary team approach means the person is being treated by medical professionals from a number of disciplines working together as a team. Though they work as a team, each professional stays within their professional boundaries. A more detailed explanation of the role of the team members is included in Gillette's *Cerebral Palsy Road Map: What to Expect as Your Child Grows* [14] (web link included at the end of this section).

---

61   The roles of physical therapy (PT), occupational therapy (OT), and speech and language pathology (SLP, also termed speech and language therapy, SLT) are explained in section 3.3.

62   Orthotics is the branch of medicine concerned with the design, manufacture, and management of orthoses (braces). An orthosis (or brace) is a device designed to hold specific body parts in position in order to modify their structure and function. It is usually made of lightweight, custom-molded plastic or carbon fiber.

63   Pediatrics is the branch of medicine dealing with children and their conditions.

64   Neurology is the branch of medicine dealing with disorders of the nervous system.

65   Neurosurgery is surgery performed on the nervous system, in particular the brain and spinal cord.

66   Orthopedic surgery is surgery performed on the musculoskeletal system: the bones, joints, muscles, ligaments, and tendons.

67   Physical medicine and rehabilitation (PMR, also termed physiatry) is the branch of medicine that aims to enhance and restore functional ability and quality of life among those with physical disabilities. PMR physicians treat a wide variety of medical conditions affecting the brain, spinal cord, nerves, bones, joints, ligaments, muscles, and tendons.

I recently came across a booklet on type 2 diabetes which outlined the members of the diabetes care team. The very first answer to the question, "Who is in your diabetes team?" was, "You, the person with diabetes, are the most vital member of the team."

The same can be said of CP. You, the parent—and, later in life, the person with the condition—are the most vital member of the team. The person with the condition "owns" it: they can seek the best help available, but at the end of the day they still own their condition. (And in the early days, the parent owns the condition on behalf of the young child.)

To use a sporting analogy, the success of the multidisciplinary team depends on the members playing as a team, not as individuals skilled in their own positions.

Specialist centers

Specialist centers, also known as centers of excellence, are on the rise in many areas of medicine across the developed world. Consider, for example, specialist centers for breast cancer. Research has shown that outcomes in breast cancer treatment improve with the number of breast cancer cases a particular center has treated (this is known as centralization). The annual number of operations per center and per surgeon (specialization) are also important, and the multidisciplinary team is of paramount importance [15].

A specialist center for the treatment of CP:
- Has a multidisciplinary team that includes the specialities described earlier.
- Treats a high volume of patients with CP on a routine or daily basis. For any health condition, there is a minimum volume of patients a center must treat in order to build and maintain expertise.
- Provides the full range of evidence-based treatment options, allowing the most suitable ones to be chosen for each individual child.
- Conducts research and publishes in peer-reviewed journals. The research should include long-term outcome studies that contribute to the evidence base for treatments.
- Ideally, offers a lifetime of care. CP is not just a "children's condition."

Unless you're lucky enough to live near such a center, visiting one will likely involve travel and expense. I advise you to seek out the best specialist center in your area (the criteria listed above may be useful) and have your child reviewed there as early as possible. This doesn't mean all services have to be delivered by the specialist center. A specialist center will work with your child's local care team, but you should be able to visit it at critical times.

Early intervention

Early intervention is essential in the management of spastic diplegia,[68] usually from birth to age five. We have already seen that:

- Early diagnosis is necessary for early intervention. Since spastic diplegia is usually mild or moderate, diagnosis may be delayed, thus intervention arrives late.
- Early intervention offers the best opportunity to tap into neuroplasticity.
- Early intervention is important for minimizing the secondary abnormalities as the child grows [16]. Remember, growth is most vigorous in the first year of life [17].

Though the emphasis is on early intervention, intervention continues to be required during childhood, adolescence, and adulthood.

Setting goals

Treatment goals should be collaboratively agreed upon between the child, parent, and professional, and the achievement of goals should be evaluated after treatment. One widely used goal-directed system is known as SMART.[69] In this system, goals are designed to be "Specific, Measurable, Achievable, Relevant, and Time-bound" [1].

---

68 Early intervention has been defined as:
   Multidisciplinary services [...] to promote child health and well-being, enhance emerging competencies, minimize developmental delays, remediate existing or emerging disabilities, prevent functional deterioration, and promote adaptive parenting and overall family functioning. These goals are accomplished by providing individualized developmental, educational, and therapeutic services for children provided in conjunction with mutually planned support for their families [18].

69 The SMART system is widely used elsewhere, for example in industry in areas like project management and employee performance. It is also used in personal development.

Let's look at each aspect of the **SMART** system in more detail.

a) **Specific and measurable:** Goals that are specific and measurable should contain five elements:
- Who
- Will do what
- Under what conditions
- How well
- By when

b) **Achievable:** The goal should match the child's prognosis and be attainable.

c) **Relevant:** Goals should hold meaning for the child and family and be related to their own goals. Goals should be functional; i.e., not based on impairment (problems with body functions and structure) alone.

d) **Time-bound:** Goals must have a specific date for achievement.

The following are some examples of SMART goals. The first three are for a younger child. The last two may be more common following a treatment like SEMLS.
- James will pull to stand with furniture support in order to participate in play activities (train table) within three months.[70]
- Guilherme will creep 30 feet independently in order to move between rooms of his home within three months.
- Emma will maintain tailor sitting independently while using both hands for play for 10 minutes in order to participate in play activities within her home within six weeks.
- Athena will use her posterior (reverse) walker to walk 300 feet over the sidewalk in order to access the playground at recess within three months.
- Jack will ascend/descend 13 stairs with one rail and minimal assistance (steadying assistance of a parent) in order to access the bedroom on the upper level of his home within one month.

---

70 Typically the goal would include a specific date for achievement, rather than the less specific "within three months."

Research has shown that:

- Therapies that focus on achieving functional goals in everyday life result in measurable improvements in gross motor skills when compared to therapies that are not goal-directed [19].
- The development of fewer and more meaningful goals is imperative for adherence, improved outcomes, and greater patient and family satisfaction [20].
- Children can be trusted to identify their own goals, thereby influencing their involvement in their own treatment programs. If the child creates their own goal, they will likely be more motivated to achieve it. Children's self-identified goals were found to be as achievable as parent-identified goals and remained stable over time [21].

Measuring outcome

Many variables can be measured, including height, walking speed, and walking ability. Some variables can be measured using equipment, others by parent report. A tape measure, timed walk test, 3D computerized motion analysis,[71] and the Gillette Functional Assessment Questionnaire (FAQ)[72] are all examples of measurement tools used to measure these variables.

A measurement can be taken at any point in time to establish a person's status (e.g., the person's current height, walking speed, or walking ability).

An outcome is defined as a result or an effect, thus "measuring outcome" means measuring a result or an effect. If a person's walking speed is measured before a treatment such as orthopedic surgery and then again afterward, one can evaluate the effect or result—the outcome—of the surgery on the person's walking speed by comparing the before and after measurements. The outcome of surgery can thus be measured using the variable of walking speed. It can also be measured using the variable of walking ability, as measured by the FAQ.

---

71 Three-dimensional computerized motion analysis (3D computerized motion analysis) provides a very detailed analysis of gait. Gait is analyzed simultaneously in three planes, hence the term "3D."

72 The Gillette Functional Assessment Questionnaire (FAQ) has a 10-level walking scale. It asks the family to rate the individual's typical walking ability with their usual assistive devices. The scale covers a range of walking ability, from level 1 ("Cannot take any steps at all.") to level 10 ("Walks, runs, and climbs on level and uneven terrain and does stairs without difficulty or assistance. Is typically able to keep up with peers.")

Variables used to measure outcome can be classified as technical, functional, or patient/parent satisfaction. For example, orthopedic surgery is commonly evaluated using many technical variables (joint ROM, gait deviations, energy consumed in walking) as well as functional variables (gross motor function, walking ability). Each variable provides different but complementary information. Variables can be measured in each domain of the ICF (body functions and structure, activity, and participation). To provide the most comprehensive evaluation of a treatment, a range of variables (technical, functional, and patient/parent satisfaction) covering different domains of the ICF should be used. Appendix 3 includes more information on measurement tools.

Conclusion

The discussion above summarizes the current generally accepted principles underpinning best practice in the management and treatment of spastic diplegia. We next look at different treatments during childhood and adolescence.

We parents want the very best for our children with spastic diplegia. We understand that it is a lifelong condition and that there is currently no cure. Our children deserve the best management and treatment to ensure the effects of their condition are no more burdensome than they absolutely need to be. We want its management to be limited only by medical science.

The reality, however, is that the quality and standard of available services varies greatly between countries, and even within a country. Some areas have much better services than others. Management of a child's (or adolescent's or adult's) condition should not be limited by zip or postal code.

Many professionals may themselves wish they could provide more and better services to people with CP. They, too, may recognize gaps in their service provision. Rosenbaum and Rosenbloom (2012) noted that both parents and professionals need to be aware of what effective services look like and lobby health policy-makers appropriately (and hopefully in concert) to improve services [22]. I agree: we parents need to know what good management and treatment looks like, and if the services in our community or country do not measure up, we need to lobby to effect change, even if this is challenging. Otherwise, our children, adolescents, and adults with CP are the ones who lose out.

Useful web links

- CanChild (2019) *Family-Centred Service.* [online] canchild.ca/en/research-in-practice/family-centred-service

- Gillette Children's Specialty Healthcare (2016) *Cerebral Palsy Road Map: What to Expect as Your Child Grows.* [pdf] gillettechildrens.org/assets/uploads/care-and-conditions/CP_Roadmap.pdf

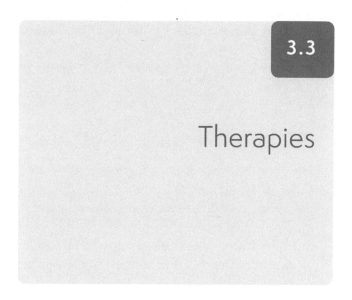

3.3

Therapies

The nice thing about teamwork is that
you always have others on your side.

Margaret Carty

Many children with spastic diplegia attend physical therapy, occupational therapy, and/or speech and language pathology (or therapy) at various points during their development. Therapy is defined by Rosenbaum, Rosenbloom, and Mayston (2012) as [1]:

> *A process of helping a family (and a child) to learn ways for a child to function optimally in their many environments. It [...] involves using the therapist's expertise to explore ways that will enable the child and the family to live as fully and functionally as possible.*

Obviously, this definition extends to the adolescent and adult with CP as well. Improvement in function should be the primary goal of therapy.

This section covers:
- **Physical therapy (PT, also termed physiotherapy)**
- **Occupational therapy (OT)**
- **Speech and language pathology (SLP, also termed speech and language therapy, SLT)**
- **Delivery of therapy services**[73]

Physical therapy (PT, also termed physiotherapy)

Physical therapists provide services that develop, maintain, and restore a person's maximum movement and functional ability [2]. Physical therapists have different titles in different countries: in many countries they are called physiotherapists. In this book, I use the terms "physical therapist" and "physical therapy."[74] PT is usually one of the first services the parent of a child with spastic diplegia encounters.

In a paper titled "Activity, Activity, Activity: Rethinking Our Physical Therapy Approach to Cerebral Palsy," Damiano (2006) made the following point [3]:

> *It becomes increasingly difficult over time for elite athletes to break individual sports records as human limits are approached. In contrast, the state-of-the-science in neurorehabilitation suggests that we are not even close to approaching the human limits for physical and neural recovery in many disorders. A growing body of scientific data [...] strongly suggests that activity-based strategies, which are within the purview of physical therapy, are one of the keys to unlocking the now far brighter potential for functional recovery.*

Three major potential outcomes were identified for an activity-based approach [3]:

---

73   There are other types of therapists; for example, play therapists, music therapists, and therapeutic recreation specialists (TRS). A therapeutic recreation specialist is a professional qualified to provide recreational therapy services in the US and Canada. There may be an equivalent professional in other countries.

74   The only confusion is that in Ireland the term "physical therapist" is used for people who are trained in the manual treatment of soft tissues, mostly massage. Thus in Ireland the terms "physical therapist" and "physiotherapist" are not interchangeable.

- Preventing secondary musculoskeletal impairments (the secondary abnormalities) and maximizing physical functioning.
- Fostering the cognitive, social, and emotional development of the child.
- Developing, maintaining, and perhaps restoring neural structures and pathways. (This relates to neuroplasticity.)

Physical therapists select treatments based on their own evaluation and the family and child's goals. Treatments are often task-specific, functional activities. For example, if the child's PT goal is to walk more independently, then the therapy might primarily involve walking and the many activities that form the building blocks for walking.

Physical therapists apply motor learning theory to guide therapy activities and help the child achieve their goals. The American Physical Therapy Association (APTA, 2012) explained the concept [4]:

> During the beginning stage of learning, the cognitive stage, the focus of practice for the child is to gain a general idea of the movement strategy. Performance will be variable, with a large number of errors. A greater amount of guidance and feedback from the PT is optimal. During the second stage of learning, the associative stage, high quantities of practice are required for the child to refine the movement pattern. Performance becomes more consistent over time, with a gradual weaning of feedback from the PT. During the third stage of learning, the autonomous stage, the focus is on practice across different environments so that automaticity of performance can occur. Practice in different environments affords the child a greater variety of meaningful learning opportunities to create motor memory and establish a learned task.

Physical therapists select treatments that aim to reduce the primary abnormalities (or impairments) and prevent secondary abnormalities. Though they may select treatments designed to improve functional activities, the treatments themselves are often not functional activities. For example, a child's goal may be to be able to get up from the floor without holding on to anything for support. During the evaluation the physical therapist may identify limited ankle range of motion (ROM) and weak hip and knee extensors as the factors (the underlying abnormalities) preventing the child from meeting their goal. As a result, the physical therapist might include casting (to address the limited ROM) and isolated strengthening exercises (to address the weak extensors) in the plan of care for that child. These treatments address the underlying abnormalities, but they themselves are not functional activities. However, as the underlying abnormalities are reduced, the treatment will shift to task-specific practice of moving from the floor to standing.

Common treatments that may be used by the physical therapist as part of the goal-directed/functional training approach include:
a) **Stretching (using multiple methods) to maintain or improve joint ROM and alignment**
b) **Strengthening**
c) **Functional mobility and gait training**
d) **Electrical stimulation, usually in combination with functional activities**

There is evidence to support this goal-directed/functional training approach [5,6].[75]

Before addressing each treatment in turn, it is important to note that the goal-directed/functional training approach and many of the following treatments (specifically stretching, strengthening, functional mobility, and electrical stimulation) are also used in occupational therapy, which we will review in the next section. Since the lower limbs are more involved in people with spastic diplegia, this section focuses on treatments in relation to the lower limbs. This is not to forget that there may also be some upper limb involvement, thus these treatments may have relevance for the upper limbs as well.

a) Stretching (using multiple methods) to improve or maintain joint ROM and alignment

We saw in Chapter 2 that two to four hours of stretching per day is required for normal muscle growth and that the typically developing child gets this amount of stretch during the day when they get up and

---

75 It is worth noting that there are and have been other therapy approaches. Some continue to be used, such as conductive education and vojta therapy [6]. The recommendation for others has been that they be discontinued, such as patterning—the Doman-Delacato technique [7]. A discussion of other therapy approaches is beyond the scope of this book.

start to move about, run, and play. We also saw that lack of muscle growth leads to contractures in people with spastic diplegia.

Stretching is required throughout growth for the young child, the older child, and the adolescent with spastic diplegia. How this stretching is achieved may vary over the years, but the need for stretching remains constant. There are also critical periods when stretching is especially important, which coincide with the periods of most rapid growth: the first three years and the adolescent growth spurt.

Traditionally, stretching was done by performing slow passive stretching of the spastic muscles. However, due to the number of hours of stretching needed to achieve muscle growth and weak evidence supporting the efficacy of passive stretching, greater emphasis is now placed on other, active methods of achieving muscle stretch [8].

Though we refer to stretching muscles, what is actually being stretched is the muscle-tendon unit (MTU), not just the muscle. Muscles in particular need of stretching include the hip flexors, hip adductors, rectus femoris, hamstrings, and calf muscles. Most are two-joint muscles that are more prone to contractures [9]. Refer to Table 2.4.1. If the person has significant upper limb involvement, the upper limb muscles may also be included in the stretching program.

The following are different methods of stretching (any number of methods may be used simultaneously):
i) **Positioning**
ii) **Orthoses**
iii) **Casting**
iv) **Active movement**

i) Positioning
A variety of positions can be used throughout the day to achieve sustained/prolonged muscle stretching in order to promote muscle growth. It is important that the child/adolescent gets a variety of positions throughout the day and does not spend too much time in one position. The child/adolescent may have favorite positions, but it is important to vary them. For the small child, moving between positions may require parental support.

"W-sitting" is the term used to describe the sitting position which the child with spastic diplegia (and other forms of spastic CP) adopts. The child's bottom is on the floor while their feet are out. Looking from the top, the legs form a "W" shape. Children with spastic diplegia like W-sitting because it is a stable position, requires no balance work, and leaves the hands free for play. The problem with W-sitting is that it may cause a loss of hip external rotation, which interrupts the typical process of bone remodeling. The child also misses out on functional opportunities to develop balance reactions. While W-sitting was traditionally not recommended, it is now thought to be somewhat acceptable provided the child gets plenty of time in other positions to balance out the less ideal elements of W-sitting.

For older children and adolescents with spastic diplegia, it is also very important not to spend prolonged time in one position, usually sitting—a particular challenge given the common overuse of electronic devices.

Appendix 4 includes information on various positions, including long sitting, side sitting, tailor sitting, prone positioning, and standing. It is important to look for lots of opportunities during the day to incorporate positioning—for example while playing, reading, watching TV, or using electronic devices.

ii) Orthoses

An orthosis (or brace) is a device designed to hold specific body parts in position in order to modify their structure and function. It is usually made of lightweight, custom-molded plastic or carbon fiber. One of the goals of orthoses is to achieve muscle stretch for a longer duration.

Night splints, such as ankle-foot orthoses (AFOs, which cover the ankle joint and foot) plus knee immobilizers, may also be used to achieve stretching. Wearing an AFO plus a knee immobilizer allows stretching of the calf muscles (both the one-joint soleus and the two-joint gastrocnemius; refer to Table 2.4.1). Night splints are worn to tolerance during sleep. Wearing one knee immobilizer each night and alternating between right and left may help if wearing both at once is too much.

iii) Casting

Casting consists of putting a joint in a plaster of Paris or fiberglass cast (such as a below-knee cast) for sustained passive stretching of the joint.

Fiberglass casts are lighter. Serial casting is usually practiced to gain further ROM with each casting.

iv) Active movement
Active movement is exactly what it sounds like. The child or adolescent needs to get plenty of active movement through the entire ROM of the joints. This is achieved through exercise and physical activity.

The method (or methods) of stretching used depends on a number of factors, including level of spasticity, muscle tightness, age, and developmental stage. The physical therapist can provide guidance, but the work has to be done at home: stretching must be built into the activities of normal life.

The research evidence for stretching is mixed, but the clinical expertise of medical professionals supports its use. In a letter titled "To Stretch or Not to Stretch in Children with Cerebral Palsy," Gorter and colleagues (2007) concluded that stretching can be helpful in children with CP if it is part of an integrated habilitation plan [10].

b) Strengthening

Muscle weakness is one of the primary abnormalities of spastic diplegia, but muscle strength is further affected by the development of the secondary abnormalities (abnormal muscle growth and bone development). We saw earlier that the strength of the major muscle groups of both legs of children with spastic diplegia was lower than that of age-matched, typically developing peers [11]. Traditionally, strengthening was frowned upon in spastic diplegia because it was thought to increase spasticity. However, strengthening has been found to increase the force-producing capability, not the spasticity, of the muscle [12].

Muscle strengthening is especially important for people with spastic diplegia because muscle weakness is a feature of the condition. Muscle strengthening is needed for all muscles, but it is particularly important for the antigravity muscles: the hip extensors (gluteus maximus) and the ankle plantar flexors (gastrocnemius and soleus). Other muscles to be considered include the hip abductors, ankle dorsiflexors, the core muscles, and the upper limb muscles, if there is upper limb involvement.

The physical therapist can determine which strengthening exercises are most appropriate for the child at their developmental stage. Muscles can be strengthened in different positions. We addressed different types of muscle contractions in section 2.4; depending on the role of the muscle, the strengthening exercises may be concentric, eccentric, or isometric. Strengthening may be functional, like sit to/from standing or stair climbing.

In addition to focused muscle strengthening exercises, as with stretching, strengthening has to be built into normal life. For the small child, a variety of positions can provide an opportunity to strengthen the muscles during play. Often, the same positions can be used to achieve both stretch and strength. The need for strengthening also applies to the older child and adolescent. Specific details on strengthening are included in Table 3.4.1 in the next section as well as in Appendix 4.

Many early studies demonstrate the benefit of strength training [13]. More recent studies have noted that although strength training increased muscle strength, the benefits did not necessarily carry over to functional improvement [14,15]. Recent recommendations include context-specific strength training for gait or other functional activities [16]. This means that the strength training should be related to actual function and that the approach may need to be more targeted to the individual muscles whose weakness is most limiting to the child or adolescent's motor task performance [9,17].

Once parents understand the key muscles that need stretching and/or strengthening, they can look for opportunities to incorporate these activities into the child's play. For example, the hip adductors (the inner thigh muscles) are often tight, while the hip abductors (the outer thigh muscles) are often weak. One can make a game of side walking on a playground or around the perimeter of the shallow end of a swimming pool. These can be fun ways for the young child to stretch the adductors and strengthen the abductors in everyday life.

c) Functional mobility and gait training

Physical therapists specialize in movement, and a significant amount of time in PT is focused on practicing functional mobility. The physical therapist selects specific mobility activities or tasks based on the child's age and function as well as the child and/or family's goals.

For very young children, physical therapists emphasize practicing developmental activities such as rolling, creeping, and crawling. Later, they may emphasize moving from one position to another, for example moving in and out of standing positions or moving with support (e.g., cruising along a surface: the child walks alongside a sofa while holding on for support). Depending on the child's function and environmental demands, physical therapists may teach children to use compensatory movements[76] or recommend the use of orthoses or assistive mobility devices[77] in order to maximize the child's independence. For older children, adolescents, and adults, functional mobility includes how a person moves in and out of bed, transfers (stands up and sits down or moves from chair to chair), and moves around in their environment (walking or using a wheelchair).

Gait training refers to treatment interventions used by the physical therapist to work on developing or improving walking skills. As with other aspects of functional mobility, physical therapists may recommend the

---

76 An example for negotiating stairs: a "normal" or preferred pattern would be to place one foot on each step (step over step). However, if a child needs to walk up or down the stairs at school independently and is unable to use this pattern safely, they may be taught to place both feet on each step. This is a compensatory pattern that allows the child to rely on their stronger leg. An example for walking: a child may be able to walk short distances at home without using a walker, but in less familiar or busy environments they may require a walker for stability and/or safety. In addition, their pattern of walking might be smoother (more fluid) with a walker. They may demonstrate more compensatory movement patterns (deviations) without the walker.

77 Assistive mobility devices (also termed assistive devices, walking aids, mobility aids, and gait aids) vary in the level of support they provide. Here they are listed in order of least to most support:
- Walking sticks (canes)
- Crutches
- Reverse walker
- Gait trainer (a device which is more supportive than a walker but less supportive than a wheelchair)
- Wheelchair

Walking sticks (canes) may be single or triple-pronged (three-point). Triple-pronged walking sticks provide more support if the person has balance issues. There are also quadruple-pronged (four-point) walking sticks for even greater support. One or two walking sticks or crutches may be used. Wheelchairs may be self-propelled or power-assisted.

use of orthoses or assistive mobility devices in order to maximize the child's independence.

Gait training is often a progression. It may initially require more assistance and more-supportive assistive devices but progress to less assistance and less-supportive assistive devices. It may also progress to increasing distances and walking in more challenging environments. Conversely, following surgery or based on environmental demands (e.g., moving between classes on a large high school or college campus), more-supportive assistive devices and orthoses might be recommended to reduce fatigue, pain, and/or falls. Physical therapists (in collaboration with other members of the multidisciplinary team) are a great source of guidance on assistive devices and orthoses to use in daily life. Though I acknowledge the difficulties involved, there is a balance to be struck between independent walking and using assistive devices and orthoses; the latter may allow the person to more fully participate in everyday life.

Specific gait training interventions used during therapy may include treadmill training, body weight support treadmill training, and various forms of assisted and even robotic training. The emphasis during these interventions is on practicing a high number of repetitions or steps, providing the opportunity to learn from errors, decreasing support, and getting practice in a variety of environments. Research evidence supports treadmill training for improving gait [5], weight bearing, and functional walking [6].

d) Electrical stimulation, usually in combination with functional activities

Neuromuscular electrical stimulation (NMES, also simply termed electrical stimulation, ES) involves the electrical stimulation of muscles with impaired motor control or weakness in order to produce a contraction. NMES uses an electrical current to stimulate the nerves and make the muscles contract. Functional electrical stimulation (FES), a subtype of NMES, involves electrical stimulation that produces a contraction in order to obtain a functionally useful movement. Electrodes are placed on the muscle and a device transmits the electrical current through a wired or wireless connection.

Electrical stimulation is used during functional activities and for muscle strengthening. It may be used during gait training (e.g., to stimulate the ankle dorsiflexor during swing phase). Research supports the use of FES in spastic CP [18–21].

Occupational therapy (OT)

An occupational therapist helps people participate in the things they want and need to do through the therapeutic use of everyday activities (occupations) [22]. Occupational therapists work with children to build confidence and independence through:

- Modification of activities or the environment to enable successful task completion
- Recommending or providing equipment (e.g., custom splinting, wheelchairs, bathing equipment) and/or technology that can increase independence when performing activities
- Completion of motivational tasks to engage in strengthening, movement, compensation, and use of technology

Areas covered in OT include, but are not limited to:

- Daily living skills such as dressing, feeding, grooming, and bathing
- Fine motor skills such as writing, using scissors, and manipulation of toys
- Cognitive skills such as sticking to a schedule, learning to play a new game, and following step-by-step directions
- Visual motor skills and visual perceptual skills such as using eye movement to explore and interact with the environment
- Participation in the day-to-day activities that motivate the person, such as play, sport, crafts, and vocational skills

Some OTs also specialize in upper limb involvement (Certified Hand Therapists [CHTs]).

Occupational therapists work with children and adolescents to increase their functional independence. They can be especially important as the child grows, when daily activities and independent living skills become more demanding and potentially more difficult to complete.

Speech and language pathology (SLP, also termed speech and language therapy, SLT)

Speech and language pathologists/therapists work with children, young people, and adults to support those with speech, language, and communication needs as well as feeding and swallowing difficulties.

The following definitions of the key elements of speech and language therapy are from the Royal College of Speech and Language Therapists [23]:

- **Speech** refers to saying sounds accurately and in the right places in words. It also relates to speaking fluently without hesitating, prolonging, or repeating words or sounds. It also means speaking with expression in a clear voice, using pitch, volume, and intonation to add meaning.
- **Language** refers to understanding and making sense of what people say. It also includes using words to build up sentences which are used in longer stretches of spoken language and to build conversations. This skill involves putting information in the right order to make sense.
- **Communication** refers to how we interact with others, such as being able to talk to people and take turns in conversation, in addition to changing language to suit the situation. It includes nonverbal communication such as eye contact, gestures, and facial expressions. Communication also relates to being able to consider another person's perspective, intentions, and the wider context.

Speech and language pathologists (therapists) are trained in strategies to help people develop these skills as well as technologies that can compensate for any skills that may require additional support. Just as there is overlap between PT and OT, there is overlap between OT and SLP/SLT. An example would be in the area of executive function. Executive function is defined as "a set of brain skills that help you plan and get things done. It is a higher cognitive process that involves communication and organization across multiple brain sites and brings all aspects of brain functioning together" [24]. I have included a web link at the end of this section to a fact sheet from the AACPDM[78] on executive function in individuals with CP and other conditions.

Tommy had delayed language development and attended SLT at an early age. He was delayed in expressive speech; his vocabulary was very limited relative to his age. (I still have the short list of his early words.)

I remember Tommy doing his SLT homework, which began with practicing the various sounds that were problematic for him. Fast-forward to age 13, when Tommy won a Best Overall Communicator award at a large national science competition for best explanation/discussion of a project in conversation with judges. It was a very sweet moment. (His project was called "What are the issues faced by children with cerebral palsy in mainstream education?") Indeed, language would become very important for Tommy. During his teenage years he wrote an award-winning blog. After completing secondary (high) school in Ireland, Tommy attended New York University and graduated cum laude in 2017 with a degree in journalism, and won the David James Burrell Prize. Those who meet Tommy as an adult would be surprised to learn of his delayed speech and language development.

His early SLT was also very important because his therapist referred him for complete review by the multidisciplinary team at the Central Remedial Clinic (CRC) in Dublin. That started our long association with the clinic.

Delivery of therapy services

Given that the delivery of therapy services is so variable, I will only address some broad points here. Having a lifelong condition such as spastic diplegia does not mean a person will need lifelong, nonstop PT (or other therapies). Nonstop PT has sometimes been referred to as the "once a week for life" model.

Guidelines were developed for determining the frequency of PT and OT services in a pediatric medical setting [25]. The guidelines were based on:

---

78 The American Academy for Cerebral Palsy and Developmental Medicine.

- The child's ability to benefit from and participate in therapy
- The parent's ability to participate in therapy sessions and follow through with activities in the home and community
- The family's decision related to available resources (time commitment, availability, transportation, and financial resources)

Four frequencies of therapy were identified [25]:
- **Intensive:** For children who are in an extremely critical period for acquiring a skill or are regressing. More than three times per week.
- **Weekly/bimonthly:** For children who need frequent therapy and are making continuous progress toward their goals. Frequency varies from twice per week to twice per month.
- **Periodic:** Best suited to children whose rates of progress are very slow but who require the skilled services of a therapist to periodically assess a home program and adapt it. Once a month or less.
- **Consultative:** Once the child has been discharged from therapy, consultative services are available as necessary.

The episodes of care (EOC) model is used for service delivery [26,27]. An EOC is a period of therapy (at the appropriate frequency) followed by a therapy break. Referring to "therapy breaks" might make it sound like getting therapy is the normal state of affairs for a person with CP, but living life, not receiving therapy, should be considered the normal state of affairs. Ideally, after an EOC the child generalizes the skills gained in therapy at home, in school, and in the community. For each EOC, the family and therapist, working together, draw up typically no more than two long-term and four short-term goals. Figure 3.3.1 shows periods when different therapies may be used, interspersed with breaks in therapy, during childhood and adolescence [26].

Web links to the following are included at the end of this section:
- Cincinnati Children's *Guidelines for Determining Frequency of Therapy* information leaflet for families
- Gillette's *Rehabilitation Therapies Episodes of Care in Childhood and Adolescence* information leaflet for families
- The APTA's *Intensity of Service in an Outpatient Setting for Children with Chronic Conditions* fact sheet for physical therapists

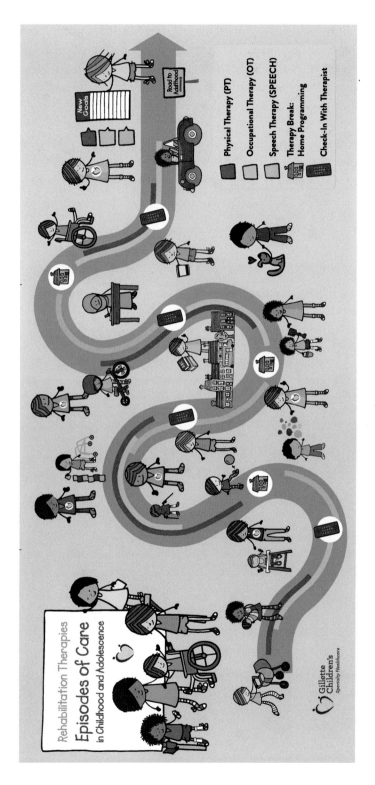

Figure 3.3.1 Rehabilitation therapies episodes of care in childhood and adolescence [26]

In addition to having formal goals, it is very important that therapists use objective measurement tools to evaluate whether therapy goals have been met. In the next section, we address the home program, which includes practicing what the child has learned in therapy at home and incorporating it into normal life.

Rosenbaum, Rosenbloom, and Mayston (2012) developed a very useful table (see Table 3.3.1) which neatly summarizes the broad focus of therapy at each life stage and serves as a useful wrap-up for this section [1].

Table 3.3.1 A life span view of general therapy goal areas for GMFCS levels I–III

AGE RANGE	FOCUS OF DEVELOPMENT AT THIS STAGE	THERAPY FOCUS
Neonatal period	Adaptation to extrauterine environment	Early intervention with focus on caregiver-child interaction/bond. Creating the appropriate environment and ways of engaging with the infant, daily life handling/holding, caring for the infant. For the extremely preterm infant, there is a need to minimize sensory experiences and handling, as preterm infants are unable to tolerate even usual levels of stimulation, e.g., touch, noise, light, etc. Early challenges with feeding may be the first sign of a problem.
Early (~0–8 months)	Self-discovery and communication	Awareness of self, the other, and discovery of own body enabled by midline orientation and self-exploration, especially early attention to hand functioning. Differentiation of cries and early communication by varied sounds/facial expressions/gestures and body movement. Developing a reference point for interaction with the external world. Early floor mobility (rolling, pivoting) and experiences of different postures; e.g., prone, sitting.

Cont'd.

AGE RANGE	FOCUS OF DEVELOPMENT AT THIS STAGE	THERAPY FOCUS
8–20 months	Early floor mobility and exploration	Many ways of moving on the floor to enable discovery of the self with respect to others and the environment. Likes/dislikes; cause/effect. Mobility and exploration mediate learning. Introduce early communication with gestures, signs, simple pictures; self-feeding. Begin to monitor musculoskeletal status and provide aids/orthoses as appropriate.
Toddler (20–36 months)	Mobility and peers	Realization that one is not the centre of the world and needs to interact with others. Provide alternative means of mobility as needed with supportive equipment to enable upright postures and participation in the world. Continue communication/musculoskeletal management as needed (this is ongoing through all life stages). Behavioral: needs to learn boundaries like any typically developing child.
Nursery school (3–5 years)	Need to fit a structure; peer interaction	Required to fit in with group activities and attend as needed. Often requires a reliable floor sitting position: needs to develop a variety of ways of doing activities, e.g., sitting postures/standing/mobility. Importance of work on standing for later standing transfers if at all possible.
School years (6–11 years)	Independence in and outside the classroom	Mobility in and outside the classroom and independence at recreational times, making friends—acceptance. Hip surveillance always very important (in GMFCS level III) but more so at this stage as more time spent sitting and greater mobility demands to keep up with the group. Recreational/physical activities important.

Cont'd.

AGE RANGE	FOCUS OF DEVELOPMENT AT THIS STAGE	THERAPY FOCUS
Puberty (~12 years)	Growth spurt: mobility challenge/ decisions	Important transition to secondary school and further development of independence and choice. Early mobility options may need to be questioned and will be again in the future. Another critical time for musculoskeletal system, especially for muscle/joint contractures due to the rapid skeletal growth. Develop recreational/ sports activities.
Adolescence (12–18 years)	Social participation; sexuality; relationships; occupation; maintain physical level	Focus on scholastic achievement and making meaningful friendships; higher education; getting ready for living away from home. Independence in all aspects. Psychosocial well-being: "talking therapies" may be of value at this time and onward. Continue with recreational activities to maintain fitness and contribute to well-being. Specific therapeutic input as needed.
Adult	Occupation; independence; relationships; "wear and tear"	Maintaining useful and fulfilling employment; relationships; childbearing. May require specific focused physical surveillance and intervention for pain, joint wear and tear, and general mobility in addition to fitness/recreational activities.

Adapted from Rosenbaum, Rosenbloom, and Mayston (2012). Reproduced with kind permission from Cerebral Palsy: From Diagnosis to Adult Life by Peter Rosenbaum and Lewis Rosenbloom, published by Mac Keith Press (mackeith.co.uk), 2012, 978-1-908316-50-9.

Spastic diplegia is managed by a multidisciplinary team. The physical therapist is likely one of the first members you will meet, and you will likely have regular contact during childhood and adolescence. Though physical therapists move jobs and change roles, your physical therapist will probably work with your family for a long time. They will get to know you and your child well.

Unless you have a health care background, raising a child with spastic diplegia involves a lot of new information. There's a lot to absorb. Therapists can be a great source of support and advice. In the acknowledgments, I include a number of therapists who treated Tommy over the years. It truly felt like the family, not just the child, was being cared for—definitely family-centered care in practice.

As noted earlier, evidence supports the goal-directed/functional training approach to therapy described in this section, but there are and have been other therapy approaches. Some, but not all, have supporting evidence.

Conductive education is an example of another therapy approach. It is based on the philosophy of Professor András Pető, who founded the Pető Institute in Budapest, Hungary. It combines treatment and education into one program. The term "conductor" is used to refer to the therapist trained in conductive education. A single conductor provides the therapies we would recognize as PT, OT, and SLP/SLT. Novak and colleagues (2013) recommended conductive education be accompanied by sensitive tools to measure outcome (i.e., tools that can evaluate whether the treatment is actually achieving its intended purpose and whether family goals are being met) [6].

We used conductive education when Tommy was two to three years old. I will briefly describe our experience with it.

A conductor from Hungary who trained at the Pető Institute worked with Tommy for about 10 three-week blocks over a period of approximately 15 months. The program consisted of exercises and activities for three hours in the morning and one hour in the afternoon. Tommy had to put everything into practice throughout the day: the way he ate, dressed, brushed his teeth, played on the playground, etc. It was intense and tiring for a small child, but the conductor, Szilvia, had a wonderful way with him. She was very firm, but also warm and friendly. While Tommy was undergoing conductive education, Szilvia stayed with our family. She was insistent on Tommy getting to bed on time each night and getting up early each morning, ready to start the program at 9 a.m. When she returned to Hungary, we continued the program until her next visit.

Conductive education provided an intensity of therapy that was not otherwise available to us at that time (now over 20 years ago), and it provided a very structured approach to developing motor function. While at that time we had not set formal goals for Tommy's conductive education, nor were we using tools to measure outcome, I can certainly say it was a successful treatment. Tommy began walking independently just after his third birthday. (I only realized while writing this book that this was earlier than predicted for him using the GMFCS.) I don't have data on how widely used this approach is today.

When we decided to try conductive education, we did so quietly. We had to: at that time, families were discharged from conventional services if they were using any other form of treatment. Nowadays I find the medical establishment is far more open, and parents can and should feel comfortable discussing other treatment options with professionals. Parents and professionals both want what's best for the child. However, I have one strong piece of advice for parents considering any alternative form of treatment: be sure there is an evidence base to support its effectiveness. We will look at alternative and complementary treatments in section 3.9.

Below are several photographs from Tommy's period of conductive education. They indicate some of the progression in his learning to walk: using a ladder-back chair, parallel bars, ropes, two tripods, single stick, and independent walking.

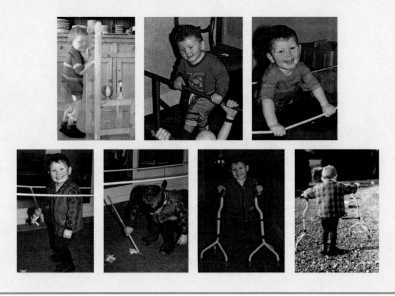

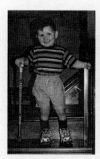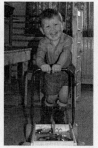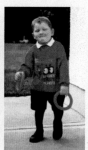

Useful web links

- American Academy for Cerebral Palsy and Developmental Medicine (AACPDM) (n.d.) *Executive Function in Individuals with Cerebral Palsy, Spina Bifida, and Brain Injury.* [pdf] aacpdm.org/UserFiles/file/ExecutiveFunctionFactSheet.pdf

- Cincinnati Children's (2008) *Guidelines for Determining Frequency of Therapy.* [pdf] cincinnatichildrens.org/-/media/cincinnati%20 childrens/home/service/o/ot-pt/patients/default/for-patients -guidelines-for-therapy-pdf.pdf?la=en

- Gillette Children's Specialty Healthcare (2016) *Rehabilitation Therapies Episodes of Care in Childhood and Adolescence.* [pdf] gillettechildrens.org/assets/uploads/care-and-conditions/Episodes_ of_Care-English.pdf

- American Physical Therapy Association (2012) *Intensity of Service in an Outpatient Setting for Children with Chronic Conditions.* [pdf] pediatricapta.org/includes/fact-sheets/pdfs/12%20Intensity %20of%20Service.pdf

3.4

The home program

Come to the edge.
We might fall.
Come to the edge.
It is too high!
COME TO THE EDGE!
And they came,
And we pushed,
And they flew.
Christopher Logue

Spirit in motion.
Paralympian motto

Exercise is medicine.
Susruta

The home program is the therapeutic[79] practice of goal-based tasks by the child, led by the parent and supported by the therapist, in the home environment [1]. Practicing what is learned in therapy is very important,

---

79 Recommended for reasons of health.

but there are other areas that also need attention at home for best management of the condition. In my opinion, it makes sense to have a broader view of the home program; it is easier to have one "package" that encompasses all areas that require attention at home. The five elements of the home program include:

- **The "homework" prescribed by therapists** (relevant when attending therapy)
- **Wearing orthoses** (relevant when prescribed)
- **Stretching** (relevant throughout childhood and adolescence)
- **Exercise and physical activity** (relevant throughout childhood and adolescence)
- **Postural management** (relevant throughout childhood and adolescence)

A child may attend therapy for one hour per week, but there are 167 more hours in the week to consider. In addition, as we saw in the previous section, there are periods when the child or adolescent is not attending therapy. The first two elements of the home program (the "homework" prescribed by therapists and wearing orthoses) are applicable at particular times. The next three (stretching, exercise and physical activity, and postural management) are constants in the life of the child and adolescent with spastic diplegia. Indeed, aside from stretching,[80] this program changes little in adulthood.

Graham and colleagues (2016) noted that [2]:

> *Strength and fitness programs should not be considered as therapy interventions but rather as crucial components of a healthy life-style for everyone, something that is even more important for those at higher risk of inactivity. The role of the therapist is mainly to help their patients with CP identify effective, sustainable strategies for incorporating intense physical activity in their lives and, perhaps, training specific capabilities that will increase their exercise capacity.*

Refer back to Figure 1.4.2, CanChild's series of "F-words." "Fitness" was one of their six areas of focus, underscoring its importance.

---

80 In adulthood, stretching is needed only to maintain flexibility. Bone growth ceases once a person reaches adulthood; thus the challenge of keeping muscle growth at pace with bone growth is over.

This section addresses each element of the home program in turn. Though they are addressed separately, they are very much interlinked.

The "homework" prescribed by therapists

The benefit of any therapy (PT, OT, and/or SLP/SLT) is only partly gained in the therapy session itself. The real benefits come from regular practice at home. It's like learning the piano: the true learning does not happen during the weekly half-hour lesson but through consistent practice at home.

Families depend on therapists to prescribe evidence-based treatments. Therapists depend on the child or adolescent (with the support of the parent) to get in the practice at home. This is a collaborative relationship. Much of what is learned in therapy has to become part of everyday life for the child or adolescent with spastic diplegia in order to be effective. Once a child has learned to read at school, it becomes a skill they can use in all situations.[81] The same can be said of the skills learned in therapy.

Working with a therapist is a partnership, and the parent and child (or adolescent) are partners with the therapist in the decision-making process. I recommend you talk with your therapist and make sure you have a good understanding of the activities you'll need to carry out at home and that it is a realistic plan.

Wearing orthoses

Orthoses are required for providing stretch and stability in the presence of muscle weakness. Wearing orthoses, if prescribed, is important. Orthoses are addressed in section 3.5.

Stretching

Stretching was addressed in section 3.3. Therapists may offer guidance on stretching during the therapy session, but the work has to be done

---

81   I am simply using reading as an example of a skill. I acknowledge that children may learn to read at home rather than at school.

at home. Stretching is one of the constants in the life of the child and adolescent with spastic diplegia.

Exercise and physical activity

Exercise and physical activity is another constant in the life of the child and adolescent with spastic diplegia. The goal of exercise and physical activity for a person with spastic diplegia is the same as for their able-bodied peers. Having a physical disability does not confer any exemption from needing to exercise and stay physically active.

Just so there is no ambiguity, let us first clarify some terms:
- **Exercise** is planned, structured, repetitive, and intentional movement intended to improve or maintain physical fitness [3]. Exercise is a subtype of physical activity. Examples of exercise include running, cycling, or attending a gym class.
- **Physical activity** is movement carried out by the skeletal muscles that requires energy expenditure, thus any movement is physical activity [3]. Physical activity varies from light to moderate to vigorous. Examples of each include:
  - Light physical activity: slow walking
  - Moderate physical activity: brisk walking, jogging, climbing stairs
  - Vigorous physical activity: fast running, fast cycling

It follows that energy expenditure is lowest while doing light physical activity and highest while doing vigorous physical activity. Recent advancements in wearable monitoring devices allow better measurement of physical activity levels [4,5].

Do children and adolescents with spastic diplegia take part in enough physical activity? No. Studies have shown that children with CP walk significantly less [6] and spend more time being sedentary [7] than typically developing children. A further study [5] found that children aged three to 12 showed a decrease in amount and intensity of physical activity with increasing GMFCS level[82] and increasing age. Participants at GMFCS level I showed the steepest decrease with increasing age.

---

82 Level I and level II were compared with levels III–V combined.

Does this reduced physical activity have health consequences? Yes. Reduced physical activity was associated with higher energy cost of walking in adolescents with mild spastic CP [8] and elevated blood pressure in children and adolescents with mild or moderate spastic CP [9].

Do studies show exercise and physical activity are beneficial for children and adolescents with CP? Again, yes. Studies have found benefits across a range of measures, including fitness, body composition, quality of life, and happiness [10–12]. A physical therapy research summit sponsored by the American Physical Therapy Association emphasized the need to promote and maintain physical fitness in children with CP to improve health, reduce secondary conditions, and enhance quality of life [13].

Verschuren and colleagues (2016) published a set of exercise and physical activity recommendations for people with CP under the following headings [14]:
- Cardiorespiratory (aerobic) exercise
- Resistance (muscle strengthening) exercise
- Daily moderate to vigorous physical activity
- Avoiding sedentary behavior (i.e., not being physically inactive)

Their recommendations are similar to (and based on) the World Health Organization's guidelines for able-bodied people [15]. Though these recommendations are relatively recent, the concept that "exercise is medicine" is not new [16]. Table 3.4.1 details their recommendations. Note that these are lifetime recommendations; it may take at least eight to 16 consecutive weeks of exercise to see the benefit.

Note that there is no lower (or upper) age limit on the exercise and physical activity recommendations for people with CP. There is no denying these recommendations are very high. However, research has found that typically developing infants can take up to 9,000 steps in a given day and travel the equivalent of 29 football fields [17]. It is important to be aware of the recommendations and aim to meet them as much as possible. And remember, any activity is better than no activity. Appendix 5 includes tips on exercise and physical activity for the younger child.

Table 3.4.1 Summary of exercise and physical activity recommendations for people with CP

FROM VERSCHUREN AND COLLEAGUES (2016)		AUTHOR'S NOTES
TYPE OF EXERCISE/ PHYSICAL ACTIVITY	**RECOMMENDATIONS FOR PEOPLE WITH CP**	
Cardiorespiratory (aerobic) exercise	• 3 times per week • > 60% of peak heart rate* • Minimum time of 20 min per session • Regular, purposeful exercise that involves major muscle groups and is continuous and rhythmic in nature	This is the type of exercise that gets the heart pumping and the lungs working.
Resistance (muscle strengthening) exercise	• 2–4 times per week on non-consecutive days	Muscle strengthening is especially important for people with spastic diplegia because muscle weakness is a feature of the condition. It is important for all muscles, particularly the antigravity muscles: the hip extensors (gluteus maximus) and the ankle plantar flexors (gastrocnemius and soleus). Other muscles to be considered include hip abductors, ankle dorsiflexors, core muscles, and upper limb muscles, if there is upper limb involvement.
Daily moderate to vigorous physical activity	• 60 minutes ≥ 5 days per week	This is the ordinary movement of everyday life. Physical activity counts as long as it is moderate to vigorous. It is less taxing than cardiorespiratory exercise but more vigorous than gentle movement. Walking, going up stairs, and household chores are all in this category.

Peak heart rate can be approximated as 220 minus age. For example, at age 15, peak heart rate is 205 (220 –15). 60 percent of peak heart rate is approximately 120 beats/minute (205 x 0.6).

Cont'd.

FROM VERSCHUREN AND COLLEAGUES (2016)		AUTHOR'S NOTES
TYPE OF EXERCISE/ PHYSICAL ACTIVITY	**RECOMMENDATIONS FOR PEOPLE WITH CP**	
Avoiding sedentary behavior (not being physically inactive)	• Sit for less than 2 hours/day or break up sitting for 2 minutes every 30–60 minutes	One can be physically active but still sedentary; they are separately measured. For example, if the person meets the recommendation for moderate to vigorous physical activity but sits for long periods watching TV or playing computer games, then they are physically active but sedentary. Prolonged sitting in one position, particularly with bad posture, is not good for any person, but it is particularly ill-advised in spastic diplegia.

For older children, adolescents, and adults with CP, the Peter Harrison Centre for Disability Sport at Loughborough University in the UK has published two excellent guides specifically for people with CP. The first, *Fit for Life*, is for people with CP who are new to exercise [18]. The second, *Fit for Sport*, is for people who want to take their athletics to a more advanced level [19]. Web links to both are included at the end of this section. Table 3.4.2 details a range of exercises suitable for people with CP.

Table 3.4.2 Types of exercise suitable for people with CP

TYPE OF EXERCISE	ADVANTAGES	DISADVANTAGES	ADAPTATIONS/ ADVICE
Aerobic gym equipment (e.g., cross-trainer, arm crank, recumbent bike)	Found in most gyms. Reduced environmental influencers, which minimizes the need for balance.	Remaining seated for long periods on a hard surface can increase the risk of pressure sores. Try using a pressure cushion to reduce this risk.	Flexion mitts or straps can be used if you have limited grip.

Cont'd.

TYPE OF EXERCISE	ADVANTAGES	DISADVANTAGES	ADAPTATIONS/ ADVICE
Aerobics	Inexpensive. Can be performed at home or as part of an adapted exercise class.	It may take you longer to master some movement patterns.	Therabands can be incorporated into the routine. Ask about public classes that can accommodate your needs.
Circuit training	A weights circuit can be interspaced with low-resistance arm cranking/ cycling/jogging.		Use a number of exercise stations and alternate between muscle groups. Rest after each activity or when the circuit is complete.
Hand cycling/ cycling	Relatively efficient form of locomotion. You can use a static bike in your home or at the gym.		Arm crank attachments can be used on everyday wheelchairs at minimal cost.
Power chair sports (e.g., boccia, football)	Competitive and social team environment. Controlled movement of the chair required.		Do as much as you are able and gradually build on it.
Pushing	Specificity training for wheelchair sports. You can wheel almost anywhere within reason (e.g., the park, a local track, or a leisure center).	Risk of overuse injuries due to increased stresses to the shoulder if training is not structured appropriately.	Use a hybrid day chair or sports wheelchair. Use a familiar circuit to monitor progression.

Cont'd.

TYPE OF EXERCISE	ADVANTAGES	DISADVANTAGES	ADAPTATIONS/ ADVICE
Rowing	Good all-around conditioning. It uses opposite muscle groups to those used during chair propulsion.	There may be safety issues for some due to the fixed position of the feet.	A stationary seat can be incorporated into the Concept Rower (found in most gyms), enabling an isolated upper-body rowing action.
Running	Inexpensive. You can run outdoors on a track, road, or trail or indoors on a treadmill.	Running is not recommended for those who are unable to balance and maintain coordination.	Always attach the emergency cord when treadmill running.
Sports/ wheelchair sports (e.g., tennis, fencing, curling, basketball, football)	Good cross-training or specific training for a given sport. Competitive and social environment.	You may have to purchase some additional equipment.	Strapping can be used to help stabilize you in your chair.
Swimming	Good cross-training as the water supports your body weight. Warm water pools can help soothe muscles.	You may need to consider how you will get from the changing room to poolside, especially if you are a wheelchair user.	Swim-jogger buoyancy vests/ floats can be used for aqua-jogging or to support impaired limbs. Check if your local pool has a hoist if you require one to enter the pool.
Tai chi/yoga	Improves balance, posture, flexibility, and breathing patterns.		A focus on slow, deliberate movements may help improve balance and coordination.

Reproduced (with minor adaptations) with kind permission from the Fit for Life *guide published by Loughborough University, Peter Harrison Centre for Disability Sport, UK [18].*

Further tips on exercise and physical activity for the older child, adolescent, and adult are included in Appendix 5.

If you think being good at exercise and sports is impossible for the person with spastic diplegia, think again. Rixt van der Horst is a Dutch Paralympian with spastic diplegia who competes in dressage.[83] Rowan Crothers, an Australian Paralympic swimmer, and Brianna Salinaro, a US Paralympian who competes in tae kwon do, also have spastic diplegia.

Daniel Dias, a Brazilian Paralympic swimmer who has won multiple medals, credits fellow Paralympian Clodoaldo Silva, who has CP, for getting him into the sport. "I only began because I saw Clodoaldo swimming on television. I didn't know people like me could swim, could do any sport at all," Dias said in an interview [20].

Paralympians include people with a range of different types and levels of disabilities. Many Paralympic athletes are able to swim, cycle, and run faster than their average able-bodied peers. It is inspirational to watch Paralympians achieve records almost equal to—and sometimes surpassing—their able-bodied Olympic athlete peers. For example, at the Brazil 2016 games, four Paralympic runners beat the time of the Olympic gold medalist in the men's 1,500 meters [21]. US Paralympians now train with Olympic athletes at US Olympic and Paralympic Committee training centers under the supervision of the same coaches [22]. Indeed, the US Olympic and Paralympic Committee recently agreed to pay equal bonuses to both Paralympic and Olympic athletes who win medals [23].

In 2018, Nike offered a contract to US runner Justin Gallegos, the first professional athlete with CP to be signed by the brand. I was delighted to be able to interview Gallegos for this book. The interview is included in Chapter 5.

These athletes' stories are proof that, though it is not easy, spastic diplegia does not have to be a barrier to achieving great levels of fitness and skill.

---

83 In dressage, a horse and rider perform a series of predetermined movements.

Postural management

Postural management is another constant in the life of the child and adolescent with spastic diplegia. "Posture" refers to the position in which a person holds their body while standing, sitting, or lying down. Good posture applies to everyone, not just individuals with CP.

To maintain good posture, a person needs to have adequate strength in their trunk stabilizing muscles and balance reactions. This is why the typically developing child cannot sit independently until they are approximately six months old [24]. People with spastic diplegia may have some challenges with posture [25]. Due to their musculoskeletal differences, it is important to support them in the most optimal position possible to promote decreased pain, musculoskeletal changes, and asymmetries. See Table 3.4.3 for a list of recommendations from Gillette.

Table 3.4.3 Ideal positioning in sitting, standing, and sleeping

GOOD POSTURE IN:	ILLUSTRATION
Sitting • Feet flat on the floor, with hips, knees, and ankles at 90 degrees and both sides of the trunk straight and symmetrical. (If feet cannot reach the floor, something firm, such as a box or book, can be placed under them to ensure they are flat and that the 90-degree angle is achieved.) • Support provided at the sides, if necessary, to ensure the trunk is straight and symmetrical. • Arms close to the body and relaxed. • Head balanced on the neck (not tilted forward or backward).	
Standing • Feet flat on the floor. • Knees neither locked nor bent. • Abdominal muscles tight and buttocks tucked in. • Shoulders back and down slightly, even and relaxed. • Head facing forward, not tilted to one side or the other. • Chin tucked and ears over the shoulders.	

Cont'd.

GOOD POSTURE IN:	ILLUSTRATION

Sleeping
- Posture is midline and symmetrical (i.e., the two sides are equal).
- Sleeping in a supine position (on the back) is recommended.
- If/when lying on one side, it can be helpful to place a pillow between the legs to keep the spine in good alignment. A pillow under the top arm can also be useful to support good alignment—often the top arm is pulled down by gravity, which can result in curving of the spine or rolling to prone position (sleeping on the front) in the night.

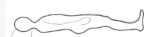

Good exercise and physical activity habits start early in life. Children are much more likely to have good habits if their parents do, and they are much more likely to have good habits as adults if they had good habits as children. The habits we parents keep, and the habits we instill in our children, have lifelong effects on our children's adult health. The good news is that it is never too late to start.

Exercise and physical activity are part of the lifelong home program for people with spastic diplegia. However, it is worth acknowledging that many people (including able-bodied people) do not meet the recommendations for exercise and physical activity. People with spastic diplegia may be at greater risk of an inactive lifestyle for many reasons, including overprotective parents (we may fear our child might get hurt) and difficulties with movement.

The concept of self-care versus expert care is an interesting one [26]. Self-care refers to what the child or adolescent (with help and support from the parent) does at home: the home program. The real gains are made by completing this day in and day out, week in and week out. Expert guidance is great, but it is only of value when it is supported by a large amount of self-care. Through self-care, the child or adolescent can do a great deal to reduce and/or minimize the effects of their condition.

In Chapter 2, we addressed the unfavorable strength-to-mass ratio that develops as the child grows. It is therefore very important that the child with spastic diplegia enter the adolescent growth spurt with no excess weight and strong muscles. The home program can help with both.

Missing a day of the home program is not a problem. Indeed, missing a week may not be a problem. However, missing a month might be a problem, and missing a year is definitely a problem. When increased intensity is required after a treatment such as selective dorsal rhizotomy (SDR) or single-event multilevel surgery (SEMLS), missing even a short period can become a problem. The elements of the home program have to become part of normal life for the person with spastic diplegia, just like brushing one's teeth.

Useful web links

- Loughborough University Peter Harrison Centre for Disability Sport (n.d.) *Fit for Life*. [pdf] lboro.ac.uk/media/wwwlboroacuk/content/peterharrisoncentre/downloads/brochures/pdfs/Cerebral%20Palsy%20guide_Fit_for_Life.pdf

- Loughborough University Peter Harrison Centre for Disability Sport (n.d.) *Fit for Sport*. [pdf] lboro.ac.uk/media/wwwlboroacuk/content/peterharrisoncentre/downloads/brochures/pdfs/Cerebral%20Palsy%20guide_Fit_for_Sport.pdf

- American Academy for Cerebral Palsy and Developmental Medicine (AACPDM) (n.d.) *We Can All PLAY: Participation in Adapted Sports and Recreation for Children and Youth with Disabilities*. [pdf] aacpdm.org/UserFiles/file/AdaptedSportsandRecreationFACTSheet3.1.18_v2.pdf

- American Academy for Cerebral Palsy and Developmental Medicine (AACPDM) (n.d.) *Walking Changes and Associated Implications across the Lifespan for Individuals with Cerebral Palsy*. [pdf] aacpdm.org/UserFiles/file/WalkingChangesFactSheet.pdf

- American Academy for Cerebral Palsy and Developmental Medicine (AACPDM) (n.d.) *Fatigue in Individuals with Cerebral Palsy*. [pdf] aacpdm.org/UserFiles/file/FatigueFactSheet.pdf

- American College of Sports Medicine (2016) *Health-Related Fitness for Children and Adults with CP.* [pdf] acsm.org/docs/default-source/files-for-resource-library/basics_youth-cerebral-palsy.pdf?sfvrsn=d3d6e067_2

- The National Center on Health, Physical Activity and Disability (NCHPAD) (2019) [online] nchpad.org (NCHPAD is a public health practice and resource center for people with disabilities. It has a selection of informative videos at nchpad.org/Videos.)

- Gillette Children's Specialty Healthcare (2019) *Protecting Your Joints.* [online] gillettechildrens.org/your-visit/patient-education/protecting-your-joints

- Gillette Children's Specialty Healthcare (2019) *Work Simplification Techniques.* [online] gillettechildrens.org/your-visit/patient-education/work-simplification-techniques

- Gillette Children's Specialty Healthcare (2019) *Ergonomics in the Home.* [online] gillettechildrens.org/your-visit/patient-education/ergonomics-in-the-home

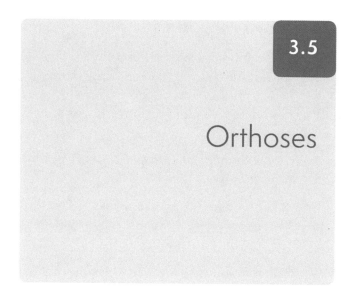

3.5

Orthoses

Determine that the thing can and shall be done,
and then we shall find the way.
Abraham Lincoln

An orthosis (plural orthoses) is a device designed to hold specific body parts in position in order to modify their structure and function. It is usually made of lightweight, custom-molded plastic or carbon fiber.[84]

The term "orthosis" comes from the Greek word "ortho," which means "to straighten or align." Orthotics is the branch of medicine concerned with the design, manufacture, and management of orthoses. The orthotist is the professional in this specialty. The word "orthotic" is sometimes used to mean the device; "orthosis" is the more correct term, but given how alike the two terms are, their interchangeability is understandable. The term "brace" is also sometimes used. Orthoses work best when a child has no contractures or bone torsions, though many children with spastic diplegia have both.

---

84 Carbon fiber is sometimes used instead of plastic because it is more lightweight and can theoretically offer some energy return due its "springy" nature.

This section addresses only lower limb orthoses, the type most commonly used in spastic diplegia, but there are also orthoses for the upper limbs.

Different orthoses have different functions. In spastic diplegia, the goals of treatment with orthoses may include some of the following (and the goals may be interlinked) [1]:

- To correct the position and movement of a joint
- To stretch the muscle-tendon unit (MTU) and thus prevent contracture by maintaining the MTU in an elongated position
- To assist with walking
- To assist with other functional activities (in the younger child, for example, they may help them get from the floor to standing)
- To prolong or enhance the benefit achieved from earlier casting
- To protect a joint

There is often a trade-off with orthoses. The best orthosis for walking may not be the best for getting up and down from the floor. Using an orthosis to protect or correctly align a body part may decrease muscle strength; it may also lead to muscle atrophy or wastage (think of the muscle shrinkage that occurs when a limb is put in a cast). For this reason, if the orthosis includes the ankle joint, the child or adolescent should also spend some time out of the orthosis since it is important to maintain plantar flexor strength (strength in the calf muscles).

Choosing an orthosis involves the collaboration of different specialists on the multidisciplinary team, who will prescribe the most appropriate one.[85] Different orthoses may be prescribed over the years as the child or adolescent grows and their body structure and function changes.

Well-fitting shoes must be worn when wearing orthoses. If shoes do not fit well, the orthoses may not be able to function correctly and may not be comfortable. In some cases, a slightly larger shoe may be needed. Athletic shoes that can be laced or fastened snugly can be a good option. Some manufacturers of athletic shoes now offer models that are specifically designed to be easy to get on and off with orthoses. Nike has two such models: the Nike FlyEase, which has a zipper and strap system to quickly and easily get shoes on and off, and the Nike FlyEase Wide, which is wide enough to fit an orthosis.

---

85 The particular specialists who choose and prescribe orthoses may vary in different countries.

Orthoses commonly used in the treatment of spastic diplegia include the following, listed in order of increasing control of structure and/or function [1]:

- **Foot orthosis (FO)**
- **University of California Biomechanics Lab (UCBL) orthosis**
- **Supramalleolar orthosis (SMO)**
- **Ankle-foot orthosis (AFO)**

Foot orthosis (FO)

Foot orthoses (FOs) are soft, custom-molded inserts. They replace regular shoe insoles and can be left in the shoes. FOs are used to support, distribute pressure, and help maintain proper alignment of the foot, especially the heel and the arch. Many athletes and older people who do not have CP also use custom-made FOs. See Figure 3.5.1.

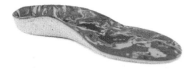

Figure 3.5.1 Foot orthosis (FO)

University of California Biomechanics Lab (UCBL) orthosis

UCBLs have the same function as FOs: they support, distribute pressure, and help maintain proper alignment of the foot. The difference between FOs and UCBLs is their structure: FOs are soft inserts, while UCBLs are usually made of plastic and provide greater support. Like FOs, UCBLs usually replace regular shoe insoles and can be left in the shoes. See Figure 3.5.2.

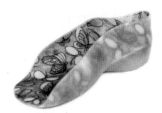

Figure 3.5.2 University of California Biomechanics Lab (UCBL) orthosis

Supramalleolar orthosis (SMO)

"Supra" means "above" and "malleolar" refers to the ankle. A supramalleolar orthosis (SMO) is therefore an orthosis that covers the ankle. As with FOs and UCBLs, the SMO controls the foot. However, the SMO also captures the ankle joint and therefore exerts greater control. See Figure 3.5.3.

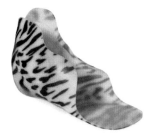

Figure 3.5.3 Supramalleolar orthosis (SMO)

Ankle-foot orthosis (AFO)

The difference between an SMO and an ankle-foot orthosis (AFO) is that the AFO has a posterior shell along the calf that supports the lower leg. AFOs minimize the amount of plantar flexion that is allowed. Most don't allow any plantar flexion.

AFOs may be subdivided into the following—the first four types of AFO are listed in order of increasing control of structure and/or function:
a) **Articulated AFO**
b) **Posterior leaf-spring AFO (PLS AFO)**
c) **Solid AFO (SAFO)**
d) **Ground reaction AFO (GRAFO, also termed floor reaction AFO)**
e) **Dynamic AFO (DAFO)**

a) Articulated AFO

An articulated AFO has a hinge at the ankle joint to allow free dorsiflexion but limits plantar flexion (i.e., the hinge is only in one direction). The hinge allows the ankle the flexibility small children need to rise to standing from the floor, transition from one position to another, and climb stairs. They are also worn by adolescents and adults. See Figure 3.5.4.

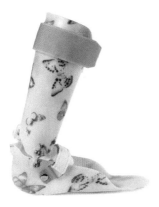

Figure 3.5.4 Articulated AFO

b) Posterior leaf-spring AFO (PLS AFO)

The posterior leaf-spring AFO (PLS AFO) has a calf cuff that tapers to a band behind the ankle (the "leaf"). The band allows some flexibility. The PLS does not have the free dorsiflexion of the articulated AFO; it restricts dorsiflexion. The width and pliability of the band behind the ankle can be varied; this affects the stiffness of the AFO and the amount of dorsiflexion that is allowed. See Figure 3.5.5.

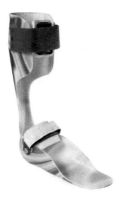

Figure 3.5.5 Posterior leaf-spring AFO (PLS AFO)

c) Solid AFO (SAFO)

The solid AFO (SAFO) is stiff and restricts dorsiflexion completely. The ankle joint does not move. See Figure 3.5.6.

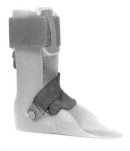

Figure 3.5.6 Solid AFO (SAFO)

d) Ground reaction AFO (GRAFO, also termed floor reaction AFO)

The ground reaction AFO (GRAFO) has a shell at the front, so it has to be put on by coming in from the back of the AFO (rear entry). The GRAFO not only controls the ankle like a SAFO, but the anterior shell (the shell at the front) provides extra input to "push" the knee back into extension. The anterior shell is more restrictive than the strap of a SAFO. See Figure 3.5.7.

The proper functioning of this AFO is dependent on the wearer having no knee flexion contracture or torsion deformity of the tibia (shinbone). When a knee flexion contracture is present, the ground reaction component cannot be effective because the knee cannot be pushed back. A twist (torsion) in the shinbone also reduces the effectiveness of the ground reaction component because of the lever-arm dysfunction.

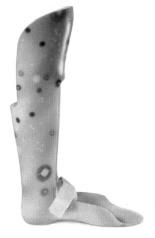

Figure 3.5.7 Ground reaction AFO (GRAFO, also termed floor reaction AFO)

e) Dynamic AFO (DAFO)

DAFO is a brand of orthosis made of lightweight, custom-molded plastic manufactured by the Cascade company (cascadedafo.com). The brand name DAFO is frequently used when referring to orthoses, much as the brand name Kleenex is used for facial tissues. Because DAFOs tend to be made of thinner plastic, they allow some movement (hence the term "dynamic"). Cascade manufactures a range of dynamic orthoses.

The above are the types of orthoses most commonly used in spastic diplegia. However, other types of orthoses may be used.

We learned about the gait cycle in section 2.5. Here are some examples of how orthoses can assist with walking:
- Providing rigidity for the foot can help make the foot a more effective lever for push-off.
- Limiting plantar flexion can help prevent toe walking (equinus gait).
- Limiting plantar flexion can also help prevent foot drop in the swing phase of gait, which causes the toe to drag along the ground.
- Limiting dorsiflexion can help restore the plantar flexion/knee extension couple. Refer to Figure 2.9.2. By preventing dorsiflexion (the tibia moving toward the foot) during the stance phase of the gait cycle, the ground reaction force (GRF) can be restored to in front of the knees to keep the knees extended (straight). It was previously thought GRAFOs had the most potential to restore the plantar flexion/knee extension couple and help straighten the knee. However, a recent study found that SAFOs and GRAFOs were equally effective at correcting crouch gait [2,3].

Overall, there is good evidence supporting use of orthoses [2–6]. Aboutorabi and colleagues (2017) concluded that the use of specific types of AFOs improved gait parameters and energy expenditure in children with spastic CP [6].

> To get a child to consistently wear an orthosis, it must be comfortable; it must not cause any rubbing or blisters, for example. You should not hesitate to speak up if you notice any problems, even minor ones.

Orthoses must also be acceptable-looking to the wearer. It helps to be able to choose from a variety of colors and designs. An orthosis would not (and should not) be prescribed unless it's necessary, so although the child may not love wearing it, they should wear it as prescribed. A child may not like being restrained in a car seat, but we don't give them the option of not wearing a seat belt. We really have to adopt the same approach when it comes to orthoses (within reason); it's what's best for the child in the long term. We have to be both good cop and bad cop at once.

Thankfully, Tommy never objected to wearing orthoses. Over the years he was prescribed different types, including FOs, UCBLs, SMOs, and articulated and solid AFOs. Being able to choose from different colors and designs certainly helped—though I didn't love the American flag design he chose for his AFOs after orthopedic surgery in the US—I wanted to be diplomatic when we returned to our home health care services after having chosen an alternate treatment route. The two American flags on Tommy's calves didn't exactly help!

The only real problem we encountered with orthoses was when Tommy left Ireland for college in the US. We tried to make sure he was well prepared, which included getting new orthoses (in this case, SMOs). The orthoses arrived just a few days before he was due to leave. He'd never had problems with new orthoses before, but this time he developed large blisters on the soles of both feet. A nurse friend dressed his feet each night to allow him to walk easily by day. Leaving for college, I was honestly more worried about the blisters on his feet than anything else. We dropped him off at his dorm and the following day we checked out the college medical center. The staff assured him (well, mostly me) that they would be available any time he needed them. Thankfully, both Tommy and his new orthoses settled in just fine. Today Tommy uses FOs only.

AFOs were recommended early on in Tommy's treatment. At the time, I had no idea what they were. The term "AFO" was new to me, and it's not exactly self-explanatory. To me, they sounded like UFOs!

3.6

Tone reduction

The good physician treats the disease;
the great physician treats the patient who has the disease.

Sir William Osler

We addressed abnormal muscle tone in section 2.6. Just to recap: muscle tone is the resting tension in a person's muscles. A range of "normal" muscle tone exists. Tone is considered "abnormal" when it falls outside the range of normal or typical. Abnormal muscle tone occurs in all types of CP. Spasticity is the main type of high tone in spastic diplegia, but dystonia may also occur. Spasticity is defined as an abnormal increase in muscle tone or stiffness of muscle, which might interfere with movement, speech, or be associated with discomfort or pain [1]. Other definitions highlight the velocity-dependent nature of the condition [2]. In a person with dystonia, sustained muscle contractions cause twisting and repetitive movements or abnormal postures [3].

Tone reduction is a high priority in the early years. However, tone reduction is only one part of the integrated treatment of spastic diplegia by the multidisciplinary team. It is usually performed in conjunction with other treatments such as PT, OT, serial casting, and orthoses. When tone reduction is included with other treatments, the effects of each treatment may be amplified: the combination of treatments may be more effective than any one treatment on its own.

Reducing spasticity helps reduce the harmful effects of high tone on skeletal growth. It also helps reduce stiffness and increase the overall ROM of joints, thus increasing the ROM the person can move through. It facilitates strengthening, working on motor control, balance, and other functional goals. It can also improve a person's tolerance for wearing orthoses.

Table 3.6.1 lists five types of tone reduction treatments commonly used in spastic diplegia.

Table 3.6.1 Tone reduction treatments

TREATMENT	GENERALIZED OR FOCAL	REVERSIBLE OR IRREVERSIBLE
Oral medications	Generalized	Reversible
Botulinum neurotoxin A (BoNT-A) injection	Focal: injected into muscles	Reversible
Phenol injection	Focal: muscles controlled by the injected nerve	Reversible
Intrathecal baclofen (ITB)	Generalized	Reversible
Selective dorsal rhizotomy (SDR)	Generalized	Irreversible

Generalized = treatment affects a large region of the body
Focal = treatment has an effect on a local area (e.g., a single muscle)
Reversible = the effects of the treatment are not permanent

Many centers have special team evaluations of spasticity because of its complexity and significance in CP. At Gillette, a spasticity evaluation involves several professionals together at a Spasticity Evaluation Clinic. There, members of the multidisciplinary team include professionals from physical medicine and rehabilitation (PMR), orthopedics, and neurosurgery. The specialists see the child together, not individually, and come to a consensus opinion on the best spasticity treatment for the child. The evaluation includes a gait analysis and functional PT assessment completed as part of the (typically) two-day evaluation. Spasticity clinics at other facilities may include additional team members from other specialities including neurology, developmental pediatrics, and rehabilitation therapy.

Different institutions have different protocols for how they perform each tone-reducing treatment. For example, the selection criteria (those for whom the treatment is suitable) and protocols (how the treatment is actually carried out) for SDR were found to vary between institutions [4–6]. This is why SDR is not a uniform procedure.[86] (Indeed, this point applies to all treatments in spastic diplegia.)

As with all treatments for spastic diplegia, clear goals for both treatment and assessment of outcome after treatment are required. Because the child has to readjust to their new, relaxed muscles, they may initially experience weakness or loss of function. Though the use of tone reduction peaks in early childhood, it can continue into adolescence and adulthood.

We now look at the different tone reduction treatments in more detail.

Oral medications

The goal of treatment with oral medications (those taken by mouth) is to achieve generalized tone reduction. There are several oral medications physicians may prescribe to reduce spasticity [7,8], including:

- Baclofen
- Diazepam
- Dantrolene sodium
- Tizanidine

These medications act at different sites within the body, with different effects on the muscles, brain, or spinal cord [7]. They may have different brand names in different countries. The challenge of treatment with oral medications is managing their side effects, and their efficacy is greater in some people than in others. They are sometimes used in

---

86 Grunt and colleagues (2014) recommended that international meetings of experts should develop more uniform consensus guidelines [4].

combination or in conjunction with focal spasticity reduction measures such as botulinum neurotoxin A (BoNT-A). They can also sometimes be used to reduce muscle spasms, particularly after orthopedic surgery.

Novak and colleagues (2013) found strong evidence supporting the use of diazepam but recommended that the use of dantrolene, oral baclofen, and tizanidine be accompanied by a sensitive outcome measure to monitor progress [8].[87] Physicians must weigh the risk-benefit ratio of each medication alongside the patient's medical history, issues, and needs.

Botulinum neurotoxin A (BoNT-A) injection

Botulinum neurotoxin A (BoNT-A), as a medication, is injected directly into a muscle and acts by blocking the release of a chemical called acetylcholine at the neuromuscular junction (where the nerve meets the muscle). Botulinum neurotoxin[88] is produced by the bacteria that causes botulism, a lethal form of food poisoning. However, as a medication the toxin is delivered at a much smaller dose. It is also used in the cosmetic industry. There are seven different types of botulinum neurotoxin, from A to G. Type A is the the main form used to reduce spasticity [9].

The effects of BoNT-A diminish with time; within a few months, the original nerves regain their ability to release acetylcholine, hence the treatment is not permanent [9]. The effects of BoNT-A become apparent approximately three to seven days after injection and last for approximately three to six months [10]. Treatment with BoNT-A can start early—as young as one to three years—and can be used every six to 12 months for several years [11]. BoNT-A can also be used to reduce muscle spasms [9].

A number of muscles may be treated in one session. Depending on age and/or the number of muscles being injected, anesthesia may be required. There is a limit to the number of muscles that can receive treatment at one time because there is a limit to the total body dose of BoNT-A that can be safely given at one time [9]. Different institutions may have different protocols for using BoNT-A (e.g., regarding dosage

---

87 Suitable to evaluate whether the treatment is actually achieving its intended purpose and family goals are met.

88 A neurotoxin is a poison which acts on the nervous system.

and frequency of injection). Typically, no overnight hospital stay is necessary.

As with any injection, there may be some pain associated with the needle puncturing the skin and the delivery of the medicine. Different centers use different methods to manage pain; these may include distraction techniques, medication, nitrous oxide (laughing gas), or general anesthesia. Some children may experience stress and anxiety from repeated episodes of injection. Temporary incontinence has occasionally been reported following treatment with BoNT-A. One limiting factor of this treatment is that children may experience diminishing effects with repeat injections, or it may stop being effective entirely [9].

Overall, there appears to be strong evidence supporting BoNT-A treatment [8,12–14]. The simultaneous use of BoNT-A and strength training was found to be successful at reducing spasticity, improving strength, and achieving functional goals over and above treatment with BoNT-A alone [15]. This is an example of combined treatment working better.

Although BoNT-A is regarded as a reversible treatment for reducing spasticity, important questions have been raised about its long-term effects, including muscle weakness, muscle atrophy (wastage), changes in the muscle structure, and atrophy of the underlying bone [16–22]. Some studies suggest there may be permanent changes. Graham and colleagues (2016) concluded that more information is needed both from animal studies and long-term clinical studies to fully assess the benefits and risks of BoNT-A [20]. Similar conclusions have been drawn elsewhere [23,24].

Phenol injection

Phenol is another medication delivered by injection. It was used as a treatment for spasticity for many decades before the advent of BoNT-A. Phenol is injected directly into the motor nerve,[89] causing a chemical reaction that prevents the nerve from sending messages to the muscle. (Note that phenol is injected into the nerve, whereas BoNT-A is injected into the muscle.) Treatment with phenol is normally done under general

---

89   A motor nerve sends signals away from the spinal cord to a muscle. A sensory nerve sends signals (about temperature, pain, touch, etc.) from all parts of the body to the spinal cord.

anesthesia to minimize discomfort for the patient and because minimal movement is required during the injection process. Usually two to four muscle groups are injected in a single session.

The only, rare side effect of treatment with phenol occurs if the injection hits a sensory nerve.[90] This may result in the patient feeling a temporary burning sensation and/or hypersensitivity to touch that may last a few weeks [9]. Medication can be given if this occurs. Again, no overnight hospital stay is typically necessary.

The effects of phenol generally last three to 12 months. Repeated injections can lead to a cumulative effect, meaning the effects may last longer than one year [9]. Because phenol acts at the level of the nerve, whereas BoNT-A acts at the level of the muscle, phenol may have a broader effect than BoNT-A.

The use of phenol differs around the world. It has become less popular for a number of reasons, including the advent of BoNT-A [9]. Sometimes it is used in conjunction with BoNT-A because it allows more muscles to be treated without exceeding the dosage recommendations for either medication [8].There appear to be no studies of phenol use in CP [8,13]. This is an example of situation where there is a lack of research evidence but clinical expertise supports the use of a treatment.

Intrathecal baclofen (ITB)

Intrathecal baclofen (ITB) is an alternative method of administering the drug baclofen. The following is an explanation of each term:
- **Intrathecal:** "Intra" means "within," and the "theca" is the sheath enclosing the spinal cord. The intrathecal area is the fluid-filled space surrounding the spinal cord; cerebrospinal fluid (CSF) flows through this area, bathing and protecting the spinal cord.
- **Baclofen:** The name of the medication.

With ITB, a pump stores and delivers baclofen directly to the CSF in the intrathecal area. Implantation of an ITB pump is a neurosurgical

---

90 This is one reason phenol is not used in more muscle groups. It can only be used in nerves that are motor only (after the sensory nerve rootlets have separated).

procedure. The pump is filled with baclofen and inserted under the skin of the abdomen. A catheter (a narrow, flexible tube) is connected to the pump and routed under the skin to the patient's back. Surgeons make an incision to position the tip of the catheter in the intrathecal space, where it delivers the baclofen directly to the CSF. The pump is programmed to slowly release baclofen over a period of time. It can also be programmed to deliver different amounts at different times during the day. It is programmed to suit the needs of the individual patient [10].

Delivering baclofen directly into the CSF means the drug can be effective at a much lower dose. This helps avoid the unpleasant side effects patients often experience when taking oral baclofen, including dizziness and drowsiness.

ITB is a tone-reducing treatment for both spasticity and dystonia. It is better at reducing tone in the lower extremities than the upper extremities [25].

Implantation of an ITB pump usually requires a hospital stay, typically five to seven days. The patient must lie flat for up to three days after pump implantation for healing. The patient wears an abdominal binder for six to eight weeks afterward to support the pump and prevent swelling [10]. The pump has to be refilled with baclofen about every three to four months in a hospital outpatient clinic. Because the pump has a limited battery life, it must be surgically removed and replaced after seven years.

Overall, evidence supports the use of ITB in CP [8,26]. It is worth noting, however, that most research on ITB is limited to measuring tone reduction—very little data is available about functional or quality of life outcomes.

Selective dorsal rhizotomy (SDR)

Selective dorsal rhizotomy (SDR) is a neurosurgical procedure that reduces spasticity by selectively cutting abnormal sensory nerve rootlets[91] in the spinal cord. SDR reduces spasticity only, not other types

---

91 Think of nerve roots like the roots of a tree, which further subdivide into smaller rootlets.

of high tone. It is the only irreversible tone-reducing treatment. The following is an explanation of each term:

- **Selective:** Only certain abnormal nerve rootlets are cut.
- **Dorsal:** "Dorsal" refers to the sensory nerve rootlets. The dorsal nerve rootlets; i.e., the sensory nerve rootlets, are cut. (The sensory nerve rootlets are termed "dorsal" because they are located toward the back of the body. The motor nerve rootlets are termed "ventral" because they are toward the front.)
- **Rhizotomy:** "Rhizo" means "root," and "otomy" means "to cut into."

Putting it all together, "selective dorsal rhizotomy" means that certain abnormal, dorsal nerve rootlets are cut.

There are two SDR techniques, the cauda and the conus, named after the level of the spinal cord at which each procedure is performed. The choice of technique is provider-specific but also depends on the patient. The cauda technique is the most common worldwide [4].

SDR involves the removal of the back of the vertebrae (the lamina) in order to access the spinal cord. This is called a laminectomy. During the operation the sensory (dorsal) nerve roots are dissected into rootlets. The rootlets are individually electrically stimulated to determine whether they trigger a normal or abnormal (spastic) response. If a rootlet triggers an abnormal response, it is cut. If not, it is left alone. The percentage of rootlets cut varies between institutions [4]. At Gillette, the percentage of rootlets cut during SDR is lower than what is typically reported in the literature. The higher the number of rootlets cut, the less "selective" the rhizotomy procedure is, and the greater the risk of inducing weakness [6].

As with many treatments, SDR is not suitable for every child. The selection criteria for SDR differs between institutions [4]. As an example, characteristics of the "ideal" candidate for SDR at Gillette include [27]:[92]

- Aged four to seven years.
- GMFCS level I–III.
- Primarily spasticity (as opposed to dystonia) that interferes with function.

---

92 Largely based on the work of Warwick Peacock, the South African neurosurgeon who repopularized and refined SDR in the 1980s and '90s.

- Preterm birth history or injury in the late second or early third trimester of pregnancy.
- Periventricular leukomalacia (PVL) confirmed by neuroimaging (see section 2.2).
- Energy-inefficient gait.
- Satisfactory muscle strength, generally defined as antigravity muscle strength at the hips and knees.
- Fair or good selective motor control at the hips and knees. This means the child should be able to partially isolate joint movement (not move the joint in a complete pattern). This requires sufficient strength and motor control; the child shouldn't be reliant on increased spasticity for their stability or movement.
- Good ability to cooperate with rehabilitation.

Children who fit all of the selection criteria are rare, so physicians use their judgment to determine whether a particular child is a good candidate for SDR [6]. Your provider will assess whether SDR is suitable for your child based on their specific circumstances. (The thinking behind the ideal age of four to seven years is that gait is relatively stable and it is possible to decrease spasticity while the child is still young enough to learn new motor patterns; secondary contracture development is minimal at this point; and the child is old enough to complete the assessment and cooperate with the rigorous rehabilitation program.)

Children for whom SDR is not recommended include those with a predominance of dystonia, less severe spasticity, established contractures (typically in older children and adolescents), weakness, and poor selective motor control [27]. Though SDR is most effective in childhood, it can sometimes be performed in adolescents and adults.

Gait analysis is very important for evaluating whether SDR is appropriate for a particular child and for assessing outcome after surgery. We examine gait analysis in the next section.

SDR reduces spasticity only. Any secondary deformities that are present, including muscle contractures and bone deformities, will remain after SDR. These may be treated by orthopedic surgery. SDR is for tone reduction; orthopedic surgery is for bone alignment and residual muscle tightness. It is important to note that as tone-reducing procedures, neither SDR nor ITB negates the need for orthopedic surgery—they are complementary procedures. The expectation should be that both tone reduction and orthopedic surgery may be needed. However, tone reduction can allow the orthopedic surgery to focus more on bone realignment than on tendon lengthening.

As with any treatment, prior goal-setting and being able to formally evaluate outcome is essential.

SDR is a major operation, and the better the rehabilitation, the better the outcome is likely to be. Just as the operation itself varies between institutions, different institutions have different rehabilitation protocols post-SDR. A review of rehabilitation protocols post-SDR found that patients undergo intensive PT lasting approximately one year starting in the first days after surgery. Patients remain hospitalized anywhere from six days to six weeks [5].

As an example, at Gillette, rehabilitation begins three days post-SDR and usually involves a four- to six-week hospital stay. The benefit of being an inpatient rather than an outpatient is that it allows the patient to attend twice-daily therapy (PT, OT, and other therapies if necessary) and focus on rehabilitation in this early postoperative period. Whether inpatient or outpatient, the aim is to achieve the intensity of postoperative rehabilitation required to maximize functional outcome. Appendix 6 details post-SDR rehabilitation at Gillette. A detailed description of the rehabilitation plan is generally provided wherever SDR is carried out.

Overall, there is good evidence supporting SDR from both short-term and long-term studies (up to 26 years post-SDR) [6,8,28–30]. Improvements included reduced spasticity and improved gait and function. Long-term follow-up of SDR indicates that over half the patients underwent orthopedic surgery in the follow-up years [28,29]. In their long-term follow-up study (10 to 17 years after SDR), Munger and colleagues (2017) reported that non-SDR patients underwent significantly more orthopedic surgery and anti-spasticity injections than SDR patients [30].

Conclusion

No one treatment meets every child's needs, which is why a range of tone-reducing treatments exist. Tone reduction to manage spasticity (and dystonia, if present) is tailored to the individual child's needs. Which treatment is recommended depends on many factors, including age, GMFCS level, and type of high tone. An individual child may receive different treatments as they grow. For example, they may start with BoNT-A and then undergo SDR in later childhood when their gross motor function is more mature and their ability to participate in rehabilitation has improved [6]. Some tone-reducing treatments (such as SDR and ITB) are available only at specialist centers. To be able to choose the most appropriate treatment for each individual child, access to the specialist center to supplement what is available locally is needed. Though the use of tone reduction peaks in early childhood, it can continue into adolescence and adulthood.

This is the current situation with regard to tone-reducing treatments. As with all areas in the management and treatment of spastic diplegia, best practice may change as more research emerges.

Tommy had BoNT-A injections on two or three occasions as a young child. We didn't notice any major changes following these injections. Unfortunately, however, it was not clear to me back then how to best use the time after injection. BoNT-A was the only tone-reducing treatment Tommy had. I regret the fact that by the time I learned of SDR, when he was nine years old, he had missed out on what would have been a treatment of choice. At an earlier age, he would have met the "ideal" candidate criteria for SDR, but by age nine he already needed orthopedic surgery to address his muscle and bone problems. SDR can be carried out in older patients and this may be a consideration in the future, but to date there are few outcome studies of SDR in adults.

Today, Irish children who meet defined selection criteria are able to access SDR in the UK. It's great the treatment has become accessible to Irish children, but traveling abroad still places a considerable burden and expense on families. Hopefully it will become available in Ireland in the future.

Useful web links

- Gillette Children's Specialty Healthcare (2014) *Spasticity Treatment Options for Cerebral Palsy.* [video] youtu.be/ ejgnqoelW6A

- UK National Institute for Health and Care Excellence (NICE) (2016) *Spasticity in Under 19s: Management.* [online] nice.org.uk/guidance/cg145

3.7

Orthopedic surgery

Fractures well cured make us more strong.
Ralph Waldo Emerson

He jests at scars that never felt a wound.
William Shakespeare, from *Romeo and Juliet*

I have been struck again and again by how important measurement is in improving the human condition.
Bill Gates

There are two main peaks in the management of the musculoskeletal problems of spastic diplegia. The first occurs in early childhood, when tone reduction (in conjunction with other treatments such as PT and orthoses) is very important. The second occurs in later childhood (at approximately eight to 12 years), when orthopedic surgery may be needed to address the secondary abnormalities, the muscle and bone problems that have developed [1].

Delaying orthopedic surgery allows motor patterns to mature, and by this stage the gains from tone reduction have largely been achieved. Delaying orthopedic surgery is also important because it helps avoid the unpredictable outcomes of early surgery [2]. Orthopedic surgery becomes necessary when the muscle and bone deformities (the secondary abnormalities) are having a marked adverse effect on gait and function, and when they can no longer be treated by more conservative means. Because children at GMFCS level III are more involved, they may reach the point of requiring orthopedic surgery earlier than children at lower GMFCS levels.

Single-event multilevel surgery (SEMLS) involves multiple orthopedic surgical procedures performed on the lower limbs during a single operation [3–6]. Surgeons try to correct all the bone and muscle abnormalities in the same surgical event to avoid multiple hospital admissions, repeated anesthesia, and multiple rehabilitations. SEMLS is now considered best practice for orthopedic surgery in CP [7].

This section addresses:
- **Gait analysis**
- **Single-event multilevel surgery (SEMLS)**
- **How research and assessing outcome change treatment (example: plantar flexor lengthening)**
- **Our personal experience with SEMLS**

Gait analysis

SEMLS in spastic diplegia is guided by gait analysis [8–10], which provides detailed information about a person's manner of walking and how far it deviates from typical walking. Gait analysis is simply a measurement tool that uses some of the same technology used in the movie industry. Gait analysis allows treatment to be individualized (i.e., tailored to each individual child). Two children with spastic diplegia may walk in a similar manner, but the mechanisms behind their walking may differ. Analyzing those mechanisms allows treatment to be tailored to each individual child or adolescent. This is why gait analysis prior to SEMLS is so important.

Gait analysis is done for two main reasons:
- As a measurement tool[93] in which all gait deviations are identified

---

93   Gait analysis is a measurement tool used to evaluate gait. Within gait analysis, multiple outcome variables are evaluated using multiple measurement tools.

and a problem list is created. A treatment plan to meet the family's and surgeon's goals can then be devised. This is an example of data-driven decision-making in medicine.

- To help measure the effectiveness of treatment—in other words, to assess the outcome of treatment. This allows for a critical appraisal of the decision-making process for the individual.

Analyzing gait is a complex process involving many technologies. The precise elements of gait analysis[94] vary slightly between institutions. Gait analysis at Gillette includes the following elements:[95]

- Medical history
- X-rays
- Parent-reported functional questionnaires
- Two-dimensional video
- A standardized physical examination (which assesses bone alignment and soft tissue problems)
- Three-dimensional computerized motion analysis (3D computerized motion analysis):[96]
  - Kinematics: 3D measurement of motion (movement)
  - Kinetics: 3D measurement of forces and mechanisms that cause motion
- Electromyography (EMG): Measurement of the activity of muscles
- Pedobarography: Measurement of the pressure distribution under the feet
- Energy expenditure: Measurement of the energy used during walking

3D computerized motion analysis is the key part of gait analysis. The San Diego Children's Hospital (now Rady Children's) in California, Newington Children's Hospital (now Connecticut Children's Medical Center) in Connecticut, Gillette in Minnesota, the Children's Hospital of Los Angeles, and the Central Remedial Clinic (CRC) in Dublin, among others, were early adopters of 3D computerized motion analysis in the early 1980s and '90s.

---

94 When I refer to "gait analysis," I mean 3D computerized motion analysis. I do not mean merely observing gait or gait analysis done with simpler technologies.

95 Some of these elements are used at other times in the management of spastic diplegia, outside of formal gait analysis.

96 3D computerized motion analysis is the broader term because it includes other forms of motion, such as upper body motion. Gait is just one form of motion. However, the terms "3D computerized motion analysis" and "3D computerized gait analysis" can be used interchangeably.

In 3D computerized motion analysis, gait is measured simultaneously in three planes (hence the term "3D"). The three planes are:
- From back or front: the coronal plane
- From the side: the sagittal plane
- From top or bottom: the transverse plane

The list of gait deviations is derived from the elements of gait analysis listed above. The combination of information from all of these sources is very important as it provides a complete picture of a person's gait problems. Each source provides critical and unique information. When combined, data from one source can explain findings and/or complement data from another source. Comparing the gait of the individual with CP to a group of individuals with typical gait is very useful because it reveals how far the person's gait deviates from typical gait, as well as which joints are principally affected.

Once all of the gait analysis data is collected, a team of professionals interprets all the pieces of data. This team may include physicians, physical therapists, and engineers. The team identifies gait deviations from the gait analysis data, then a problem list is created from which a treatment plan can be devised. It is important to note that gait analysis provides only data; the *interpretation* of that data (i.e., to determine the gait deviations, problem list, and treatment plan) is done by the team of professionals. The family will typically meet their physician at a separate appointment to discuss the results.

I encourage all parents and people with the condition to obtain a copy of their gait report and read it. It is not a simple report by any means, but the explanations in this book will aid your understanding. Gait analysis is important when planning treatment. Given that parents and people with the condition are co–decision makers with professionals when planning treatment, a good understanding of the gait report is helpful and necessary in this role.

Repeat gait analysis after treatment assesses the treatment's outcome. This closed-loop approach (plan, treat, evaluate) is very important for each individual patient because it objectively assesses whether the decisions and treatment (data interpretation, treatment plan, SEMLS, and rehabilitation) were effective. This closed loop leads to continuous improvement in the standard of treatment offered by an institution over the long term. For example, gait analysis can be used to evaluate the outcome of a group of children who had a particular procedure. Gait analysis may also be repeated many years after a procedure to evaluate the long-term outcome of that particular procedure. These evaluations inform practice at an institution. In addition, shared learning and research lead to treatment improvements on a national and international level.

Reasons for referral for gait analysis vary between institutions, but a referral is usually made when a person reaches a plateau in their treatment (including therapy) and previous treatments are no longer effective. The age at which gait analysis is recommended varies, but it is usually recommended for children above three years of age; before age three, children are too small and would likely have difficulty cooperating. The ability to cooperate remains a consideration even in slightly older children. Gait analysis is most often performed in children and adolescents with spastic diplegia, GMFCS levels I–IV.

Further information on gait analysis is included in Appendix 7 available online, www.GilletteChildrensHealthcarePress.org/sdbook.

Single-event multilevel surgery (SEMLS)

The number of procedures performed during SEMLS varies but is typically eight to 16 [7]. (A procedure is a single treatment for a muscle or bone. For example, lengthening of the gastrocnemius muscle is one procedure. If it is carried out on both legs, it counts as two procedures. A femoral derotation is one procedure if it is carried out on one leg and two if it is carried out on both legs.) The number of procedures may seem overwhelming to the patient and family, but the purpose of the surgery is to correct all secondary abnormalities in a single operation.

Before gait analysis was common, orthopedic surgery for children with CP typically involved carrying out procedures on a yearly basis followed by intensive rehabilitation. Mercer Rang, an English orthopedic surgeon, coined the phrase "birthday syndrome" to refer to this type of orthopedic surgery: the child had an operation each year, followed by rehabilitation for the rest of the year [11]. Thankfully, orthopedic surgery for CP has progressed significantly since those days.

As we have seen, many muscles span more than one joint. Thus, for example, a procedure at the ankle also affects the knee. A procedure at the knee also affects the hip and foot. This is another reason why SEMLS has replaced the "birthday syndrome" approach.

The overall goal of SEMLS is to improve or maintain gait over the long term. Secondary goals may include improvements in gait efficiency[97] and appearance, gross motor function, independence, and quality of life [12]. Improving gait efficiency might mean that the person doesn't tire as easily while walking. Improving the appearance of walking can have huge effects on self-esteem, particularly during the adolescent years.

The typical surgical team that performs SEMLS consists of two experienced surgeons with two assistants [7]. Having two surgical teams means one team can operate on one lower limb while the other team operates on the other, minimizing the amount of time the patient spends under anesthesia. The child normally remains in the hospital for about four to five days after SEMLS. A web link to Gillette's SEMLS information booklet, *All about Your Single-Event Multilevel Surgery (SEMLS)*, which includes common procedures performed as part of SEMLS, is included at the end of this section.

As with all treatments, goal-setting is an important part of SEMLS. The expectations and goals of the surgeon and the family (both the parent and the child or adolescent) must be aligned. The Gait Outcomes Assessment List (GOAL) questionnaire is a newer measurement tool directed specifically at gait outcomes [13,14]; it is used in children and adolescents with CP aged five to 18 years. This parent or self-report tool asks questions across seven different categories, including function, pain, and self-esteem. One of the unique aspects of this tool is that for each question, the individual or parent can indicate whether it is an important goal area for improvement. This is useful because it can help

---

97 Gait efficiency can be measured by how much energy is consumed during walking. Think of energy expenditure during walking like the fuel efficiency of a car: a more efficient car will consume less fuel while traveling a set distance.

the surgeon understand the family's priorities and expectations and ensure their goals are aligned.

We saw in Chapter 2 that three longitudinal studies found deterioration in gait over time in children and adolescents with untreated spastic diplegia [15–17]. The time interval for deterioration was as low as 1.5 years. The aim of SEMLS is to counteract this deterioration and improve gait or maintain walking function. Because the natural history of gait in adolescence is of deterioration, even maintenance of gait should be viewed as success.

Although SEMLS is increasingly popular, Vuillermin and colleagues (2011) noted that many orthopedic surgeons still perform single-level surgery because of the limited availability of 3D computerized motion analysis, as well as differences in surgical philosophy [18].

SEMLS, like SDR, is usually followed by an intensive rehabilitation program to gain the maximum benefit from orthopedic surgery. Most centers will contemplate this surgery only if the child, with their family, is capable of completing the rehabilitation program. As with any orthopedic surgery, the better the rehabilitation, the better the outcome is likely to be.

Following SEMLS, the child does not return to their presurgical level of function for nine months to a year (or longer, depending on age and other factors). Thus full recovery following SEMLS can take up to one year, and the full benefit may not be seen for up to two years. Short-term outcome after SEMLS is generally assessed no earlier than one year after surgery.

Though the rehabilitation may commence with a hospital physical therapist, it is likely to be continued with the child's community physical therapist. Good liaison between physical therapists is very important to ensure a smooth handover of care. Although there is no agreed-upon consensus on optimal rehabilitation post-SEMLS [19,20], work is being done to achieve this, and protocols have recently been developed [20,21]. Each person who undergoes SEMLS will receive a detailed rehabilitation program; the program will vary depending on the procedures carried out during the surgery. Gillette's SEMLS information booklet includes details on rehabilitation.

Implants (plates and/or screws inserted during surgery), if used, may require subsequent removal approximately one year after surgery. Some institutions remove the implants, while others do not. At Gillette the practice is generally to remove them.

Though SEMLS is a major undertaking, it should not be seen as an end point. It is just a treatment along the journey to adulthood for the child or adolescent with spastic diplegia. SEMLS cannot alter the primary abnormalities (the underlying cause of impaired bone and muscle growth), and a gradual recurrence of deformity may occur post-SEMLS. Until the body reaches skeletal maturity, it is important to keep muscle growth at pace with continuing bone growth through stretching. Puberty is a period of very active bone growth; stretching and strengthening are as important in the years after SEMLS as they were in the years before.

Overall, there is good evidence supporting SEMLS [10,12,19,22–24]. The benefits include improvements in gait 12 months after surgery and improvements in gross motor function and quality of life 24 months after surgery [12]. Two studies were longer-term—up to nine years after the original SEMLS—and showed that the improvements were maintained [10,23]. However, in these studies, 39 percent [10] and 67 percent [23] of adolescents required additional orthopedic surgery (other than implant removal) in the years after their initial SEMLS. It should be noted, however, that the subsequent surgeries were less invasive (an average of two procedures, compared with eight to nine procedures for the original SEMLS) and required a shorter and easier period of rehabilitation than the original SEMLS.

Thus it must be emphasized that SEMLS reduces, but does not eliminate, the likelihood of further surgeries. Dreher and colleagues (2018) suggested the term SEMLS might be misleading because of the possibility of further surgery; they suggested removing the words "single-event" and using the term "multilevel surgery (MLS)" for the initial surgery [10]. Regardless of the precise term (SEMLS or MLS), the initial surgery is designed to correct the muscle and bone problems in one surgical event. If further muscle and bone problems arise during subsequent adolescent growth, then further surgery may be required.

A report published by Gillette provided information on how gait analysis guides decision-making and is incorporated into a person's care (web link included at the end of this section). It followed a group of 391 children for just over three years and reviewed outcomes [25]. The report concluded that:

- Gait analysis is a valuable tool for diagnosis and treatment planning.
- By receiving appropriate data-guided diagnoses and treatment planning, children had good outcomes.
- Children and their families reported that treatment was worth the difficulties encountered and their expectations were met.

How research and assessing outcome change treatment (example: plantar flexor lengthening)

In section 2.9, we saw that any treatment that weakens the ankle plantar flexors (the soleus/gastrocnemius) may contribute to crouch gait [7]. Preserving plantar flexion strength is important for preventing crouch gait.

Research has shown that the soleus is very sensitive to lengthening [26]. A 1 cm lengthening of the soleus reduces its moment-generating ability by 30 percent, and a 2 cm lengthening reduces it by 85 percent. Graham, Thomason, and Novacheck (2014) noted that even a small error in over-lengthening the soleus may be disastrous and recommended gastrocnemius lengthening only when there is no contracture in the soleus [7]. They further reported that there is usually a delay between this lengthening and the development of crouch gait: the lengthening is often done between three and six years of age, and it may take another three to six years before crouch gait becomes a significant problem. It may only be when the adolescent growth spurt occurs that the full extent of the crouch gait develops. (The reason why the lengthening was commonly performed between three and six years of age was because toe-walking —the first pattern seen in spastic diplegia—becomes very prevalent at that age [27]. The lengthening was to address the toe-walking. Toe-walking is a noticeable gait deviation and an unstable form of walking.)

In a study of the prevalence of severe crouch gait over a 15-year period, severe crouch gait was found to be precipitated by lengthening of either the Achilles tendon or the gastrocnemius and soleus in combination[98] that was not part of an SEMLS [18]. This is consistent with earlier studies [28,29], which found that the majority of those who develop more severe crouch gait had previous Achilles tendon lengthening. It may be necessary to lengthen the short two-joint gastrocnemius, but the single-joint soleus is generally not short [7]. It appears severe crouch can largely be avoided if lengthening of the soleus is avoided and in a setting where consistent, timely, and appropriate management occurs.

Thankfully, nowadays surgeons usually lengthen the gastrocnemius alone, but I caution readers that the old procedure may still be carried out in some parts of the world and at less specialized institutions. I encourage readers to always understand what lengthening is being done if surgery for the calf muscles (the gastrocnemius and soleus) is being proposed. It is important to know which muscle is being lengthened.

Our personal experience with SEMLS

Our story refers to Gillette because that is where our son underwent SEMLS, but other specialist centers around the world offer this treatment. As with all treatments, different institutions and different providers may have different protocols.

In 2001, just after 9/11, Dr. Gage, an orthopedic surgeon at Gillette, presented at a conference I attended at the Central Remedial Clinic (CRC) in Dublin. That day I made a mental note that if Tommy ever needed orthopedic surgery, I would contact Dr. Gage. Unbeknown to me, that day would arrive sooner than I realized. In 2003, orthopedic surgery was recommended for Tommy. I wrote to Dr. Gage, sending him Tommy's records (including his recent gait analysis, carried out at the CRC) and asking if he would be willing to see Tommy. We brought Tommy to Minnesota, where Dr. Gage recommended SEMLS. To support my own understanding, I decided to complete a research master's: a

---

98 The Achilles tendon is the tendon common to both the gastrocnemius and soleus muscles. The lengthening of the soleus and gastrocnemius in combination is performed closer to the where the muscles join the tendon but still includes both muscles.

case study providing a detailed picture of SEMLS and rehabilitation and evaluating outcome (up to two years post-SEMLS) using a comprehensive range of measurement tools.

My husband and I traveled from Ireland to Minnesota in 2004 with 10-year-old Tommy. Everyone at home was terribly worried about us taking Tommy abroad for orthopedic surgery. Neither professionals nor friends supported our decision. The most support we had was from our family physician, who said the amount of surgery the SEMLS would entail was akin to a very bad road traffic accident, but at least the surgery would be planned and they would not be picking glass fragments from Tommy's muscle tissue. Positive, but not exactly a ringing endorsement! And those were the only words of "encouragement" we heard amid a lot of well-meaning discouragement, including, "They cut too much in America."

Despite all the worry and lack of support back home, we—Tommy, my husband, and I—were not at all worried. We had complete confidence in Dr. Gage and the surgical team at Gillette.

In writing this book I have reflected on why I felt so confident in our decision to pursue SEMLS despite the negative reactions of so many people, including many for whom I had and still have a huge amount of respect. It really came down to:

- The logical explanation of the primary, secondary, and tertiary abnormalities in spastic diplegia and the logic of the treatment plan.
- Understanding that SEMLS required pediatric orthopedists who were specialists in analyzing gait in CP and well versed in 3D computerized motion analysis, that planning this type of orthopedic surgery was not like planning a knee or hip replacement, and that the complexity and skill involved in the surgery lay in the choice of which procedures to perform. I recognized that Gillette had developed this expertise.
- At that time (2004), SEMLS was supported by research from a number of international centers [3,4,6,30,31]. An early 2001 research study from Gillette [31] was followed by a more detailed study in early 2004, just prior to Tommy's SEMLS [6]. The 2004 outcome study included 66 patients with an average age of nine with a

diagnosis of spastic diplegia and no prior surgical procedure—exactly the same as Tommy. This study showed that gait pattern, gait efficiency (energy consumed while walking), community walking, and higher-level functional skills improved after orthopedic surgery for the majority of those patients. (Since that time, studies from many international centers have supported SEMLS, including the first randomized controlled trial of SEMLS in CP [12]).

- The attitude of humility, care, and respect for children with CP at Gillette was extraordinary. I have visited a number of times in the intervening years and this still hits me every single time. The combination of world-class expertise and world-class care is amazing.

Tommy's operation lasted six hours. He had 13 procedures in all, nine on his right leg and four on his left. Despite all the procedures, he refused to take any pain medication once he left the hospital four days later. (Having left the hospital, his only "medication" if he woke in pain during the night was having his dad sing him back to sleep or watching videos.)

An intensive, year-long rehabilitation back in Ireland (based on Gillette's rehabilitation plan) followed the surgery. No one should underestimate the amount and intensity of rehabilitation required after SEMLS: it took a lot of work on Tommy's (and our) part. Rehabilitation post-SEMLS is a lot longer than rehabilitation following, say, knee replacement surgery.

I would advise each parent and patient to understand what they are signing up for when they plan to undergo SEMLS. Surgery is only the start of a long road. In a sense, once you've driven away from the hospital following the surgery, the hard work (for the child and the parent) is only just beginning. However, the long rehabilitation will likely be very much worth it.

Surgery can be regarded as a three-part process: good surgical planning, good surgery, and good rehabilitation. The surgeon is responsible for the first two parts, and the parent and child, in conjunction with the physical therapist, are largely responsible for the third. A successful outcome requires all three.

We stayed in the US for six weeks. Ideally, SEMLS and the period immediately following discharge from the hospital requires the support of two adults; in my opinion it is too much work for just one. The surgery wasn't easy for Tommy, nor for us. It was difficult leaving our other children at home and being away for so long. But without a shadow of a doubt, we would do it all again.

Rehabilitation from SEMLS can take up to one year, and the full benefit of the surgery may not be seen for up to two years. I remember how surprised people were to see how much less functional Tommy was after his SEMLS. Without understanding what was involved, they expected to see near-immediate improvements. Tommy had his implants (the plates and screws inserted during surgery) removed in Dublin one year later.

In my research study, SEMLS was judged to have been successful by all stakeholders (surgeon, researcher, teacher, child, and parent).[99] Objective measures of change included improvements in gait, endurance, gross motor function, muscle strength, and flexibility. Patient and parent satisfaction were evident in interviews conducted by my research supervisor with Tommy and his dad. One of the most noticeable findings from the interviews with Tommy was how unconcerned he was about the surgery, both before and after, and how positive his outlook was throughout. (To keep his mind off surgery and later as pain medication, we used distraction techniques: Tommy had asked for a particular box set of videos, which we bought but didn't allow him to start watching until he was in the hospital. As a result, he couldn't wait to get to the hospital. Heading to the operating room on the morning of the surgery, he wasn't anxious; he was just disappointed he had to press pause on the DVD player.)

Once we made the decision to proceed with SEMLS in the US, the staff at the CRC and our community physical therapist could not have been more helpful. They provided information to the team in the US in advance, stayed in touch with us while we were away, and supported Tommy's long rehabilitation afterward. In addition, the CRC gait lab and our community physical therapist provided data and other assistance to help me complete my master's.

---

99 Because I was the researcher, my husband completed the parent evaluations.

When Tommy was 16 years old, he developed severe knee pain. He has a high pain threshold, but the pain was so bad that it interfered with his sleep. We tried a number of treatments without success.[100] We contacted the surgeons at Gillette, who immediately recognized the cause and advised further orthopedic surgery. Tommy had two additional orthopedic surgeries when he was 16 and 18. By this time Dr. Gage had retired and Dr. Novacheck was at the helm. Tommy's surgery at age 16 included five procedures on his right leg to address the knee pain and other issues that had arisen during adolescence. The later surgery, at age 18, was an adjustment to one of the earlier procedures.

His surgery at age 18 coincided with a cycling trip through France my husband and I had planned for our 25th wedding anniversary. Our three sons insisted the cycling trip continue, and the older boys, now living in the US, decided they would accompany Tommy to the surgery. While I wanted to postpone the trip, I was totally outnumbered by the men in my life. In the end, we took the cycling trip, and I felt relaxed and not at all worried because of my confidence in Dr. Novacheck and our three boys.

Based on our journey and everything I have read, I can honestly say Tommy would not be walking as well or living as independently as he is today without the surgeries he had in his adolescent years. In the early days we had been told that Tommy would likely need to use a wheelchair by the time he was in college. I mentioned earlier that my favorite photograph from Tommy's graduation is a shot of him and the family walking to dinner that evening. I felt compelled to send a copy of it, with huge gratitude, to the many professionals who helped Tommy reach that day.

---

100 One of the treatments was to put the knee in a cast for six weeks. Although he was in severe pain, Tommy would only agree to go ahead with the leg cast if it would not prevent him from auditioning for a lead role in the musical *Rent*. As it happened, we had to cut the cast off at home after only three weeks because the pain had become intolerable. We discovered that a bad knee infection had developed underneath the cast. Despite it all, a few weeks later Tommy thoroughly enjoyed playing Mark in *Rent*.

Useful web links

- Gillette Children's Specialty Healthcare (2018) *All about Your Single-Event Multilevel Surgery (SEMLS)*. [online] flipsnack.com/95B5CFFEFB5/all-about-your-single-event -multilevel-surgery-semls.html

- Gillette Children's Specialty Healthcare (2014) *Gait and Motion Analysis for Treatment Planning and Outcomes Assessment*. [pdf] gillettechildrens.org/assets/uploads/care-and-conditions/Gait_Lab_ Outcome_Report_-_Final.pdf

3.8

The overall musculoskeletal management plan to age 20

When there is no turning back,
then we should concern ourselves only
with the best way of going forward.

Paulo Coelho, from *The Alchemist*

In the journey to skeletal maturity (i.e., adulthood), reflecting the ICF model, the overall goal is to promote optimal participation in daily life by enhancing activities and minimizing problems with body functions and structure. We want to prevent or delay the onset of muscle contractures and bone deformities and allow the child the typical experience of activity and participation at any stage of life.

Treatment in spastic diplegia depends on the person's age and GMFCS level. Age is important because the musculoskeletal and gait problems develop with growth and therefore with time. GMFCS level is important because generally the higher the GMFCS level, the greater the extent of the musculoskeletal and gait problems. Because growth is a major factor in spastic diplegia, once growth ceases at around age 20, a certain stabilization of the condition occurs. The challenges of spastic diplegia in adulthood are addressed in Chapter 4.

In the early years, treatment focuses on the development of skills, achieving motor milestones, and stretching to achieve muscle growth. Therapies are planned throughout the child's life as episodes of care, and orthoses are prescribed as required. Different treatments, when used together, can amplify the effect of individual treatments (e.g., attending PT to achieve a new functional goal following BoNT-A injections). The saying, "The whole is greater than the sum of its parts" certainly applies here. Despite best efforts in the early years, the development of some muscle and bone problems is largely inevitable. Depending on their severity, they may require correction by SEMLS. Minimizing the amount of orthopedic surgery needed is, however, an important goal. Figure 3.8.1 summarizes the musculoskeletal management plan, with two peaks in early and late childhood

With reference to Figure 3.8.1:
- The first peak in management occurs in early childhood, up to approximately age six, when management of high tone (spasticity and dystonia) is the priority. This is achieved through oral medications, BoNT-A or phenol injections, SDR, and ITB [1,2].
- Currently, BoNT-A is the most commonly used tone-reducing treatment [2].
- Generally, the only orthopedic surgery required in the early years is for the prevention of hip displacement [2]. The risk of hip displacement increases with GMFCS level, and the frequency of hip surveillance is linked to the child's GMFCS level [3].
- The term "transition" refers to the period when tone-reducing treatment may become less effective, but it is not yet time for orthopedic surgery. It occurs at approximately six years of age.
- The second peak in management occurs between the ages of six and 12, which is when SEMLS is best carried out for the one-stage correction of all the muscle and bone abnormalities. "Fine-tuning" may later be required. Research has found that a significant percentage of children with spastic diplegia, GMFCS levels I–III required additional surgery in the nine years after their original SEMLS [4,5].
- Spasticity management is still relevant as growth continues. SEMLS does not alter the primary abnormalities of CP, and a gradual recurrence of deformity may occur post-SEMLS. Until the body reaches skeletal maturity, it is important to keep muscle growth at pace with continuing bone growth through stretching. Puberty is a period of very active bone growth.

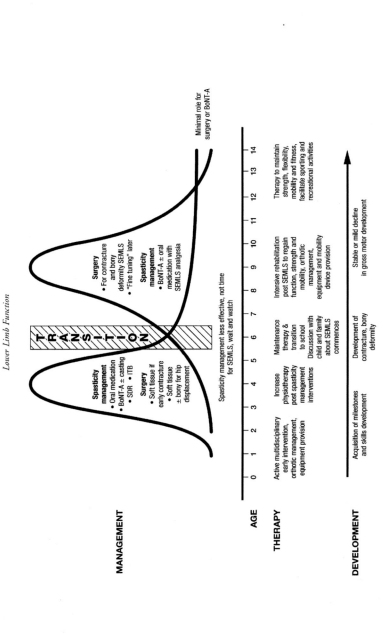

Figure 3.8.1 Musculoskeletal management plan for children and adolescents with CP. Reproduced with kind permission from *Cerebral Palsy: Science and Clinical Practice*, edited by Bernard Dan, Margaret Mayston, Nigel Paneth, and Lewis Rosenbloom, published by Mac Keith Press (mackeith.co.uk) in its Clinics in Developmental Medicine Series, 2014, 978-1-909962-38-5.

No treatment (e.g., BoNT-A, SDR, SEMLS) should ever be viewed as an end point. They are aids in the pursuit of the overall goal of getting to skeletal maturity (i.e., adulthood) with the fewest possible effects of the brain injury. In the case of both SDR and SEMLS, long periods of rehabilitation can help achieve a higher level of function following the surgery.

Finally, the home program (addressed in section 3.4) is a constant in the life of the child and adolescent with spastic diplegia.

3.9

Alternative and complementary treatments

It is possible in medicine, even when you intend to do good, to do harm instead. That is why science thrives on actively encouraging criticism rather than stifling it.

Richard Dawkins

Alternative (as a substitute) and complementary (in addition to) treatments are treatments that are not part of current standard conventional medical or rehabilitation treatments and care [1].

We parents want only the best for our children, and for a number of reasons we may consider alternative and complementary treatments. These reasons can include:

- We hear about a treatment option in the media (internet, radio, TV, newspapers, magazines) or from well-meaning family and friends.
- We want to try all treatment options in case the one we haven't tried is the one that works.
- We want to complement or increase the effectiveness of present treatment.
- We want to relieve symptoms (such as pain).
- We believe our child can do better.

Often, alternative and complementary treatments are expensive. If the parent-professional relationship is good, we parents should be able to discuss these treatment ideas with the medical professionals who treat our child. We—both parents and professionals—should be guided by the best research evidence available. This principle guided the writing of this book.

Table 3.9.1 lists a number of common alternative and complementary treatments and the available research evidence.

Table 3.9.1 Alternative and complementary treatments

TREATMENT	DESCRIPTION OF TREATMENT	EVIDENCE (OR LACK OF) SUPPORTING TREATMENT
Hyperbaric oxygen	The person inhales 100 percent oxygen in a pressurized hyperbaric chamber. The theory behind its use in CP is that there are inactive cells among the damaged brain cells that have the potential to recover.	The evidence indicates that hyperbaric oxygen is ineffective and adverse events can occur [2].
Massage	Massage involves applying pressure to muscles, generally using the hands, to relieve pain and tension. A massage therapist is a person who is professionally trained to perform massage.	The evidence indicates that massage does not achieve specific therapy goals, but it may improve the feeling of well-being in children with CP and their parents [3].
Cranial osteopathy	Cranial osteopathy involves using the hands to perform small movements that ease musculoskeletal strain and treat the central nervous system.	The evidence indicates that cranial osteopathy is ineffective [2].
Acupuncture	Thin needles are inserted into the skin at specific points.	There is insufficient evidence supporting its use. If used, it should be accompanied by sensitive tools to measure outcome to monitor progress [2].

Cont'd.

TREATMENT	DESCRIPTION OF TREATMENT	EVIDENCE (OR LACK OF) SUPPORTING TREATMENT
Stem cell therapy	Stem cell transplantation is a regenerative therapy that has the potential to replace damaged and nonfunctional nerve cells in the brains of people with CP, in addition to providing support to remaining nerve cells [4].	Stem cell therapy is still an experimental technique that is not ready to be adopted as the standard of care for patients with CP [4]. In the next few years, the role of stem cell therapy in CP will be clarified as further studies are undertaken to determine efficacy and the best stem cell type, as well as the most appropriate dose and mode of delivery [5]. If stem cells have the potential to enrich the nervous system, they may add to the therapeutic options available to facilitate functional gains, even if they cannot achieve a cure [5]. Similar opinions have been expressed elsewhere [6–8].

Of the five therapies reviewed above, two were found to be ineffective and there was insufficient evidence to support the remaining three.

Hopefully stem cell therapy will continue to be an area of active research so its potential in CP becomes clearer. A web link is included at the end of this section for people who would like to read more about stem cell treatment. Graham (2014) noted that many parents delay or refuse conventional treatments because they have unrealistic expectations of the potential outcomes of stem cell treatment. He explained that although Australia has an efficient hip surveillance program, the most common cause of a dislocated hip in a child with CP is delayed intervention because parents expect stem cell treatments to cure the child [9]. We parents cannot afford to abandon conventional treatments with their evidence base for an unproven treatment.

A Canadian study looked at the extent to which adolescents with CP across all five GMFCS levels had used alternative and complementary treatments in the past year.[101] Most (73 percent) did not currently use any. The most commonly used services were massage (15 percent), hyperbaric oxygen (10 percent), and osteopathy (6 percent) [1].

Useful web link

- Beldick S, Fehlings MG (2017) *Current State of Stem Cell Treatments for Cerebral Palsy: A Guide for Patients, Families, and Service Providers.* [online] canchild.ca/en/resources/276-current -state-of-stem-cell-treatments-for-cerebral-palsy-a-guide-for -patients-families-and-service-providers

---

101 Options offered were hyperbaric oxygen, acupuncture, herbal therapy, chiropractic intervention, osteopathy, reflexology, massage therapy, homeopathy, high-dose vitamins, lifestyle diets, folk remedies, spiritual healing, hypnosis, and other interventions. Other interventions included conductive education, the Alexander technique, amino acids, hippotherapy (horse riding for reasons of health), and faith.

3.10

What the parent can do to help the child, what the adolescent can do to help themselves

The Child is father of the Man.

William Wordsworth, from "My Heart Leaps Up"

When it comes to the overall management of the person with spastic diplegia, no matter how hard we try, we cannot mitigate the effects of the brain injury. No matter how much we might want to, we cannot "treat and fix" our child, as Lach and colleagues (2014) so aptly put it [1]. Spastic diplegia cannot (currently) be cured, but with good management its effects can be reduced. As a parent, it is important to be clear on what you can and cannot do to make a difference in your child's life.

Looking back, I wish I'd had a much clearer sense of what we could and could not change and how I, as a parent, could best contribute to Tommy's management and care. Spastic diplegia is very complex, and I am still learning. In retrospect, I see a number of things I would have done differently.

The following are some thoughts on the management of spastic diplegia in childhood and adolescence. They are largely gleaned from my personal experience, particularly of the "make mistakes and learn from them" variety. They are presented in no particular order.

Thinking philosophically

Play to the strengths of your child. Focus on strengths rather than deficits, on what your child can do rather than what they can't do. Focusing on strengths means fostering your child's interests. One of our duties as parents is to help our child discover their passions by allowing them to try different things and then supporting them in what they choose to pursue.

Having a glass-half-full attitude serves us so well in life. With effort, so much is possible. One of my overarching beliefs is that the person with spastic diplegia can largely be anything they want to be. The sky's the limit. I also think the child with spastic diplegia has to be a "despite it" kid—they have to know that despite their spastic diplegia, they will succeed. Indeed, we all need to be "despite it" people in life.

I have always felt that the greatest gift you can give any child is the gift of self-confidence. Your child with spastic diplegia may have a higher hill to climb to achieve it, but you, the parent, can greatly help them on their way.

It is worth keeping in mind that scientific studies generally present the average of outcomes. The gross motor development curves, for example, are based on averages. Be realistic in your goals for your child, but do not limit your aspirations to the average. Aim for the top of the range. It may or may not be possible to get there, but, as with any field of endeavor, the first step toward success is aiming high. Do not let your knowledge of averages limit your child's potential.

You may not see improvement day to day, or even week to week, but when improvement does happen it is very sweet. These improvements are skills that able-bodied children acquire when you're not even looking, and—aside from the big milestone of walking—they are often taken for granted. With Tommy, I stopped taking things for granted and began to notice and appreciate every little change.

We go to great lengths to help our child walk and keep them walking, in other words, to achieve ordinariness. One has to go to extraordinary lengths to achieve ordinariness. Sometimes friends and extended family members may not fully understand.

In the very early days after Tommy's diagnosis, I remember a family physician explaining the conundrum of degree of disability versus effort. She said moderate CP demanded the most effort because a person with moderate disability has good potential to improve. If the disability is more mild, the person might not need to put in as much effort. If it is more severe, the person might not benefit as much from the effort. I could see her point, but as technology develops, more effort and input may be beneficial for children at higher GMFCS levels as well.

Having spastic diplegia does not define the person, be they a child, adolescent, or adult.

We need to be careful about how we view our children with spastic diplegia. We need to be careful not to see our child as any more challenged than they actually are. How we view and treat our child is important because we provide the leadership for how others will view and treat them, from extended family to friends and teachers.

Drs. Rosenbaum and Rosenbloom advised parents to take the long view when it comes to the life of a child with CP [2]:

> We encourage [parents] to take a long-term view of their child's journey through childhood. We remind them that the adult world imposes on all children the expectation (at least in school) that they try to perform in a wide range of areas. Adults expect children to learn and hopefully demonstrate skills in many activities—be they social, physical, intellectual, artistic—that are much more demanding than what the adults ever expect of themselves, or even perform, on a day-to-day basis. We want to help parents to recognize that [...] they can help their children weather the childhood years with these many and varied demands (demands which often challenge many children without disabilities) [...] We should encourage parents to strive to help their children, in the course of their developing years, to develop competencies,

interests, and a sense of self-confidence despite their "disabilities," because after the childhood years they will have many more opportunities to find their niche in life.

I think this is excellent advice.

The importance of the home program

If you take just one thing away from this book, I hope it will be the importance of the home program (detailed in section 3.4). Life with spastic diplegia is a great balancing act. Completing the program without either the child or parent experiencing burnout requires skill. As a parent, I felt conflicted between supporting and encouraging Tommy and firmly insisting that he do his home program. The parent has to be a parent, not a therapist, but this is sometimes a challenge. As parents we have to protect our child and help them achieve a normal childhood, yet at the same time attend many appointments and complete the home program.

I encourage parents to get as much help as they can in carrying out the home program. For example, someone can take your child to the playground or swimming pool. My husband very much shared the load with me, and our two older sons were a great help. Over the years we also had two excellent sisters who helped out as babysitters—Sinead and Clodagh Killeen. Interestingly, they both went on to study and qualify as physiotherapists, and they both credited their interest in the field to their early days working with Tommy.

Exercise and physical activity can be done with family and able-bodied friends in regular rather than therapy settings. Indeed, the child's need to exercise may motivate the whole family to get moving. Choose activities the child and the family really enjoy; this increases the likelihood that you will all stick with it. Exercise and physical activity are also fantastic ways to make friends and develop a good social network. We humans are pack animals: we need our pack (our family and friends) for good mental health. Strong social connectedness is important at all stages of life, and anything that increases social connectedness is good.

The concept of regarding the child or adolescent with spastic diplegia as an elite athlete is useful. The elite athlete's program is designed to help them win competitions; the child/adolescent's home program is designed to minimize the effects of their spastic diplegia. The elite athlete leaves nothing to chance: they optimize all aspects of their life, from training to rest to diet. Indeed, this precise formula (physical activity, adequate sleep, and good nutrition) is recommended for the health and well-being of individuals with CP [3]. Even if the reasons are different, many of the requirements are the same for the elite athlete and the person with spastic diplegia. The other major advantage of this is that it shifts the management of the condition from a medical context to a sports context. And, as we saw earlier, there's nothing to stop the person with CP from actually becoming an elite athlete!

Resisting the urge to be overprotective

Children learn by making mistakes, as we all do. The typically developing toddler learns to walk while (and by) toppling a lot: they get a sense of their limbs in space, threats to their balance, and how to negotiate obstacles. Because a child with spastic diplegia has difficulty with fluid movement and may have balance issues, we should be careful not to become overprotective and unintentionally stifle their opportunities to learn from movement mistakes. We have to let them fall and learn from falling.

In Tommy's early days at school, he could sense that the staff supervising outdoor play were always very close by. Even as a young child, he sensed they were being overprotective. I asked the school to allow him to play freely, adding that we would not hold them responsible in any way for falls or fractures. It worked. Tommy played much more freely after that, and as it happened, he never did get injured.

Guarding against being overprotective applies throughout life. We need to swing the pendulum the other way and foster independence right from the start. Again, others will take their cues from us. The principle of patient-centered care is one we parents must emulate at home: it encourages us to actively involve our child in decision-making related to their care and foster their independence in all areas of life from an early age. Indeed, this principle should apply to all of our children.

Resisting the urge to do too much for the child

I would encourage parents to resist the temptation to do too much for your child. It is much faster, for example, to dress the young child than to allow them to do it themselves. (This was an impulse I very much had to resist.) But it is important the child learn to perform movements and practice the skill, even though the task will take longer. Breaking down dressing tasks and doing each movement correctly, ensuring both hands are involved if one hand is stronger, is an excellent exercise.

We have to develop patience. This applies to parenting across the board, but the temptation to do things for your child is even greater when they have spastic diplegia. Most parents are time-poor, but recognizing the importance of giving your child these opportunities to practice and learn will pay dividends down the line.

The importance of good nutrition

Good nutrition (and hydration) is important for the child with spastic diplegia, as it is for all children. No special diet is needed so long as your child is eating a good, balanced diet. I encourage parents to get advice on this if necessary. The whole family might benefit.

Monitor your child's bone health throughout childhood and adolescence. Good nutrition, ensuring no deficiencies in calcium and vitamin D, and physical activity, especially weight-bearing or impact activities, can help promote good bone health [4]. A review found some evidence of lower bone mineral density in ambulant children (and adults) with CP at GMFCS levels II and III [5].

We often read about the increasing prevalence of obesity, including childhood obesity, in many developed countries. Obesity has many negative effects, including increasing the risk of conditions such as type 2 diabetes. As important as good weight management is for all of us, it is even more important for people with spastic diplegia because muscle strength is already compromised and excess weight can limit walking.

As with exercise, good eating habits start early in life, and children are much more likely to have good habits if their parents do. In addition, parents' influence on a child's eating habits can have an impact long after the child has left home. It is never too late to recognize unhealthy eating habits and make the decision to change.

Getting the most out of appointments

Life with a diagnosis of spastic diplegia involves many appointments, particularly in the early years. I encourage parents to ensure they're getting as much as possible out of these appointments. I suggest you come to appointments with a written list of questions. I found it very useful to write notes after each appointment, including what I'd learned and what I needed to do next. If I didn't take notes, I couldn't be sure I would remember everything.

To get the most out of appointments on a practical level, try to ensure your child isn't tired or hungry when you arrive. (For that matter, make sure you aren't tired or hungry either!) We tried to make Tommy's appointments as much fun as possible by tying them in with some other activity, like visiting with extended family so he could play with his cousins. When they involved travel, these appointments felt like a little adventure for the family.

Throughout childhood and adolescence, the parent and child work together in partnership with medical professionals. Neither can achieve best management of the condition on their own. Nurture the relationship with the professionals treating your child—they are your allies. You may be angry about aspects of your child's diagnosis or treatment, but don't put professionals on the receiving end of any misplaced anger. The expression "Don't shoot the messenger" comes to mind. You might be dissatisfied with the range of services provided to your child, for example. However, frontline staff are rarely the policy-makers—indeed, they may silently agree with you.

Good communication between disciplines is vital for the functioning of the multidisciplinary team. The parent and child are the constants in this relationship, thus the parent can support communication between the different team members. No matter how good services are, things can go wrong: for example, a referral might be forgotten and an appointment might not get scheduled. Supporting communication between team members is particularly important when the child is getting a large part of their care in the community but travels to a specialist center at intervals. The parent can play an important role in the smooth coordination of care. It's helpful to stay organized and keep medical reports together and to hand. This coordinator role can later fall to the adolescent themselves.

Being a juggler

Balancing all the requirements of the family is quite a juggling act: you might be attending regular appointments and completing the home program while also holding a job, being a partner to a spouse or significant other, parenting other children, and looking after aging parents. The needs of siblings must not be neglected when so much attention is focused on the child with the disability. Parents have to look after themselves, too. To help others, we have to help ourselves. Think of the safety advice on an airplane: you must put on your own oxygen mask before putting on your child's. Do not create a "disabled family."

Managing education and transitions

Employment is one of the keys to achieving independence. We will see in the chapter on adulthood that the rate of employment among people with spastic diplegia does not match that of able-bodied peers. You, the parent, have to be forward-thinking.

Damiano (2006) considered activity to be very important in CP—the title of her paper was "Activity, Activity, Activity: Rethinking Our Physical Therapy Approach to Cerebral Palsy" [6]. I would add a further mantra: "Education, Education, Education." A person with a physical impairment is unlikely to be employed in a role requiring physical prowess; they will have to rely on other skills. It is important to maximize your child's cognitive and intellectual abilities to maximize their opportunities for employment. A good education is important for every child—indeed, education is included in the United Nations Convention on the Rights of the Child [7]. The range of career options open to people with spastic diplegia is large; their disability places only a small limit on their choice. Today, technology has created jobs that didn't even exist 10 years ago.

Change is the one constant in life. Transitions are a big step for any child, and they keep coming: from home to daycare, to preschool, to elementary school, middle school, high school, and on to college, higher education, or work. Transitions can be more challenging for the child with spastic diplegia because of, for example, difficulties with mobility or difficulties participating in some activities at school.

I would advise parents to plan ahead at each school stage to ensure sufficient accommodations are made to ease transitions and maximize your child's opportunity for a good school experience and education. In Tommy's case, accommodations at school included being allowed to use a laptop in class (because of his difficulties with handwriting), extra time in exams, and extra time to move between classes.

Health care professionals can be a good resource for planning ahead and problem-solving if or when challenges arise. Practicing skills that might be needed in the next phase of life at home with time, supervision, and someone with whom to problem-solve is highly beneficial, both for activity completion and to boost the child's self-confidence. An example might be practicing dressing skills for changing in the locker room.

Regrettably, school bullying continues to affect significant numbers of children and adolescents, and those with disabilities are at higher risk [8]. A study found that children and adolescents with CP experienced bullying and social exclusion at school [9]. What was interesting were the strategies suggested by the children and adolescents to help improve social inclusion at school [10]. These included:

- Creating awareness of their disability by disclosing their condition to peers and teachers. (It was suggested that health care professionals could help with this.)
- Being vocal about incidents of bullying and exclusion (to peers, teachers, and parents).
- Building quality friendships as an effective peer support network.

They also emphasized the importance of teachers paying close attention to the needs of students with disabilities. Tindal (2017), a student teacher who has mild CP, created a tip sheet for teachers of students with mild CP [11]. A web link is included at the end of this section.

Given that teachers have such a profound influence on the lives of their students, parents should speak with their child's teacher to ensure they understand the child's disability. This is not a one-off conversation—as the child progresses through school, teachers change. If the student has multiple teachers, talking with a key staff member may work best. Thankfully, Tommy did not experience any problems with bullying at school. (I checked in with him again at the time of writing, just in case he'd been reluctant to tell us about it at the time.)

Reassuringly, a large European quality of life (QoL) study reported that children with CP aged eight to 12 have similar QoL to other children [12]. A follow-up study found that adolescents with CP aged 13 to 17 had significantly lower QoL than the general population in only one area: social support and peers [13]. Pain in childhood or adolescence was strongly associated with low QoL [12,13].

It is heartening to see QoL is similar for children and adolescents with and without CP. However, the studies make evident that we must support children and adolescents with CP in developing peer relationships. If pain is present, pain management is also important because of its association with low QoL.

Adolescence and achieving independence

When does adolescence actually begin? The World Health Organization defines adolescence as the period between 10 and 19 years of age. The great majority of adolescents are, therefore, included in the age-based definition of the child adopted by the UN Convention on the Rights of the Child, which defines a child as a person under age 18 [7]. Adolescence can thus be viewed as that vaguely defined period between childhood and adulthood. The adolescent is gaining independence from the parent, but is not yet there.

Independence is an important goal in life, and parenting is the one relationship in which separation is a successful outcome. The bird's work is done when the fledglings fly the nest. Parents play a huge role in the life of their child but (assuming the child achieves independence) a much smaller role in the life of their adult son or daughter. At some point in adolescence, we parents have to facilitate this change. This is a transition for both the parent and the adolescent, and it ideally happens gradually, over time. Indeed, increasing independence ought to begin early in childhood: we need to be preparing for this separation from the cradle.

The parent has to learn to cut the cord at the end of adolescence, but the adolescent also has to be ready for the cord to be cut. It is a two-way process. As with exercise and good eating habits, the foundations for becoming an independent adult are laid early in childhood.

Leaving the security of home is daunting for any adolescent, and they need to leave home equipped with the skills to look after themselves. The adolescent with spastic diplegia also needs to be able to manage their own health care. Health care for the person with spastic diplegia usually changes from pediatric to adult services at the end of adolescence, and this is another daunting change. Loss of services from professionals the adolescent has effectively grown up with can be a big challenge. We will see in Chapter 4 that adult services are much more fragmented than pediatric services. I encourage adolescents to fully understand their condition, how to manage it, and how to get the best from their bodies.

Being able to practice independence in a safe environment is important. For example, the adolescent can start running their medical appointments with a parent there as a safety net and support, or complete chores or cook at home with the parent there to help if something goes wrong. Practicing these skills at home, in a familiar environment, and learning from mistakes in a safe setting makes the transition to independence less difficult, less scary, and more successful. OT is a great resource in this area.

Self-determination refers to a person's ability to act as their own primary decision-maker. Independent of cognitive level, young adults with disabilities who demonstrate increased levels of self-determination were found to fare better across multiple life categories, including employment, access to health care and other benefits, financial independence, and independent living [14]. It is also useful to instill an aptitude for self-advocacy, the ability to represent oneself or one's views or interests.

Thomason and Graham (2013) made the very interesting point that the decision to proceed with SEMLS for younger children is largely made by parents, but adolescents must be given the freedom to make their own informed decisions about surgery and rehabilitation [15]. They added that an adolescent who feels they have been forced into SEMLS against their will or without their full consent is likely to be resentful and may develop depression and struggle with rehabilitation. Indeed, this advice may be applicable to other areas in the life of the adolescent.

A study of older adolescents with CP (aged 18–20) defined success in life as being happy. Three key psychosocial factors related to this success were being believed in, believing in oneself, and being accepted by others (a sense of belonging) [16]. The seeds of these factors are sown early in life, and we parents do the sowing.

Going through the normal changes of puberty, graduating from high school, choosing the next life stage, leaving home, assuming responsibility for one's own health care, and transitioning from the familiar and more organized setting of children's health services to the unfamiliar and more fragmented adult services—putting it all together, there is a lot going on in the life of an adolescent with spastic diplegia packed into a short amount of time. I have included web links to videos and information relevant to adolescents with CP at the end of this section.

In conclusion, the child becomes the adolescent, who in turn becomes the adult. How we look after the child with spastic diplegia will have repercussions long after childhood has ended. Recall the quotation at the beginning of this chapter: the child truly is the father of the man.

Useful web links

- Tindal SR (2017) "Students with Mild Cerebral Palsy in the Classroom: Information and Guidelines for Teachers." [pdf] digitalcommons.northgeorgia.edu/cgi/viewcontent.cgi?article =1198&context=papersandpubs

- CanChild (2009) *"If I Knew Then What I Know Now..." Tips for Parents of Children and Youth with Cerebral Palsy, from Parents.* [pdf] canchild.ca/system/tenon/assets/attachments/000/000/448/ original/ASQMEmajor_advicefinaltipsheetjan112010final.pdf

- CanChild (2013) *The Doctor Switch: Shane's Story.* [video] vimeo.com/69747752

- Cerebral Palsy Foundation (2016) *Letting Go (at Least a Little Bit).* [video] youtube.com/watch?v=h2yLYpT9QqM& feature=youtu.be

- CP-NET (2015) *These Six F-Words Won't Fill Up Your Swear Jar: What Do the F-Words Mean to Youth with Impairments?* [video] vimeo.com/236235559

Key points Chapter 3

- It is important to understand best practice and know what it looks like in the management and treatment of spastic diplegia. The generally accepted principles underpinning best practice to date include family-centered care and patient-centered care, evidence-based medicine, data-driven decision-making, a multidisciplinary team approach, specialist centers, early intervention, setting goals, and measuring outcome. Best practice will likely continue to evolve over time.

- Different institutions and providers may have different protocols for how they perform each treatment.

- Different treatments, when used together, can amplify the effects of any individual treatment: the whole is greater than the sum of its parts.

- The main therapies for spastic diplegia include physical therapy (PT), occupational therapy (OT), and speech and language pathology/therapy (SLP/SLT). These are usually delivered as episodes of care at appropriate frequencies during childhood and adolescence.

- The importance of the home program cannot be overemphasized. It is a constant in the life of the child and adolescent (and adult) with spastic diplegia. The home program includes the "homework" prescribed by therapists, wearing orthoses, stretching, exercise and physical activity, and postural management.

- The most appropriate orthoses for the child/adolescent are prescribed as needed.

- There are two main peaks in the management of the musculoskeletal problems of spastic diplegia. The first occurs in early childhood, when tone reduction (in conjunction with other treatments such as PT and orthoses) is very important. The second occurs in later childhood (at approximately eight to 12 years), when orthopedic surgery may be needed to address the secondary abnormalities, the muscle and bone problems that have developed.

- Tone reduction treatments to manage spasticity (and dystonia, if present) may be focal or generalized. They include oral medications, botulinum neurotoxin A (BoNT-A) injection, phenol injection, intrathecal baclofen (ITB), and selective dorsal rhizotomy (SDR).

The tone-reducing effects of each are reversible, except for SDR. No one tone-reducing treatment meets every child's needs, which is why a range of options exists. Tone reduction is tailored to the individual child's needs. Which treatment is recommended depends on many factors, including age, GMFCS level, and type of high tone.

- Although the use of tone reduction peaks in early childhood, tone reduction treatment can continue into adolescence (and adulthood).
- Orthopedic surgery becomes necessary when the muscle and bone deformities (the secondary abnormalities) are adversely affecting gait and function and can no longer be treated by more-conservative means.
- Single-event multilevel surgery (SEMLS) involves multiple orthopedic surgical procedures performed on the lower limbs during a single operation. Best practice is that it is guided by gait analysis. Surgeons aim to correct all the bone and muscle abnormalities in the same surgical event to avoid multiple hospital admissions, repeated anesthesia, and multiple rehabilitations. SEMLS is now considered best practice for orthopedic surgery in CP.
- SDR and SEMLS are normally followed by an intensive rehabilitation program after surgery to gain the maximum benefit.
- SEMLS reduces, but does not eliminate, the likelihood of further surgeries until the child is finished growing.
- Some treatments (including SDR, ITB, and SEMLS) are typically available only at specialist centers.
- No treatment (e.g., BoNT-A, SDR, SEMLS) should ever be viewed as an end point. They are aids along the way in the pursuit of the overall goal of getting to skeletal maturity (i.e., adulthood) with the fewest possible effects of the brain injury.

CHAPTER 4

The Adult with Spastic Diplegia— Bilateral CP

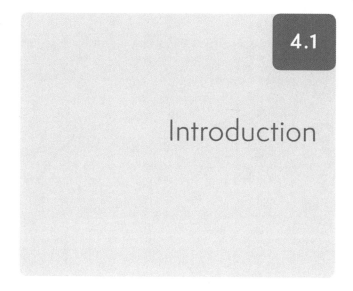

4.1

Introduction

I don't think motor neurone disease can be an advantage to anyone, but it was less of a disadvantage to me than to other people, because it did not stop me doing what I wanted.

Stephen Hawking

CP is often thought of as a children's condition, but it is not. People with CP who walk during childhood tend to have a relatively normal life expectancy [1]. If one considers a normal life span, for every child and adolescent with CP there are approximately three adults with the condition. In the Preface we saw that worldwide there are an estimated 6 million people with spastic diplegia [2,3].

The World Health Organization (WHO) defines an adult as a person older than 19 years of age [4]. But what does being an adult really mean? Being an adult was described as including the following accomplishments [5]:

Completing formal education, entering the labor force, living independently, having romantic relationships and sexual experiences, getting married and having children, establishing peer and family relationships, participating in recreation/leisure, driving a car, and enjoying group social encounters. Well-being has been defined to include these factors, and that well-being and success also includes the individual's own goals, aspirations, and values, such as leading a life in accord with one's religious values.

Everybody's path in life is different. Preparing our children to become independent adults is the ultimate goal of most parents.

Once a person with spastic diplegia reaches adulthood and skeletal growth has ceased, a certain stabilization of the condition occurs. The rate of change of the condition is slower in adulthood, assuming the adult remains physically active. People with spastic diplegia may, however, develop secondary conditions in adulthood.

The Center for Disease Control and Prevention described secondary conditions as follows [6]:

People with disabilities often are at greater risk for health problems that can be prevented. As a result of having a specific type of disability, such as a spinal cord injury [...] other physical or mental health conditions can occur. Some of these other health conditions are also called secondary conditions [...]

The specific secondary conditions that may develop depend on the primary condition. For example, eye problems are secondary conditions that may develop as a result of having diabetes; osteoarthritis, pain, and fatigue are secondary conditions that may develop as a result of having spastic diplegia. This chapter addresses the secondary conditions associated with spastic diplegia.

The development of secondary conditions is not inevitable. Good management can help prevent and/or minimize their development. Though they are addressed in this chapter on adulthood, some secondary conditions may appear earlier in life. Secondary conditions should not be confused with the secondary abnormalities addressed in Chapter 2.

In childhood and adolescence, growth is the major challenge for the person with spastic diplegia. In adulthood, typical aging becomes the main challenge. Though there are far more adults than children with CP, most of the efforts of health care providers are directed at children and adolescents. Meeting the needs of young people with CP is absolutely essential, but given that CP is a lifelong condition and further issues may arise with age, the medical establishment must better address the lack of service provision for adults with CP.

There are huge personal, societal, and economic costs associated with suboptimal health. We will see in section 4.3 that adults with spastic diplegia are underemployed. If the moral argument for improving service provision and thus quality of life for adults with spastic diplegia is not sufficiently persuasive, then perhaps the economic argument will be. The cost of care, loss of income, and tax revenue losses from CP were reported to cost the Australian and American economies $87 billion per year [7].

In addition to reduced service provision, much of the limited research in CP to date has focused on children. An analysis of National Institutes of Health (NIH)[102] funding for CP research from 2001 to 2013 found that only 4 percent went toward studies of CP in adulthood [8]. Earlier in this book we saw that although the prevalence of CP is three times higher than that of Down syndrome, the amount of funding allocated to CP research in 2018 ($26 million) was significantly lower than Down syndrome research ($60 million) [9]. Thus research on CP in adulthood receives only a small percentage of an already small budget. (Based on these numbers, I estimate it receives approximately $1 million annually —enough to fund only about three or four studies.)

Thorpe (2009) reported that federal funding agencies in the US (including the NIH, CDC, and NIDRR)[103] are very interested in funding research on aging [10]. They recognize that adults with developmental disabilities face similar—if not more devastating—age-related changes and see the need for interventions to protect function and prevent secondary conditions. This is a positive development.

More research is needed to fully understand how spastic diplegia changes in adulthood and what can be done to prevent or minimize

---

102   The National Institutes of Health (NIH) is the primary US body responsible for health research.

103   NIH = National Institutes of Health. CDC = Centers for Disease Control and Prevention. NIDRR = National Institute on Disability and Rehabilitation Research.

the problems that arise as adults with CP age. Many research studies involve "adults"—yet adults, ranging in age from 20 to 80-plus years, are not a homogenous group. It is necessary to have a better sense of how health care challenges evolve across the decades. Longitudinal research studies that follow adults with CP as they age would offer valuable information.

A workshop to define the challenges of treating and preventing secondary complications in adults with CP concluded that [11]:

> *The same sense of responsibility and compassion that motivated the research that led to such advances as increasing the survival rates of very low birth weight infants must now be applied to developing the best means of caring for children with CP as they reach adulthood [...] The medical and research communities have helped these individuals survive. It is now our responsibility to help them thrive and live productive lives, as uninhibited as possible by the chronic pain and secondary conditions associated with CP.*

This is a very worthy goal.

This chapter covers:
Section 4.2   Aging in the typical population
Section 4.3   Aging with spastic diplegia
Section 4.4   Management and treatment of spastic diplegia in adulthood

Writing earlier chapters of this book, I was familiar with the material: having raised a child with spastic diplegia, I had experienced many of the issues I was writing about. But as I wrote this chapter on spastic diplegia in adulthood, I, too, was learning. I was surprised by some of what I learned about spastic diplegia in adulthood.

This chapter is the result of extensive reading of the research and discussions with staff at Gillette Phalen Clinic, which provides lifelong specialty care to adolescents and adults who have conditions that began in childhood.

4.2

Aging in the typical population

Send me a postcard, drop me a line
Stating point of view
Indicate precisely what you mean to say
Yours sincerely, wasting away
Give me your answer, fill in a form
Mine for evermore
Will you still need me, will you still feed me
When I'm sixty-four.
The Beatles, from "When I'm Sixty-Four"

With mirth and laughter let old wrinkles come.
William Shakespeare, from *The Merchant of Venice*

The Oxford English Dictionary defines aging as "the process of growing old." But that doesn't give us much information. The fact that decline occurs with age is obvious from observing those around us and from seeing how the performance of elite athletes declines relatively early in life. Before addressing aging in adults with spastic diplegia, let us first look at aging in the typical population.

Examples of the decline that occurs with age include sarcopenia (loss of skeletal muscle mass and strength), joint pain, dementia, osteoarthritis (the breakdown of cartilage in the joints; for example the hip joint), osteoporosis (greater bone loss than normal), falls, and low-trauma fractures (easily acquired bone breaks). Many conditions become more prevalent as people age, including cardiovascular disease, cancer, respiratory disease, and diabetes. These conditions are termed noncommunicable diseases (NCDs).

Some of the above can be considered part of "normal" aging (e.g., sarcopenia and osteopenia),[104] but most are diagnosable medical conditions. Diagnosable medical conditions occur in the typical population, but they are not "normal." This section explains these conditions.

Sarcopenia

Sarcopenia is the loss of skeletal muscle mass and strength [1]. Typically developing adults achieve peak muscle mass by their early 40s and progressively deteriorate from that point on, resulting in as much as 50 percent loss by the time they are in their 80s. As we saw earlier, muscle strength is related to muscle size. Losing muscle mass has consequences for maintaining the level of function we need to carry out activities of daily living as we age, for example lifting and carrying objects or even just getting up from a chair. By performing simple muscle strengthening exercises, adults can offset the natural loss of muscle mass that commonly occurs with age.

Protein is required for muscle growth. Older people are less efficient than younger people at extracting protein from food, thus older people need to be especially vigilant about meeting their daily protein needs [2]. For adults over age 65, an average daily intake of at least 1 to 1.2 grams of protein per kilogram of body weight is recommended [3].[105]

---

104   Osteopenia refers to bone density that is not normal but is not as low as osteoporosis [4].

105   For example, a person over 65 weighing 57 kilograms (126 pounds) requires 60 grams (just over 2 ounces) of protein per day.

Osteoporosis

The term "osteoporosis" means "porous bones" (i.e., bones with low bone density). Bone is a living tissue that is constantly being removed and replaced. Low bone density arises when the rate of absorption of bone is greater than the rate of formation of new bone.

As people age, more bone is naturally lost than replaced. People with osteoporosis, however, have greater bone loss than is normal for their age. Figure 4.2.1 shows a normal bone and one with osteoporosis; the latter has much less bone material (i.e., less bone density).

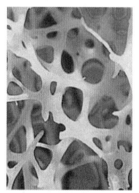 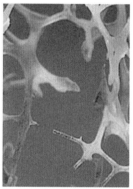

Normal bone   Osteoporotic bone

Figure 4.2.1 Cross-section of normal and osteoporotic bone. Reproduced with kind permission from the Irish Osteoporosis Society.

Bones can become so weak that a break (fracture) may occur with stress (such as a fall). A break may even occur spontaneously. Osteoporosis is a "silent" disease in that it is often only diagnosed when a bone fracture occurs. It is the most common cause of bone fractures among the elderly.

Older women have a much higher risk of osteoporotic fractures than older men [5]. In many developed countries, women above a certain age (or with known risk factors) are screened for osteoporosis. The condition can be diagnosed by a bone mineral density scan (called a DXA or DEXA scan) of the spine and hips.

Osteopenia is the term used to define bone density that is not normal but is not as low as osteoporosis [4]. It can be regarded as the midpoint between healthy bone and osteoporosis. Having osteopenia places a person at risk of developing osteoporosis. To promote optimum bone health throughout life, good nutrition, ensuring no deficiencies in calcium and vitamin D, and physical activity, especially weight-bearing or impact activities, are important [6].

Falling, osteoporosis, and bone fractures are closely linked. The risk of falling increases with age due to factors such as decreasing muscle strength and balance. Maintaining muscle strength and balance is therefore very important for preventing falls. The consequences of a fall can be grave, and they can go on to have further impact—for example, a broken leg may lead to much-reduced activity, or a broken wrist may lead to difficulties with self-care. Either may lead to reduced independence. Fear of falling can be another consequence of falling, which may lead to self-imposed restrictions on activity.

Noncommunicable diseases (NCDs)

A noncommunicable disease (NCD) is a medical condition not caused by an infectious agent.[106] NCDs, also known as chronic diseases, tend to be of long duration. The WHO reported that NCDs are the cause of over two-thirds of deaths worldwide. The following four conditions account for 80 percent of all deaths due to NCDs [7]:
- Cardiovascular disease (e.g., heart attack and stroke)
- Cancer
- Respiratory disease (e.g., chronic obstructive pulmonary disease [COPD] and asthma)
- Diabetes

In section 1.2 we examined the difference between causes and risk factors. (As a reminder, a risk factor is "any attribute, characteristic, or exposure of an individual that increases the likelihood of developing a disease or injury" [8]). NCDs share four behavioral risk factors [9]:
- Tobacco use
- Unhealthy diet
- Physical inactivity
- Excess alcohol consumption

---

106 A communicable disease is caused by an infectious agent such as a bacterium or virus.

We have control over each of these risk factors—they are lifestyle choices. Very often multiple combinations may be present, such as an unhealthy diet combined with physical inactivity.

Cardiometabolic risk factors ("cardio" refers to heart disease and "metabolic" refers to biochemical disorders such as diabetes) include:
- Unhealthy levels of blood cholesterol (a type of fat in the blood)
- High levels of triglycerides (another type of fat in the blood)
- High blood pressure (also termed hypertension)
- Insulin resistance or diabetes
- Being overweight or obese[107]
- Metabolic syndrome (a person is diagnosed with metabolic syndrome if they have at least three of the five risk factors above)
- High levels of C-reactive protein (CRP, a protein in the blood; high levels are a sign of inflammation in the body)

The WHO reported the five leading global risk factors for mortality and the percentage of deaths globally due to each (indicated in parentheses) [10]. They are:
- High blood pressure (13 percent)
- Tobacco use (9 percent)
- High blood glucose (6 percent)
- Physical inactivity (6 percent)
- Being overweight or obese (5 percent)

Note that these five mortality risk factors are included in the two lists of risk factors above.

In addition to good lifestyle choices, regular health checks with a primary care provider are important for managing our health as we age. A primary care provider will check many of the above risk factors. Most developed countries also have screening programs for many cancers, such as breast and colon cancer. Appropriate health checks and screening can lead to early identification and treatment of conditions.

---

107 Measured by BMI and/or central obesity. Body mass index (BMI) is calculated by dividing a person's body mass by the square of their body height. A large waistline ($\geq$ 40 inches for men and $\geq$ 35 inches for women) is a measure of central obesity. This body type is also known as "apple-shaped," as opposed to "pear-shaped," in which fat is deposited on the hips and buttocks. Apple-shaped people are known to be more at risk for cardiometabolic disease than pear-shaped people. A web link to a CDC resource on weight is included at the end of this section.

The book *Younger Next Year,* written by a specialist in internal medicine and preventive health care and his patient, emphasizes the importance of good nutrition, aerobic exercise, strength training, and good social connectedness for healthy aging [11].

Finally, not everything goes downhill as we age. Wisdom, sense of self, and comfort in one's own skin generally increase as we get older. Happiness appears to follow a U-shaped trajectory (also known as a "happiness curve"), declining from the optimism of youth to a slump in middle age, then rising again around age 50 [12].

Generally, we all hope to live a long life, but we also want the quality of those later years to be good. In other words, we want quantity *and* quality. Whether we like it or not, we all age—but how we age differs. Good lifestyle choices play an important role in preventing many of the health conditions of typical aging described above. Aging is inevitable, but how we age is not—we can choose how we age.

Useful web link

- Centers for Disease Control and Prevention (CDC) (2015) *Assessing Your Weight.* [online] cdc.gov/healthyweight/assessing/index.html

4.3

Aging with spastic diplegia

You are never too old to set another goal or to dream a new dream.

C.S. Lewis

When discussing adults with spastic diplegia, it is important to recognize they are not a homogenous group. For one thing, they range in age from 20 to 80-plus years. For another, they vary in how their condition was managed during childhood and adolescence. They also vary in personality, level of drive, determination, perseverance, and interest in self-care. This is no different from typical adults or those with other primary conditions such as diabetes.

Adults with spastic diplegia have had their condition since childhood, but they are also susceptible to the same challenges of aging as their able-bodied peers. For the person with spastic diplegia, it is almost as if, on entering adulthood, two roads converge: the challenges of growing up with the condition meet the challenges of typical aging. The adult with spastic diplegia must manage these two sets of challenges in combination. It is important to note that the problems of aging are likely to occur at a younger age and with more severity in adults with CP than in those without the condition [1]. But we will see in this chapter that this does not have to be the case; much can be done to prevent or minimize many of the secondary conditions that arise as a result of having CP.

As in almost all areas of medicine, the management and treatment of spastic diplegia in childhood and adolescence has improved in recent decades. This influences how today's children and adolescents will fare as tomorrow's adults. For example, single-event multilevel surgery (SEMLS) has replaced the original approach of annual surgery and rehabilitation—also known as "birthday syndrome"—commonly practiced in the 1980s and earlier. Use of gait analysis also commenced in the early '80s. Good hip surveillance programs are a recent addition to the management of the condition. The general public's awareness of many health issues has also improved. For example, people today are much more aware of the downsides of smoking and the important contribution of physical exercise to overall health.

As in childhood and adolescence, spastic diplegia in adulthood affects not only the individual with the condition but also their family and those in their immediate circle.

I reviewed the research relevant to adults with spastic diplegia, GMFCS levels I–III. The lack of research on aging with CP requires that we include earlier studies from a time when health care and our knowledge of health were not what they are today. While the findings of earlier studies are still relevant, they may in some cases be less informative for people now entering adulthood.

On a philosophical note, don't be discouraged when you read statements like, "Nearly one-third of adults with CP had chronic pain." Remember, this means more than two-thirds of adults with CP did *not* have chronic pain. That's just as significant. The research tends to focus on the negatives, so it's up to the reader to recognize the unstated positive findings.

If we were to look at the body mass index (BMI) of a group of adults, we would see a normal distribution: a few people might be classed as underweight, some would be normal weight, some overweight, and some obese. The fact that many people are not at the ideal weight does not mean *you* cannot be. Similarly, as you read about the results of studies in this chapter, please use them to inform but not limit you.

This section addresses the following challenges of aging with spastic diplegia:
- **Musculoskeletal decline**
- **Mobility**
- **Falls**
- **Fractures**
- **Pain**
- **Noncommunicable diseases (NCDs) and risk factors**
- **Fatigue, depression, and anxiety**
- **Quality of life and health-related quality of life**
- **Participation**
- **Areas of unmet need**

Though these challenges will be addressed separately, they are very much interdependent.

Musculoskeletal decline

Chapter 2 addressed the primary, secondary, and tertiary abnormalities of spastic diplegia. Chapter 3 addressed the optimal management of the condition in childhood and adolescence. The aim is to arrive at adulthood (when bone growth ceases) with the best possible musculoskeletal alignment. If correction of the muscle and bone deformities is not addressed (or not fully addressed) during childhood and adolescence, they may persist into adulthood [2]. These muscle and bone deformities may cause further decline in mobility as well as pain, fatigue, and other problems in adulthood. As people age, further coping responses (tertiary abnormalities) may develop to compensate for decreased muscle strength and deterioration in balance. However, as we will see in the next section, orthopedic surgery to address muscle and bone problems is still possible in adulthood.

The conditions that occur in typically aging adults can have even greater implications for adults with spastic diplegia. For example:
- **Sarcopenia** (loss of skeletal muscle mass and strength): For individuals with spastic diplegia, muscle mass and strength have been challenges

since childhood. In adulthood, these individuals acquire the added challenge of loss of muscle mass and strength due to aging. Hip and knee extension strength was found to be considerably lower (less than 75 percent of normal) among adolescents and young adults with spastic CP [3]. Plantar flexor strength was found to be approximately 50 percent less in young adults with spastic CP (average age 25) than in typically developing young adults, and approximately 35 percent less than in typically developing adults above age 70 [4].

- **Osteoarthritis** (breakdown of cartilage in the joints): The age-adjusted prevalence of arthritis was found to be significantly greater among adults with CP than among those without CP: 31 percent versus 17 percent [5].
- **Osteoporosis** (greater bone loss than normal): Adults with CP had a higher incidence of osteoporosis (and osteoarthritis) compared with adults without CP [6].

Mobility

Retaining the ability to walk (independently or using mobility aids) for at least household distances is important for independence. A 2014 review found that approximately 25 percent of adults with CP experienced a decline in walking over time [7]. Those with worse initial gait ability, bilateral (rather than unilateral) motor impairment, older age, and higher levels of pain or fatigue were at higher risk of gait decline. The decline occurred earlier in adults with CP than in typically aging peers. The studies included in this review were conducted between 1995 and 2010 and involved adults up to their eighth decade.

Self-reported factors perceived as causes of decline in walking in adulthood included balance problems, pain, increased spasticity, decline in muscle strength, contractures or joint deformity, stiffness, fatigue, knee problems, fractures due to falls, fear of falling or falls, and reduced fitness and endurance [7]. The reasons for decline in walking in adulthood may differ from those in adolescence. (We examined reasons for decline in walking in adolescence in section 2.9, including the unfavorable strength-to-mass ratio that develops as the child grows.)

People who engage in regular physical activity were found to be at lower risk of experiencing decline in mobility. Deterioration in gait was strongly associated with inactivity [7]. In other words, mobility and physical activity are intricately linked. Thorpe (2009) reported that a disabling condition such as CP frequently causes a "cycle of deconditioning" (loss of fitness) in which physical function deteriorates, followed by a further decrease in physical activity and a cascade of increasing functional decline [8]. All of the above emphasizes how critical it is to remain physically active throughout adulthood.

Elsewhere it has been noted that individuals at GMFCS levels I and II are at lower risk of gait deterioration and generally continue to walk in their 60s [9]. Loss of walking skills in the adult with CP appears to occur at two peaks [9]. The first, at around age 20 to 25, is commonly associated with progressive crouch gait and an inability to keep up with one's peers in the community, workplace, and academic settings. The second peak, around age 40 to 45, is commonly associated with progressive fatigue, pain, and possibly accelerated joint degeneration, which prevents further functional walking.

Preserving mobility in adulthood might require the use of mobility aids the person may not have needed before.

Falls

Earlier we saw that balance, particularly posterior balance, is affected in spastic diplegia. Although adults with CP may have become somewhat used to falling (and are more aware of situations where they are at risk of falling and how to protect themselves when falling), it tends to be more socially uncomfortable when a fall occurs. In addition, for various reasons of physics, an adult is more likely to be injured from a fall than a child. A study found that 56 percent of adults with spastic bilateral CP had fallen at least once in the past month and 81 percent had fallen more than five times in the past year [10].

Falls occur naturally with aging, but they usually occur later in life in adults who do not have a disability and who have better health and fitness. The incidence of falls is higher for people with CP at younger ages and may be more common if they do not use assistive devices.

Ironically, as I wrote this section, Tommy had just had a bad fall. He fell backward and hit his head against a glass coffee table, which broke on impact. The resulting cut required stapling at the local emergency room. Falling continues to be a challenge for Tommy. Thankfully, he is aware of the risks and takes precautions—he is particularly careful around stairs or traffic.

Fractures

A recent study found that adults with CP had a higher prevalence of fractures compared with adults without CP: 6 percent versus 3 percent [11].

Pain

Studies report higher levels of pain among adults with CP compared with the general population: 28 percent versus 15 percent [12]; 75 percent versus 39 percent [13]; and 44 percent versus 28 percent [5]. (Pain was variously defined as daily pain for one year or more [12] or pain lasting more than three months [13]).

Pain is a major determinant of quality of life and affects physical and mental functioning. It leads to reduced productivity and concentration [14]. Pain may be acute or chronic, and it may have many causes. It may lead to problems with sleep, which causes fatigue, which can further exacerbate pain.

Noncommunicable diseases (NCDs) and risk factors

There is ample and very recent evidence to suggest that the burden of noncommunicable diseases (NCDs) and risk factors is higher among adults with CP compared with the general population [5,15–22].

Using data from 2002–2010, Peterson and colleagues (2015) reported the age-adjusted prevalence of chronic conditions in adults in the US with and without CP [5]. See Table 4.3.1. The prevalence of eight chronic conditions was higher among adults with CP. One can understand why adults with CP might have a higher burden of joint pain and arthritis, but the remaining conditions do not have a direct link to the condition. However, as we will see, lower levels of activity due to CP leads to lower fitness. Since people who are less active and less fit have a higher incidence of diabetes, hypertension, and cardiovascular disease, it makes sense that CP puts people at increased risk of these conditions. Interestingly, in this study 49 percent of adults with CP self-reported their level of physical disability as "none" or "minor."

Table 4.3.1 Age-adjusted prevalence of chronic conditions in adults with and without CP

CHRONIC CONDITION	WITH CP	WITHOUT CP
Diabetes	9%	6%
Asthma	21%	9%
Hypertension (high blood pressure)	30%	22%
Other heart conditions	15%	9%
Stroke	5%	2%
Emphysema (a condition in which the air sacs of the lungs are damaged and enlarged, causing breathlessness. It is also known as pulmonary emphysema.)	4%	1%
Joint pain	44%	28%
Arthritis	31%	17%

Data from Peterson and colleagues (2015) [5].

A recent UK study found that adults with CP have an increased risk of death due to diseases of the circulatory and respiratory systems [21]. Another study found that adults with more severe CP (GMFCS levels II and III) showed increased cardiovascular disease risk factors (specifically waist circumference, waist-to-hip ratio, insulin levels, and blood pressure) compared with individuals with less severe CP (GMFCS level I) [20]. The authors deduced that a person's level of mobility may play an important role in reducing these risk factors, once again underscoring the importance of physical activity.

Fatigue, depression, and anxiety

a) Fatigue

Fatigue is described as "extreme tiredness resulting from mental or physical exertion or illness." It may involve feeling exhausted, tired, weak, or lacking energy [23]. A study found that adults with CP had significantly more physical fatigue, but not more mental fatigue, than the general population [23]. Additionally, adults with a moderate grade of CP had a higher prevalence of fatigue than adults with mild or severe CP, suggesting that those with moderate CP may try to minimize their disability to keep up with their peers [23]. Crouch gait was associated with high fatigue in adults with spastic diplegia [24]. One study emphasized the importance of physical activity and good weight management to both prevent and treat fatigue in adults with CP [25]. This was consistent with the findings of earlier fatigue studies [23,26,27].

b) Depression

Depression is a common but serious mood disorder. It causes severe symptoms that affect how a person feels and thinks, and influences daily activities such as sleeping, eating, and working [28]. Signs and symptoms of depression include a persistent sad, anxious, or "empty" mood; feelings of hopelessness or pessimism; irritability; and feelings of guilt, worthlessness, or helplessness. To be diagnosed with depression, the symptoms must be present for at least two weeks. Adults with spastic bilateral CP in the Netherlands were found to have a higher prevalence of depressive symptoms than the general population (25 percent versus 12 percent) [13]. However, a US study found no such difference between adults with CP and the general population (where the rate of depression in both groups was 20 percent) [29].

c) Anxiety

Occasional anxiety is a part of life. One might feel anxious when faced with a problem at work, before taking a test, or before making an important decision. But anxiety disorders involve more than temporary worry or fear. For a person with an anxiety disorder, the anxiety does not go away and can get worse over time. The symptoms can interfere with daily activities, such as job performance and schoolwork, and with relationships [30]. Adults with CP were found to have a higher risk of developing anxiety and depression than adults without CP [31].

Quality of life and health-related quality of life

Quality of life and health-related quality of life are two different concepts.

a) Quality of life (QoL)

Quality of life (QoL) is defined as "the individual's perception of their position in life in the context of the culture and value system in which they live, and in relation to their goals, expectations, standards, and concerns" [32]. Very little research has been conducted on QoL in adults with CP [33], and the research that does exist does not paint a clear picture. Reduced QoL has been reported among adults with bilateral CP compared with the general population [24]. Long-term studies of adolescents and young adults with CP found similar QoL regardless of whether they had undergone specific surgeries earlier in life [34,35].

b) Health-related quality of life (HRQoL)

Health-related quality of life (HRQoL) is defined as "the way in which a condition (almost always a chronic condition) affects a person's well-being" [33]. A person may have reduced HRQoL because of the impact a condition has on their physical and/or mental functioning, but they may still have a high QoL because they are perfectly happy with their life. In other words, there are factors beyond health that make up a person's perception of their QoL. A study showed low perceived HRQoL for physical functioning but not mental functioning among individuals with CP [36]. Higher general self-efficacy (a greater willingness to expend effort to achieve behavior) was related to higher physical and mental HRQoL.

Participation

Participation refers to involvement in a life situation. It is one of the three levels of human functioning identified in the ICF (addressed in section 1.4). Participation restrictions are problems an individual may experience in their involvement in life situations. Employment, civil status, and having children are indicators of participation in society.

a) Employment

Employment is important for many reasons, including financial independence, social interaction, self-esteem, and sense of self, but it may also have implications for future health care and retirement costs. A study found that 68 percent[108] of Dutch adults with bilateral spastic CP were in paid employment compared with 77 percent of the general population [36]. Similar employment figures were reported in another Dutch study [37]. In a Norwegian study, 45 percent of adults with spastic CP identified paid work[109] as their source of income [38]. However, the study did not offer a comparison figure for the general population. A Canadian study reported that 26 percent of adults with CP[110] were in employment [39], describing the financial situation of the majority of the group as "precarious." A review of Healthy People 2010, a US health initiative, reported that the employment rate among adults with disabilities aged 18–64 declined 14 percent between 1997 and 2008 from 43 percent to 37 percent (moving further away from the 2010 target of 80 percent employment) [40]. Barriers to employment as well as accommodations that facilitate employment for people with spastic diplegia need to be addressed in research and public policy.

b) Civil status

Civil status describes a person's family situation: it includes being single, living with a partner, being married, in a civil union, divorced, and widowed. A study found that 27 percent of Dutch adults with bilateral spastic CP were married or living with a partner compared with 70 percent of the general population [36]. In a Norwegian study, that figure was 43 percent for adults with spastic CP (without any general population comparison) [38]. A Canadian study reported that 83 percent of adults with CP were single and 52 percent lived with parents [39]. However, a large US study found no significant differences in marital status between adults with and without CP [5].

---

108 Fifty-four percent in competitive employment and 14 percent in sheltered employment; 93 percent GMFCS levels I–III.

109 Defined as more than 20 percent of income; 85 percent GMFCS levels I–III.

110 Work not defined; 64 percent GMFCS levels I–III.

c) Having children

A study found that 11 percent of adults with bilateral spastic CP had children compared with approximately 50 percent of the general population [36]. Another study found that young adults with CP had less experience in romantic and sexual relationships than their age-matched peers [41]. It noted that being involved in peer group activities and creating a context for arranging dates could help young adults with CP develop romantic relationships and become sexually active. Further research found that young adults with CP may experience various problems or challenges with sexuality [42].

The above are indicators of participation in society, and in general, adults with CP had lower rates. Higher general self-efficacy was found to be related to better participation [36]. Participation in society is very important and more research is needed in this area, particularly in the area of participation restrictions.

Areas of unmet need

The greatest area of unmet need reported by young adults with CP was information (79 percent), followed by mobility (66 percent) and health care (66 percent) [43]. Lack of information included information on complications, consequences, and causes of CP. The study authors suggested that while parents may receive information, they might not be communicating it adequately to their children, leaving them with unanswered questions. Furthermore, a person's questions about CP might change over time as their needs change during adolescence and adulthood. Other studies have reported a similar lack of information during the transition to adulthood [44], underscoring the need for a book like this one, as well as more research on adults with CP.

There is strong evidence that adults with spastic diplegia encounter more and earlier health problems than their typically aging peers. Aging with spastic diplegia affects a broad range of areas: musculoskeletal decline, mobility, falls, fractures, pain, NCDs and risk factors, fatigue, depression, anxiety, QoL, HRQoL, and participation. These areas span all ICF levels. But much can still be done to prevent, minimize, or deal with these challenges, as we will see in the next section. However, we will also see that because of limited specialist health services for adults with CP, they must take great personal responsibility for their own health and well-being.

Finally, while the most recent definition of CP is very useful, I'm not sure it sufficiently alerts us to the secondary conditions that may arise in adulthood. As O'Brien, Bass, and Rosenbloom (2009) explained, the definition was developed to be used in childhood—it was not intended to imply that progressive problems might not appear in adult life [45].

4.4

Management and treatment of spastic diplegia in adulthood

The way we are living, timorous or bold, will have been our life.
Seamus Heaney, from "Elegy"

Keep interested in your own career, however humble;
it is a real possession in the changing fortunes of time.
Max Ehrmann, from "Desiderata"

This chapter addresses the management and treatment of spastic diplegia in adulthood. Specifically, we look at:
- **Health services for adults with CP**
- **Treatments**
- **The home program**
- **How the adult with spastic diplegia can help themselves**

Health services for adults with CP

The general consensus in the literature is that services for adults with CP are extremely limited. Multidisciplinary care teams in place for children and adolescents with CP largely do not exist for adults at a time when their needs are becoming ever more complex. This disparity has been observed in many different countries, including Norway, the

Netherlands, the US, Ireland, Germany, and Canada [1–6]. Scandinavian countries are known for their well-developed social health systems, yet they too experience this fall-off in services. It is very unfortunate that care for people with CP becomes fragmented just as they enter adulthood.

In their 2009 report following a workshop to define the challenges of treating and preventing secondary complications in adults with CP, Tosi and colleagues noted that pediatric facilities are starting to extend their mandate to include adults. They cited Gillette's model of lifetime care.[111] Gillette provides lifelong specialty care to adolescents and adults who have conditions that began in childhood. This specialization means that even though it is a lifetime care provider, it does not treat lifelong conditions that develop after early childhood [7].[112]

For the adult with CP, three different components of health need monitoring [8]:

- Acute health problems (e.g., infections)
- Lifestyle health risks
- Secondary conditions related to CP

The first two components also apply to typically aging adults, while the third relates specifically to adults with CP. The AACPDM[113] has published two useful fact sheets in relation to primary care providers. One, intended for people with the condition, is titled *Why Do Adults with Cerebral Palsy Need a Primary Care Provider?* A separate one is for primary care providers themselves. Web links to both are included at the end of this section. Cassidy and colleagues (2016) suggested that physical medicine and rehabilitation (PMR, also termed physiatry)[114] is the most appropriate specialty to provide disability-related care to adults with CP [6].

---

111 Gillette Phalen Clinic is a lifelong outpatient clinic for those aged 16 and older. It includes access to an inpatient unit for adults aged 18–40. Specialists may provide care to adults whom they previously treated as children. (The Gillette Phalen Clinic was formerly known as Gillette Lifetime Specialty Healthcare.)

112 This relates to the point of damage to an immature versus a mature brain.

113 The American Academy for Cerebral Palsy and Developmental Medicine.

114 Physical medicine and rehabilitation (PMR, also termed physiatry) is the branch of medicine that aims to enhance and restore functional ability and quality of life among those with physical disabilities. PMR physicians treat a wide variety of medical conditions affecting the brain, spinal cord, nerves, bones, joints, ligaments, muscles, and tendons.

It has been reported in the literature that health care providers often blame CP for just about all of the symptoms and problems that develop in the adult with CP [9,10]. Rosenbaum (2019) noted [10]: "We hear too many stories from adults with cerebral palsy whose abdominal pain, for example, was assumed to be 'part of (your) cerebral palsy,' when in fact they had treatable Crohn's or gall bladder disease." The AACPDM also has a useful publication on identifying the root cause of pain; a web link is included at the end of this section. It is important to ensure that the cause of a health problem is not wrongly attributed to CP when there may be another cause.

All adults—able-bodied and those with disabilities—should attend regular screenings (for example for cancers, bone health, and sexually transmitted infections) and have an annual medical checkup with their primary care provider. Research has found that many adults with CP do not receive adequate health checks and screening [7,11,12]. Referring to individuals with CP, Murphy (2018) succinctly summarized the situation: "It should be a humbling revelation to all caregivers that this population of adults is almost certainly under-studied, under-screened, and under-diagnosed [9]."

Because of their higher risk of osteoporosis, people with spastic diplegia need to be attentive to bone health. It is recommended that adults with CP have at least an annual bone health assessment (including medical history, lifestyle review, nutrition, and, as needed, evaluation for any concerning changes in bone health, such as new fractures or medications that affect bone health) with appropriate blood testing and imaging. DXA scans may be used for surveillance every three to five years [13].

Finally, it is heartening to read this optimistic conclusion from Murphy (2018) [9]: "Much improvement in specialty health care for adults with CP has occurred over the past three decades. Surely the best is yet to come."

Treatments

The goals of treatment or intervention for adults with CP are inclusion and participation in major life areas [3]. Objectives include minimizing impairments in body functions and structure, preventing secondary conditions, and optimizing activities and participation.

We reviewed the different treatments for spastic diplegia in Chapter 3, so they are not repeated here. Here we focus on what these treatments look like in adulthood. When planning any treatment, it is important to set realistic functional goals. Note that the goal for a particular treatment may be different in adulthood than it was in childhood.

a) Physical therapy and occupational therapy

Physical therapy (PT) and occupational therapy (OT) remain very relevant in adulthood and are usually delivered as an episode of care (EOC).[115] Rosenbaum, Rosenbloom, and Mayston (2012) summed up the focus of therapy for adults with CP as follows [14]: "Maintaining useful and fulfilling employment; relationships; childbearing. May require specific focused physical surveillance and intervention for pain, joint wear and tear, and general mobility in addition to fitness/ recreational activities."

Therapists at Gillette Phalen Clinic provided the following examples of EOCs for adults with CP. In these examples the therapist is acting as an educator in prevention and giving guidance rather than providing intervention.

- Instruction in balance, gait, strength-training exercises, and the home program.
- Fall assessment. Therapists can assess the reasons for falls and offer instruction in balance and strengthening exercises for fall prevention. They can also offer guidance on appropriate walking aids or orthoses and footwear to prevent falls.
- Pain education and instruction in ways to decrease pain. Certain therapists have advanced training in pain management. Many research studies show pain education can greatly decrease chronic pain [15,16].
- Advice on gentle postural exercises and possible affordable adaptations (for example, changing the angle of a keyboard or the height of chair or desk for optimal posture).
- Driving assessment. Driving specialists can assess driving ability, including behind-the-wheel and car adaptations if needed to allow independent driving.

---

115 A period of therapy (at the appropriate frequency) followed by a therapy break.

- Instruction in preservation and strengthening exercises to help prevent overuse injuries, for example when using a manual wheelchair. (Power-assist wheelchairs can also help prevent overuse injuries.)
- Mobility assessment. Therapists can offer assessment and training on ways to continue to be as independent as possible throughout the day in the home, at work, and in the community.
- Equipment provision. There are many different types of equipment; for example, a walker or other gait aid to maintain safe walking and prevent falls, a manual or power-assist wheelchair for long distances, or bathroom equipment for safe showering.
- Recommending home and environmental adaptations (such as adding handrails, removing throw rugs, or improving lighting).

A PMR physician at Gillette Phalen Clinic offered the following pointers on mobility:

- Assistive mobility devices are "tools," and people might benefit from having a variety of options available. For example, a walker or wheelchair may be used occasionally for longer distances, in certain environments, or when feeling fatigued. A person may choose to use a mobility aid in a way that suits their needs; the decision to use one does not have to be "all or nothing." Part-time use may help with participation.
- A crutch is not a "crutch"—mobility aids are tools that can help the person participate more in everyday life.
- Deciding to use a mobility aid can be a positive rather than a negative step, allowing for greater participation and less pain and fatigue. A wheelchair or motorized scooter can help a person with CP conserve energy, which they can then use to engage with peers and/or become more involved at school or at work. O'Brien and colleagues (2009) noted that [17]:

> The decision to become a regular wheelchair user is often a positive, not a negative step. People typically report not only reductions in pain and fatigue, but also associated improvements in initiative and self-esteem as a result of their decision to use a wheelchair, rather than to struggle on painfully and awkwardly, trying to walk.

- A mobility aid can help prevent falls, unusual or excessive sway through the trunk, or overreliance on one extremity at the expense of the other. It may help lessen age-related musculoskeletal changes and pain over time.

- Adults with CP sometimes lie awake at night imagining where they will have to walk the next day. It is a shame they have to waste so much mental as well as physical energy on walking.
- The design of mobility aids has improved over time. Wheelchair design and function, for example, has greatly improved in recent years: modern wheelchairs are smaller, faster, and better designed. There are also sports wheelchairs.
- Mobility aids can include the use of balance dogs. Balance dogs (or service dogs) are dogs trained to wear a particular harness or handle. The person can use the dog and harness as a gait aid or for other tasks as needed. These dogs also know how to brace their backs so that if the person falls or is on the floor they can push off the dog to stand up. A web link to a video about a student and her balance dog is included at the end of this section. There's a lot of work involved in caring for a dog, but they can also serve as emotional support animals and are often perceived as more socially acceptable than a gait aid. Dogs are also great icebreakers for getting to know other people.

b) Tone reduction

Tone reduction may include oral medications, botulinum neurotoxin A (BoNT-A) injection, phenol injection, intrathecal baclofen (ITB), and selective dorsal rhizotomy (SDR). A randomized controlled trial found that while BoNT-A injections in adults did not improve gait or HRQoL, they did help muscle stiffness and spasticity in the short term [18].

SDR has been carried out more frequently in children than in adolescents or adults. A study of 21 adults with spastic diplegia who underwent SDR concluded that SDR can be an effective treatment for adults with spastic diplegia who are unresponsive to medical therapy and should be considered as an option in carefully selected patients. Though the study represented the largest series of adult patients with spastic diplegia treated with SDR to date, the authors noted that the data needed to be validated in a larger study [19]. Rehabilitation after SDR progresses more slowly in adulthood than in childhood; this is discussed in more detail below under "orthopedic surgery."

c) Orthopedic surgery

Orthopedic surgery may be carried out in adults to address individual or multiple musculoskeletal problems. Multilevel surgery may be performed in adults. While bilateral (two-sided) surgery is generally carried out in a single operation in children, in adolescents and adults it may be performed sequentially, one side at a time [20]. This approach facilitates rehabilitation. It allows the person to bear weight on one side, allowing them to be more functional after surgery. Orthopedic surgery to address degenerative joint disease with possible joint replacement can be performed as an isolated procedure or as part of multilevel surgery.

Rehabilitation after surgery (of any type) is more prolonged in adults than in children because adults heal more slowly and their lives are generally busier than children's. Children are already dependent on their parents: after SEMLS, they return home to an environment where their needs are already being met by others. This isn't the case for the adult. Since rehabilitation takes considerable time, once the initial rehabilitation is over the adult may be trying to juggle further rehabilitation with work, caring for family, and other responsibilities.

The most difficult challenges for independent adults following multilevel surgery include loss of independence, loss of ability to care for others (such as children or a spouse), and loss of income. Can the adult even "go home"? If going home is not an option (because, for example, there is no one to care for them), where do they go? They can't go to a rehab facility right away because they are non-weight bearing. A nursing home is often the answer, but this is far from ideal because the adult generally has little in common with typical nursing home residents. Transitional care units (TCUs) are an option: they are typically set up for people whose medical needs are too intense for home but not intense enough for an acute hospital setting.

Thomason and Graham (2013) reported that rehabilitation after multilevel surgery can be an "order of magnitude"[116] more difficult for adolescents and adults than it is for younger children, and that adolescents and adults are more prone to anxiety, depression, and functional regression [20].

---

116 Strictly speaking, an "order of magnitude" more difficult means 10 times more difficult.

In addition to the age-dependent difference in rehabilitation time, rehabilitation for the same procedure (e.g., knee replacement surgery) can take longer for adults with CP than for their able-bodied peers. This is important to note because adults with CP may expect a rehabilitation period similar to that of their able-bodied peers.

Multilevel surgery was found to be an effective and safe procedure to improve gait in adults with bilateral spastic CP and in those who had undergone previous SEMLS in childhood [5]. (The study analyzed short-term outcomes at two years.) Total hip replacement was found to be safe and effective in selected individuals with CP with severe degenerative arthritis [21]. Long-term follow-up studies have shown pain relief of more than 90 percent and improved function with time even in adults as young as 30. Wear and tear to the replacement hip joint was found to be minimal [21].

Because research funding is limited, very few outcome studies on adults with CP exist. Medical professionals treating adults with CP must rely on their clinical skill and experience rather than the results of research studies.

The home program

This section needs to be read in conjunction with section 3.4. The details of the home program for the adolescent with CP included in that section apply equally to the adult with CP.

The five major elements of the home program for the adult with CP are the same as those for the child and adolescent, with some minor modifications:

- **The "homework" prescribed by therapists** (relevant when attending therapy)
- **Wearing orthoses** (relevant when prescribed)
- **Stretching** (relevant throughout adulthood)
- **Exercise and physical activity** (relevant throughout adulthood)
- **Postural management** (relevant throughout adulthood)

The first two elements of the home program (the "homework" prescribed by therapists and wearing orthoses) are applicable at particular times. The next three elements (stretching, exercise and physical activity, and postural management) are constants in the life of the adult with spastic diplegia. Reading section 3.4 will refresh your memory on the details of the home program.

The following are some points specific to adults.

During childhood and adolescence, prolonged stretching is needed to achieve the daily hours of stretch required to keep muscle growth at pace with bone growth until bone growth ceases at around age 20. In adulthood, stretching is recommended for the same reasons as for able-bodied adults: to keep muscles flexible, maintain joint range of motion (ROM), and avoid injury. Going about their normal daily lives, even able-bodied people do not fully stretch out their muscles. A study of adults with CP found that decreased hip flexion ROM may contribute to an increased risk for low back pain [22]. Stretching exercises two to three times per week are recommended for both able-bodied people and those with CP.

The WHO notes that participating in regular physical activity reduces the risk of many health conditions, including coronary heart disease and stroke, diabetes, hypertension, colon cancer, breast cancer, and depression. Additionally, physical activity is a key determinant of energy expenditure and thus is fundamental to energy balance and weight control [23]. Consistently strong evidence demonstrates that people with CP participate in less physical activity and spend more time engaged in sedentary behavior than their able-bodied peers throughout the life span [12]. Studies have shown that:

- Adults with CP who reported preserved mobility throughout adulthood attributed it to regular physical activity, participation, and maintenance of strength, balance, and overall fitness [24].
- Adults with CP who engaged in regular physical activity were at lower risk of decline in mobility. Deterioration in gait was strongly associated with inactivity [25].

Details of the exercise and physical activity requirements for people with CP, as recommended by Verschuren and colleagues (2016) [26], are included in Table 3.4.1 and are summarized below. The first four are the same as in childhood and adolescence; the fifth, neuromuscular exercise, is an addition to the list for adults:

- Cardiorespiratory (aerobic) exercise.
- Resistance (muscle strengthening) exercise.
- Daily moderate to vigorous physical activity.
- Avoiding sedentary behavior (i.e., not being physically inactive).
- Neuromotor exercise (training balance, agility, and coordination): neuromotor exercise is important for all adults, not just those with CP [23,27]. It is particularly important for avoiding falls, which we know can be a problem for adults with CP. A therapist can recommend suitable neuromotor exercises.

In summary, the elements of the home program for the adult with spastic diplegia are the same as in childhood and adolescence, with two exceptions:
- The reason why muscle stretching is important is different in adulthood.
- Neuromotor exercise is an additional requirement in adulthood.

Finally, it is worth remembering that Paralympians are proof that spastic diplegia does not have to be a barrier to achieving great levels of fitness and skill.

How the adult with spastic diplegia can help themselves

I have thought a lot about this. Having read the literature on aging with spastic diplegia, I gave the following advice to Tommy (who now lives independently) to help him maximize his health and function as he ages:
- Try to understand spastic diplegia as much as possible, as well as the possible changes that may occur with aging. In a sense, forewarned is forearmed.
- Because services for adults with CP are, unfortunately, extremely limited, I encourage you to build your own team. Do not wait around for services for adults with CP to improve. As we saw in Chapter 3, it is important to recognize that you, the person with the condition, are the most vital member of your team. You are responsible for putting your own care team in place. Find and connect with a center that provides services to adults with CP. There may not be one in your area, but take the time to research the best options available. An adult physical medicine and rehabilitation

(PMR) specialist will be able to help you prevent problems and deal with those that may arise. Try to find a good local primary care provider who understands CP for routine general health checks. Find a PT and/or OT (again, preferably one who has experience working with people with CP) who will be able to support you if and when you need it.

- Completing and maintaining an exercise and physical activity program is a crucial aspect of self-care. It is something each person has to do for themselves. The benefits of exercise and physical activity accrue at so many levels, from preserving function to cardiometabolic health to preventing secondary conditions. Think of exercise and physical activity as a powerful medication that is available for free. (How many more people would "take" it if they thought of it this way?) The concept of "exercise is medicine" has been recognized since ancient times.

- Getting adequate rest is important. Walking is more demanding for an adult with spastic diplegia than for an able-bodied adult. Additionally, the amount of exercise and physical activity required demands a lot of energy. It's important to achieve the right balance between activity and rest.

- A healthy diet is important for all adults, able-bodied and those with a disability. This includes adequate hydration. Get dietary advice from a specialist if you need it. Excess weight is not good for anyone, but it is especially taxing for a person with spastic diplegia. Weight management is important not only for reducing the risk of NCDs but also for better musculoskeletal health and to help maintain walking. Because of their smaller and weaker muscles, people with spastic diplegia cannot afford to be carrying excess weight. Keeping track of your BMI and central obesity is important. Try to keep your BMI in the healthy range and your waist circumference within recommended limits. A weighing scale and a measuring tape are all you need to monitor these. It is worth monitoring both metrics because some people with a "normal" BMI can still have an unhealthy level of body fat. Finally, regarding diet, keep in mind that older adults require more protein. Read food labels and be mindful of the amount of protein in what you're eating. It can take some effort to achieve the recommended protein intake.

- Prevent, prevent, prevent. Think of aging with spastic diplegia like taking care of your teeth. Brushing and flossing every day and visiting the dentist or hygienist regularly are the best ways to prevent tooth decay, but problems may still arise, and when they do, a dentist can help address them. The outcome may not be perfect, but problems can be dealt with. Take the same approach to the management of aging with spastic diplegia. Be aware of the problems which may arise and work hard to prevent or minimize them. Time spent preventing problems is generally much more effective than time spent dealing with problems. However, if problems do arise, medical professionals can help.

- We each "own" our health. We can get people in to clean our house, pack its contents for a move, walk our pets, and perform many more of life's chores, but we cannot get people to do our walking, cycling, or swimming for us. We have to own our fitness, BMI, and cardiovascular health. We can call in experts to help, and they may provide valuable guidance, but they do not own our health.

- All adults should strive to maintain participation in society as they age. Try to add friends as you age; our peer groups tend to diminish later in life.

- Some additional pointers for adolescents (listed in section 3.10) may remain relevant in adulthood and are not repeated here.

Finally, as C.S. Lewis put it: "You are never too old to set another goal or to dream a new dream."

Although Tommy was already doing many things to promote his own well-being in a mature and thoughtful way (for instance in employment, nutrition, and social life), his response was to up his level of exercise. When he was 23 he experienced a period of back pain and attended physical therapy at Gillette Phalen Clinic. The pain resolved after intensive PT and exercise at home. He has now decided to visit annually as a preventive measure. He thinks of it like an annual tune-up on a car. He has also registered with a primary care provider where he lives.

Useful web links

Many of the web links in section 3.4 remain relevant for adults with CP and are not repeated here. The following may also be helpful:

- American Academy for Cerebral Palsy and Developmental Medicine (AACPDM) (n.d.) *Why Do Adults with Cerebral Palsy Need a Primary Care Provider (PCP)?* [pdf] aacpdm.org/UserFiles/file/fact-sheet-pcp-patient-101415.pdf

- American Academy for Cerebral Palsy and Developmental Medicine (AACPDM) (n.d.) *Care of Adults with Cerebral Palsy.* [pdf] aacpdm.org/UserFiles/file/fact-sheet-pcp-doc-101415.pdf

- American Academy for Cerebral Palsy and Developmental Medicine (AACPDM) (n.d.) *Pain in Adults with Cerebral Palsy.* [pdf] aacpdm.org/UserFiles/file/fact-sheet-pain-011516.pdf

- Can Do Canines (2013) *Amy and Mobility Assist Dog Dinger.* [video] youtube.com/watch?v=gRwevS2elxg

- UK National Institute for Health and Care Excellence (NICE) (2019) *Cerebral Palsy in Adults.* [online] nice.org.uk/guidance/ng119

- American Academy for Cerebral Palsy and Developmental Medicine (AACPDM) (n.d.) *Physical Fitness and Exercise for Adults with Cerebral Palsy.* [pdf] aacpdm.org/UserFiles/file/fact-sheet-fitness-083115.pdf

Key points Chapter 4

- People with spastic diplegia have a relatively normal life expectancy. For every child and adolescent with CP, there are approximately three adults with the condition.
- Management and treatment of spastic diplegia in childhood and adolescence have improved in recent decades. This influences how today's children and adolescents will fare as adults.
- Research in adult CP receives only a very small percentage of an already small CP research budget.
- Health services for adults with CP are generally very limited. Multidisciplinary care teams in place for children and adolescents with CP largely do not exist for adults at a time when their needs are becoming ever more complex. Hopefully, this will continue to improve.
- Once the person with spastic diplegia reaches adulthood and skeletal growth has ceased, a certain stabilization of the condition occurs. The rate of change of the condition is slower in adulthood, assuming the adult remains physically active. Adults with spastic diplegia may, however, develop secondary conditions.
- Secondary conditions should not be confused with secondary abnormalities.
- For the person with spastic diplegia, it is almost as if on entering adulthood two roads converge: the challenges of growing up with the condition meet the challenges of typical aging. The adult with spastic diplegia must manage these two sets of challenges in combination. The problems of aging are likely to occur at a younger age and with more severity in adults with CP than in those without the condition.
- The goals of intervention for adults with CP are inclusion and participation in major life areas. Objectives include minimizing impairments in body functions and structure, preventing secondary conditions (e.g., fractures), and optimizing activities and participation.
- Studies show adults with spastic diplegia have more problems than the general population in the areas of musculoskeletal decline, mobility, falls, fractures, pain, noncommunicable diseases (NCDs) and risk factors, fatigue, depression, anxiety, quality of life (QoL),

health-related quality of life (HRQoL), and participation. Many of these problems are interlinked.

● Weight management remains very important throughout adulthood.

● For the adult with CP, three different components of health need monitoring; acute health problems (such as infections), lifestyle health risks, and secondary conditions related to CP. It can be helpful to find a physical medicine and rehabilitation (PMR) specialist as well as a primary care provider.

● Treatments such as therapies (PT and OT), orthoses, tone reduction, and orthopedic surgery remain relevant in adulthood, as needed. However, the goal for a particular treatment may be different in adulthood than it was in childhood.

● There are many areas in which PT and OT services can provide help and guidance to adults with spastic diplegia.

● The importance of the home program cannot be overemphasized. It is a constant in the life of the adult with spastic diplegia. The home program includes the "homework" prescribed by therapists, wearing orthoses, stretching, exercise and physical activity, and postural management.

● Rehabilitation after surgery (of any type) is more prolonged in adults than in children because adults heal more slowly and their lives are generally busier than children's. Rehabilitation for the same procedure (for example, knee replacement surgery) can take longer for adults with CP than for their able-bodied peers.

● When planning any treatment in adulthood, it is important to set realistic functional goals.

CHAPTER 5

Living with Spastic Diplegia— Bilateral CP

In this chapter, people share stories of how spastic diplegia impacts their lives. Each story was written independently—yet interestingly, there are common themes running through them.

Geraldine, mother of nine-year-old Joseph, from Ireland

GERALDINE

I had the most amazing pregnancy with Joseph—everything felt wonderful and I couldn't wait for our beautiful son to arrive. He was a week overdue; all went well and I left the hospital the day after his birth, in love with this adorable baby boy. It had been 19 years since we'd had a daughter, so it was such a blessing to be bestowed with another baby.

After a week or so of relative bliss, our lives were turned upside down: Joseph began to cry for most of the day and night and was sleeping only four to six hours in 24 hours, plus he would only sleep on us. This was to last for the next 18 months to two years.

Looking back now, it all makes so much sense, but at the time we explored all avenues—colic, food intolerance—but found no relief from his ongoing crying. When Joseph wasn't sitting up unaided I knew something was not quite right, but I was hoping his development had just been stunted because of the crying. I had been a nurse in the area of intellectual and physical disability for 20 years and was filled with fear and upset for what was possibly unfolding in front of me. It was a senior physiotherapist who confirmed my worst fears: cerebral palsy, spastic diplegia. I remember my head going into a spin. In a few days I had gone into full action mode: I had begun the process of taking carer's leave from work and getting Joseph into a physiotherapy program.

I felt heartbroken for the healthy baby I had dreamed of and hoped for for so long, yet I loved this little boy with all my heart. These are very opposing and challenging emotions to live with, and I found it very difficult to integrate all these feelings on my own while I was feeling very overwhelmed and exhausted.

When Joseph was two, I looked for a support group as I really wanted to meet other parents in the same position as me—parents whose whole lives had been turned upside down. No support group existed so I began one myself. I researched online for most of the information, treatments, and supports.

Having received the diagnosis, one of the most challenging aspects is having to become an advocate for all aspects of your child's care when you are feeling so vulnerable and raw yourself. You find yourself with an uphill battle to try to obtain funding for vital equipment and/or special needs assistant's hours.

Nothing prepares you for all the ups and downs, like when Joseph became ill or had a growth spurt and regressed physically: no one told us this would happen, and we didn't know what was happening to the progress he had just made. There are so many factors, like dealing with his peers, watching them reach their milestones, and wondering why this is happening to your son.

Joseph had a lot of pain, and I found this to be the most challenging aspect of his diagnosis. The pain was due to his spastic muscles. Because he had a dynamic personality and was mad for action, this wreaked havoc for his body as he would push himself beyond his limits and suffer the consequences later. In April 2016 that became a thing of the past thanks to his SDR spinal surgery.

In the early days the nonstop appointments, intervention, physiotherapy, seating, and equipment were so exhausting. Your role as a parent changes to therapist as well as parent, and this is a difficult balancing act to negotiate—you really do develop many skills along the way that stand to you in all areas of your life.

Disability, to me, feels like you are entering a different world from planet Earth. In this world of disability you are profoundly changed. The experience is like seeing with new glasses. People can tell you what it's like in this other world, but until you are touched by the experience —that is, wearing new glasses—you cannot understand what it's like.

Joseph has taught me so much. One of the most touching things, which I admire, is how he doesn't ever behave like he is restricted in any way—

he believes he can do anything he sets his mind to. He is teaching me to live like this because often all I can see are restrictions all over the place to a new challenge.

Joseph touches the lives of everyone he meets. A physical disability is an obvious challenge to others you meet, yet Joseph presents as a warm, friendly, and always positive boy despite all the challenges he regularly encounters.

Looking back I feel it's so important to prepare yourself for the marathon ahead. In the first few years we spent so much of our savings on therapies, looking for cures and trying to find someone to "fix" Joseph. We didn't realize that the real healing for us and for Joseph was in accepting him exactly as he is and providing him with as many opportunities as possible, to allow him to spread his wings and fly in this world.

I would summarize by saying I feel blessed, challenged, and privileged to have had a child with spastic diplegia.

JOSEPH
It's hard being a boy with spastic diplegia.

When I was younger, I wished I could have been more independent, especially at home, but since the operation on my spine in Leeds three years ago, I am getting stronger and this is becoming more of a possibility. I am very, very happy about this because being more independent is what I have been waiting for all my life. I have to give credit to Mam and Dad as they have been a big support on this massive journey.

I suppose I should talk about the operation because that was a big thing for me. I was very scared because I was small, but Mam talked to me a lot about it and I finally accepted the fact that I had to do it. I thought the operation would fix me straight away and I would be able to walk on my own after the operation. I found out that it wasn't as simple as that, and then I suppose I had to do huge amounts of physiotherapy. ☹ One of the things about me you should know is that I hate physio and at times I was very resistant, but I knew it had to be done. There are two big, big factors: I no longer have pains in my legs and I don't have to get Botox injections any more.

Having this condition doesn't change my confidence. I see myself as an ordinary person with hopes and dreams. My motto is: "Nothing is impossible, only challenging."

Tina, mother of twin 11-year-old boys, from Iowa

I will never forget the day we received the official diagnosis. "Both of your boys have cerebral palsy." That simple sentence set off a roller coaster of emotions as I spent the next several days and weeks processing what we had just learned.

First, there was heartbreak. Our greatest fears had just been confirmed. The boys were born seven weeks early and had spent eight weeks in the NICU, so their doctor had warned us that they may experience developmental delays. But of course we were hoping that wouldn't be the case. Next came confusion. What is cerebral palsy? What exactly does that mean? I had barely heard the term before, let alone knew what it actually was. Then the fear kicked in. Will my boys be able to walk? What will their lives look like? And lastly, there was anger. Why me? Why my boys?

Little did I know our journey was just beginning. We have spent the last 10 years navigating countless doctors' and physical therapy appointments, preparing for and recovering from multiple surgeries, and helping our boys navigate life with a different set of challenges. I have also spent a lot of time reading about cerebral palsy, learning about other health conditions that often coincide with it, and exploring different treatment options. It is important to me to understand everything I can to help my boys live a happy, healthy, and fulfilled life. Not knowing what their future looks like terrifies me, but I am determined to do everything I can to make sure they get the care and services they need. We are so much more than parents at this point. We are their voices, their advocates, their champions.

But as much as we want to take care of our children, we can't forget about ourselves. Having twins means that my experiences as a mother are very different from those of my friends and family members with kids. Add in the fact that my boys have cerebral palsy and it's a whole different ball game. It is very difficult for me to connect with moms of "typical" children. They don't understand my daily struggles and constant fears. They don't realize that our life is different from theirs. Joining a local support group for parents of kids with disabilities was one of the best decisions I've made. Although our kids all have different diagnoses and medical conditions, we all understand each other. We learn from each other. We support each other.

One of the most important things I have learned over the years is that cerebral palsy affects everyone differently. We can't listen to the stereo-types or statistics. And as difficult as it may be, we shouldn't compare our children to other kids. Every child is unique, regardless of whether they have a disability. I have also learned that cerebral palsy doesn't define who my boys are. They are so much more than their diagnosis. They are happy, healthy 11-year-olds who love to play baseball, hit golf balls with their dad, and swim whenever they have the opportunity. They just happen to walk with the assistance of a walker. Yes, they have endured more than any kid should, but they are also much stronger and more resilient than other kids. They have overcome just about every obstacle that's been thrown at them, and the next one barely seems to faze them anymore.

I sometimes think about what life would be like if my boys didn't have CP. Things would definitely be easier, but at the same time I am grateful for the experience. My boys have completely changed my perspective and have taught me so much about what is really important. They have made me stronger than I ever thought possible. I continue to be amazed at how well they adapt to what life has given them, and I look forward to seeing what their future holds.

Christine, mother of 14-year-old Aaron, from Texas

CHRISTINE

Aaron was born 10 weeks early. I was a first-time mom, so I listened to the doctors when they said, "Premature babies develop slowly," or,

"He's a premie so he's just delayed." When Aaron's physical therapist recommended we see a neurologist, I was confused and shocked, since we had been under several physicians' supervision for the first two years of his life. A few tests and several visits with a neurologist later and yes, Aaron had cerebral palsy (CP). Aaron was almost three years old when he was diagnosed with spastic diplegic CP. I had no idea what that was or what it meant. No one really talks to you about the grief and loss associated with a medical diagnosis.

Shock and denial: I was not willing to accept the diagnosis from one doctor, so I sought another opinion, and it was confirmed.

Pain and guilt: Did I do something wrong in my pregnancy? You run through every little thing from the beginning, trying to figure out what you might've done wrong.

Anger and bargaining: Anger because you can't understand—if you didn't do anything wrong during your pregnancy, why is this happening to your baby? Is it hereditary? You bargain with your higher power over how you can "fix" things.

Depression, reflection, and loneliness will be places you visit constantly on your journey with CP. A sadness sets in the first time your child doesn't get invited to a birthday party. Or the day your child comes home from school upset that he got picked on at the playground. Loneliness when you have no one to ask about the questions you have except Google. Everyone deals with grief differently. I ran a marathon to deal with my grief that year. I had my legs and my health, and my baby might never be able to run like that, so I had to run. Maybe that was the turning point for me. To train, and hurt through something hard and survive—not win, but finish the race—was when I think things changed, slowly. Just like my race, I had to come up with a plan and execute. (**Tip:** find a healthy outlet for stress.)

For the next 10 years, I attended conferences on CP and googled everything. (**Tip:** take all information on the internet with a grain of salt.) I kept a notebook of all of our appointments and what doctors said so I could keep up with what we were doing. (**Tip:** initially a notebook for notes is very helpful, especially if there is a possibility of changing doctors.) I became Aaron's case manager, always asking questions and seeking out the advice of professionals. My general rule of thumb was that so long as it didn't harm Aaron, we would try anything. And we did. We tried casting, several AFOs, physical therapy (PT), occupational therapy (OT), home exercises, Botox, and finally a tendon lengthening. Once we started with surgery, I knew there was no going back. It was only a matter of time before the next one. It was a race against time and Aaron's own growth for when that surgery would come. For us it was SEMLs at Gillette, while I stumbled my way through second and third opinions. (**Tip:** trust your instincts.) You see your child every day. The doctors are brilliant and caring and have good intentions, but you see and know your child in a way a doctor cannot. The SEMLS surgery turned Aaron onto a path of positive outlook and endless possibilities. It was by every measure a success.

The final stage of grieving is acceptance. Acceptance happens slowly and evolves. Each time we went into a children's hospital and saw other kids who were not going home that day, it was a gentle reminder that everything was going to work out. Be tenacious in your quest to give your child the best outcome. And it is most important to listen. At some point you and your doctor cannot talk around your child. They hear everything and will understand: listen to their concerns and help them get involved in their care as early as you can. Aaron's questions went from, "What flavor of popsicles will I have?" to, "Do I have to wear my braces all the time?" and, in his teenage years, "Can I wear normal shoes?" As a teen now, Aaron still has physical limitations, of course, as there is no cure for CP. But day to day, when I have to tell my teen to stop playing video games and clean his room or do his homework, it's a reminder that he's not very different from other teens.

AARON

As a teenager in high school you are around a lot of judgmental people. When you have CP as a teenager it's a little bit more of all of that. Pretty much every day I get a lot of people assuming I'm mentally disabled or that I'm faking it. They also assume I can't run or get a drivers' license or that it's impossible for me to do sports. I get an unbelievable amount of people who think I'm lucky because I don't always have to do as much in PE. I also have people who think the reason I walk differently is because I'm lazy. In school there are a lot of jokes and rude comments, too. For a while I made jokes back, but most of the time I just joined in and made fun of myself. Lately I have just been quiet and I don't respond.

Before the SEMLS surgery I was extremely negative. I had decided that my case was hopeless. I thought, even after having all these surgeries, my feet aren't pointed straight, so what's the point? I'm always going to be different, so why even care about my physical health? Since SEMLS I have never been happier. I can't think of anything that makes me regret getting this procedure. I am a lot more positive and I have more confidence. I still get lots of rude comments and I still get made fun of. But I think it was 100 percent worth it.

Giving advice for parents is kinda hard. I'm just a kid; I don't know how to help because parents usually know what is best for their kids and already have their kids as their main priority/focus. So I guess the only advice I can give is this: though all of the surgeries and procedures go a long way, sometimes the best thing is an "I love you" and a hug. Also just a small reminder to your kid that they are in no way alone.

There is a lot of advice I could give to teens, but I am just going to give a few pieces. For some reason, and I don't know why, I think people are actually jealous of us. I don't know if your parents ever told you that people who make fun of you are just doing it because they're jealous, but I think they really wish to have CP for the attention and because they think it's the easy way in life.

This may sound crazy, but your parents actually do understand what you are going through. It's not easy for them to hand you over to doctors and just hope that something is going to help your condition. It hurts them just as much to watch you go through this. The thing I regret most is all the times I told my mom how wrong she was when she said she understood how I felt.

If you find someone with CP and they aren't busy, try to talk to them—it helps a lot just to understand that someone has to go through everything you do or worse.

Lastly, I promise it will get better. You may think you're living the worst life and that your CP/gait will never improve, but I can guarantee you that life will get better. All of those things you thought you could never accomplish are possible, and you will prove so many people wrong.

Justin Gallegos, age 21, from California

Justin Gallegos is the first professional athlete with CP to be signed by Nike. He is currently a junior at the University of Oregon's School of Journalism and Communications in Eugene. Justin's running career began in high school when he ran on a home treadmill for a high school class's recommended three exercise periods at home each week. On his dad's suggestion and with the support and encouragement of his high school coach, he started cross-country running. In the beginning he dragged his feet and fell a lot while running, but he persevered and improved to the point where he hardly fell at all. As a senior in high school he set a cross-country three-mile personal record of 23:58 minutes and a single-mile personal record of 7:08. In June 2016 he won gold in the 400 meters in the Paralympic ambulatory division at the California State Track and Field Championships. He then moved on to half-marathon running. In 2017 he was featured as one of Runner's World *magazine's Heroes of Running. In April 2018 he crossed the finish line for his first half-marathon in just over two hours. In April 2019 he achieved his goal of completing a half-marathon in under two hours (1:56:36).*

The following is an interview I did with Justin for this book.

What's your typical exercise schedule?
I typically run 30–60 minutes each day and do a set of stretches after running. I also go to the gym a few times a week, where I do weights and resistance work.

What footwear do you wear?
I wear Nike FlyEase running shoes.

Do you wear orthotics?
No.

What's your current athletic goal?
To complete a full marathon.

Do you find that you're more fatigued than your peers?
Yes, sometimes.

One group of researchers advised a formula for health and well-being in individuals with CP: physical activity, sleep, and nutrition. Apart from physical activity, do you follow a similar formula?
Yes. I try to eat healthily (well, as healthily as one can in college!). I try to get plenty of rest. I try to listen to my body.

What treatments have you had in the past for your CP?
Just therapies.

Did you ever experience discouragement as you grew up with a disability?
Yes, in academics but not in running. I was discouraged from going to college. I was the only kid with a physical disability in the athletics program at high school. Athletics is one of the hardest programs for a person with CP. People didn't really expect me to succeed at it. I put in the miles. When I succeeded at running I found that people changed their attitude toward me. Running is very important for me. Running is my safe space. I became somebody in running. I feel like one of the guys. Running empowered me as a person. People sometimes think just because you have a physical disability, you also have an intellectual disability. This is so wrong.

How many people were at your high school?
2,100.

So I doubt you were the only person with a physical disability?
No, I wasn't.

Yet you were the only one with a physical disability in the athletics program. Were you always interested in sport growing up—that is, before high school?
Yes, I grew up always interested in sports. I loved football especially, but I wasn't much of an athlete. I took karate classes for a few years and did equestrian for special needs kids from when I was 18 months until I was 13.

Outside of your personal attributes, to what do you attribute your success?
My parents, my athletics coach at high school, John Truax at Nike. I give my dad a lot of the credit because he has always pushed me to do

my best and to new challenges. He suggested distance running to me in the beginning and it changed my life forever.

Did your disability ever bother you as you grew up?
No, it's just part of who I am.

Do you hope to take part in future Paralympics?
I'd love to, but unfortunately there are currently no events longer than 400 meters for people with CP at the Paralympics. This is a shame. I would love it if a half-marathon or full marathon became available.

What are your aspirations for the future?
I'd like to be a spokesperson for Nike. I'd like to be a motivational speaker.

WEB LINKS TO SOME VIDEOS FEATURING JUSTIN:
- *Justin Gallegos* (2018) [video] youtu.be/x4KC0nUmY4Y
- *Justin Gallegos: Stronger Every Mile* (2018) [video] youtu.be/Mp5SPZyeyps
- *Overcoming Cerebral Palsy Justin Gallegos 7:21.34!* (2018) [video] youtu.be/Uf13_L11ieU

Rachel, an adult, from Minnesota

As I write this, I have just celebrated my 60th birthday. I have been blessed with the resources to lead an independent and productive life, even though I was born six weeks early in the late 1950s in rural Minnesota. My preterm birth resulted in spastic diplegia, which primarily affects my walking and balance. I have been an independent walker for my entire life, though I recently started using walking sticks in the community, finding them more practical than crutches.

There are several reasons why I have a successful and fulfilling life. First and foremost is the love and support of my family and friends. I have always known that there were many people in my corner, and I have always tried to pay forward their generosity. I am a lifelong learner both inside and outside the classroom. I have also held continuous employment throughout my adult life, serving in senior leadership roles in government, higher education, and health care. Finally, I have experienced very few episodes of pain related to my disability thus far.

I have been able to develop routines that support my lifestyle. I regularly work with a personal trainer, physical therapist, and massage therapist, and have been doing so consistently for the past 15 years. In addition to the discipline of regular exercise, these professionals have provided me with excellent advice to help me pursue my goals.

In addition to working full-time, I have many interests, I am actively involved in my community, I swim, bike, and ski, I manage my own home, I maintain an active social life, and I travel internationally.

I have had some bumps along the road. I had some back issues in my late 20s and early 30s which prompted me to discover Pilates and massage, which have largely erased the problems. I experienced some knee pain in my mid-50s. Traditional and specialized medical professionals were quick to say that it was a result of my CP; I needed to advocate for myself and not be satisfied that blaming my CP for acute issues would become a way of life for me. As it turned out, my knee pain was due to osteoarthritis. I underwent successful knee replacement surgery, which eliminated the knee pain. One point to note: the post-surgery rehabilitation took longer than would typically be expected for this type of surgery. I successfully regained the ability to walk after the surgery, and my clinician now uses me as an example of successful interventions in older adults at international conferences.

When dealing with problems, I have found the following to be useful: persistence, patience, "out-of-the-box" problem-solving, and remembering that what might look like a "no" is merely a "not yet" or a "not this way."

My advice to a younger person is to remember that you are your own best advocate. I believe in taking the best information and professional advice and doing your best to make it work for you. Frequently, well-meaning individuals wanted me to direct my efforts toward disability. A vocational rehabilitation counselor suggested I abandon my pursuit of a degree in political science and change schools to become a vocational rehabilitation counselor. I ignored his "What would you ever do with a degree in political science?" In fact, my first job out of college was working for the governor of Minnesota. I found someone to make me custom boots that provide great support for my ankle and foot but are also stylish and functional; they did a lot to boost my self-confidence as a young adult.

My advice to readers of this book is to remember that this is just one point in time. The field of gait and motion management, physical therapy, and rehabilitation continues to change and advance.

The proudest moments of my life have been gaining recognition for achievements that have nothing to do with having spastic diplegia. Examples include my election to several leadership positions in high school and college, appointment to senior management and cabinet-level positions in areas unrelated disability, and completing my doctorate.

While I am proud of those accomplishments, I would be remiss if I said that living with spastic diplegia did not play a part in those successes. Living with this condition has helped me to develop a broader and bolder vision, creativity, and a willingness to persevere toward a desired outcome. I believe that my diagnosis is one aspect of my personhood that makes me fully human.

CHAPTER 6

Further reading

We read to know we are not alone.

C.S. Lewis

Education is not the filling of a pail,
but the lighting of a fire.

William Butler Yeats

The times, they are a-changin'.

Bob Dylan

Reading and evaluating the evidence

We discussed the importance of evidence-based medicine in Chapter 3. Evidence is collected by carrying out scientific studies (also called research studies), the results of which are published as papers (or articles) in journals (in print and/or online).[117] Scientific studies may also be presented at conferences and educational meetings whose proceedings are usually published. All of this is collectively known as the scientific literature (or research). Nowadays research is also discussed on various social media platforms such as Twitter, Facebook, and LinkedIn.

You may have familiarity with searching the scientific literature. If not, search engines such as PubMed (ncbi.nlm.nih.gov/pubmed) and Google Scholar (scholar.google.com) are good places to start. They provide abstracts (short summary versions of articles) which can be very useful.

In the past, one generally needed to belong to an institution to have access to full-text articles. These days, many journal articles are available online for free. Google Scholar provides links to many full-text articles. You can also check if a full-text version of an article is available online by pasting the title into the search bar. (It's helpful to include "filetype:pdf" in front of the article title.) You can also request full-text journal articles through some community libraries.

You might have heard the phrase, "Just because someone says it, doesn't mean it's true." This is worth remembering in all aspects of life, but it's especially relevant when it comes to reading scientific literature. Read research studies with a critical eye. You should always be asking yourself,

---

117   Some online journals are subscription-based. Others are open-access.

"How confident can I be in the conclusion of this research study?"

There are several different types of research studies. They are:

- **Systematic review:** The highest level of evidence is a systematic review of randomized controlled trials. A systematic review summarizes the results of a number of scientific studies. The Cochrane collaboration is a worldwide association of groups that publish systematic reviews for particular topic areas; a web link is included at the end of this section.
- **Randomized controlled trial (RCT):** The randomized controlled trial (RCT) is the gold standard in research. An RCT is a scientific experiment that has very strict guidelines to ensure that the only aspect that makes the two groups different is that one receives the treatment and the other does not. In an RCT, people are randomly assigned to either the group receiving the treatment or the non-treatment group (also known as the control group). Comparing the outcome of the two groups allows the researcher to determine whether the treatment was effective. RCTs can be hard to achieve in CP and other areas of medicine: if a professional perceives a treatment to be beneficial, then how can it be denied to the control group, morally speaking? A clever study design overcame this problem in the first RCT to evaluate SEMLS in children with spastic diplegia, conducted by Thomason and colleagues in 2011 in Australia. Children were divided into a surgery group and a control group. The control group underwent the same intensive PT as the surgery group for one year, then underwent the surgery. A comparison of outcomes at the one-year mark allowed researchers to determine the effect of the SEMLS.
- **Cohort study:** In the absence of RCTs, researchers may conduct cohort studies. A cohort study is a form of longitudinal study that samples a cohort (a group of people who share a defining characteristic, for example a group of children with spastic diplegia), collecting data at intervals over time.
- **Case series:** A case series is a group of case reports on patients who were given a similar treatment. Single-subject research is emerging as a study design that may provide valuable evidence, and it can be more easily completed than group studies.

Useful web links

- CanChild (2019) *What Is Research?* [online] canchild.ca/en/
  research-in-practice/knowledge-translation-exchange/what-is
  -research

- Cochrane (2019) [online] cochrane.org

- Oxford Centre for Evidence-Based Medicine (Oxford CEBM)
  (2011) *Levels of Evidence: Introductory Document.* [online]
  cebm.net/2011/06/2011-oxford-cebm-levels-evidence
  -introductory-document/

- Oxford CEBM (2019) *Glossary.* [online] cebm.net/2014/06/
  glossary/

Further reading: books

The following books are very useful, and they all include parents in
their intended readership.

- *Cerebral Palsy: A Complete Guide for Caregiving*
  2017, John Hopkins University Press
  Freeman Miller and Steven Bachrach and The Cerebral Palsy
  Center at Nemours/Alfred I. duPont Hospital for Children

- *Cerebral Palsy: From Diagnosis to Adult Life*
  2012, Mac Keith Press
  Peter Rosenbaum and Lewis Rosenbloom

- *Cerebral Palsy: Science and Clinical Practice (Clinics in
  Developmental Medicine)*
  2014, Mac Keith Press
  Edited by Bernard Dan, Margaret Mayston, Nigel Paneth,
  and Lewis Rosenbloom

- *Developmental Disability and Aging*
  2009, Mac Keith Press
  Edited by Gregory O'Brien and Lewis Rosenbloom

- *Finnie's Handling the Young Child with Cerebral Palsy at Home*
  2009, Butterworth Heinemann Elsevier
  Edited by Eva Bower

- *Physiotherapy and Occupational Therapy for People with Cerebral Palsy*
  2010, Mac Keith Press
  Edited by Karen Dodd, Christine Imms, and Nicholas Taylor

Further reading: websites

The following are websites which I found useful (listed in alphabetical order). Many others were included throughout the book and are not repeated here.

- *American Academy for Cerebral Palsy and Developmental Medicine (AACPDM)*
  The AACPDM is an academy of health professionals "dedicated to providing multidisciplinary scientific education and promoting excellence in research and services for the benefit of people with and at risk for CP and other childhood-onset disabilities."
  aacpdm.org

- *BlazeSports America*
  This US national sports organization supports people with physical disabilities.
  blazesports.org

- *CanChild Centre for Childhood Disability*
  CanChild is a nonprofit research and educational center at McMaster University in Ontario, Canada. It offers resources for both professionals and families on a variety of developmental conditions.
  canchild.ca

- *Centers for Disease Control and Prevention (CDC)*
  The CDC is the leading national public health institute in the United States.
  cdc.gov/ncbddd/cp/index.html

- *Cerebral Palsy Alliance*
  The Cerebral Palsy Alliance is an Australian treatment and research center.
  cerebralpalsy.org.au

- *Cerebral Palsy Daily Living*
  An educational resource for families of children with CP.
  cpdailyliving.com

- *Cerebral Palsy Foundation*
  Its mission statement is "leading research, innovation, and collaboration that changes lives for people with cerebral palsy—today." Its resources include a video library with a collection of videos on different aspects of CP that is well worth exploring.
  yourcpf.org/expert-videos-cp/
  It also publishes useful fact sheets.
  yourcpf.org/fact-sheet-library/

- *Cerebral Palsy Research Network (CPRN)*
  CPRN is a group of doctors, therapists, and patient advocates "collaborating to improve treatments and outcomes for people with CP."
  cprn.org
  The network hosts MyCP for the CP community to participate in research and discussions.
  mycp.org

- *Cerebral Palsy Sport*
  This UK national sports organization supports people with CP and other physical disabilities.
  cpsport.org/

- *Childhood Disability LINK*
  Childhood Disability LINK is a Canadian organization "Linking Information and New Knowledge" on childhood disability to service providers and families.
  childhooddisability.ca

- *CP Now*
  CP Now is a US organization whose mission is "to optimize the lifelong health, wellness and inclusion of people with cerebral palsy and their families."
  cpnowfoundation.org

- *Developmental Medicine & Child Neurology*
  This journal publishes many papers relevant to spastic diplegia.
  Papers are freely available online one year after publication.
  onlinelibrary.wiley.com/journal/14698749
  The journal also publishes plain-language summaries to make the
  research more accessible.
  onlinelibrary.wiley.com/page/journal/14698749/homepage/
  VirtualIssuesPage.html#PLS

- *Everyday Health: Cerebral Palsy*
  Everyday Health produces content related to health and wellness.
  It includes a section on CP.
  everydayhealth.com/cerebral-palsy/resources/

- *Kids Brain Health*
  Kids Brain Health is a Canadian network of researchers and health
  professionals dedicated to helping children with neurodisabilities
  and their families.
  kidsbrainhealth.ca/

- *Peter Harrison Centre for Disability Sport*
  The Peter Harrison Centre for Disability Sport is an internationally
  renowned disability sport research center located at Loughborough
  University in the United Kingdom.
  lboro.ac.uk/research/phc/about/

- *Scope UK*
  Scope is a disability equality charity in England and Wales.
  scope.org.uk

- *Surveillance of CP in Europe (SCPE)*
  This group aims to "develop best practice in monitoring trends in
  CP and to disseminate knowledge to health professionals, policy
  makers, patients, and families, to provide information for resource
  planning, and raise standards of care for patients with CP."
  scpenetwork.eu

- *United Cerebral Palsy (UCP)*
  UCP is a US organization that "educates, advocates, and provides
  support services to ensure a life without limits for people with a
  spectrum of disabilities."
  ucp.org/resource-guide/

Epilogue

I'll leave the last words to Tommy.

For as long as I can remember, I've thought most clearly while writing. When I was a teenager, I kept a blog and wrote about 1,200 posts in the space of three years. I wrote about everything and nothing at all: the classes I was taking at school, the books I was reading, the latest Broadway show I was obsessing about.

Growing up, I spent a lot of time thinking about how to be disabled without letting that one fact take over my life. As a teenager, I found it easiest to ignore my disability as much as I could. I wouldn't mention it, and people mostly did the same. I hated those moments when I couldn't ignore it—when I fell, when I got injured, or when I dropped something.

Of course, I couldn't ignore it entirely: large portions of my teenage years were consumed by joint pain and sleepless nights. I spent hours in physical therapy and had two major surgeries. When I was 18, I realized I wanted to write something about it. So over the course of a summer, I holed myself up in my room and wrote a short book. It was autobiographical in the sense that it charted the various surgeries and treatments I'd had, but more than that, it allowed me to work through what it meant to be disabled. There's no user manual for having a disability, but I was trying to write the next best thing for myself. I named that thing *Consider This*, in part because it was what I was doing (consider this disability, if you will), and in part because of a line in R.E.M.'s "Losing My Religion," one of my favorite songs.

I remember lying awake with joint pain one night in August. I couldn't sleep, and, more annoyingly, I couldn't figure out how to finish the short book I'd written. I was about to start my last year of high school, and the narrative of the book ended a few months before that. On the one hand, it felt like a natural stopping point, but on the other, it still felt like the middle of the story. What had I learned writing the book? What would I take from it?

I got up and wrote a letter, a sort of what-I-wish-I'd-known letter to the Tommy of a decade ago. I wrote about how to keep a disability in perspective and concentrate on what actually matters in life. I framed it as the letter I'd write if I had a child with spastic diplegia. It became the epilogue to my short book; I've included it below.

A lot has changed in the seven years since I wrote that piece. I can't ignore the fact that I'm disabled, no matter how much I try (and I tried!). But I've gotten much better at knowing my own limitations and being comfortable enough to ask for help when I need it. Instead of staying quiet and struggling with something, I'm more comfortable around people, and I get more done.

I'm still missing the user manual for how to get through life with a disability. I'd write a very different book if I were starting it today, but I'm proud of how *Consider This* stands on its own.

When I was writing it, I had no idea that my mother would one day write a book about spastic diplegia. In a lot of ways, the two books are in conversation with one another across time. I hope *Consider This* is as useful for you to read as it was for me to write.

August 17, 2012

I owe everything I am today to my parents, so I can only hope to live up to half of what they are. They're the most loving, caring, and dedicated parents anyone could ask for, and I hope I can be the same to you. Having a disability is tough, but you can handle it. I did. It was hard—probably the hardest thing I've had to do—but I did it. And so can you. Some days it's unimaginably difficult to get out of bed and face the world, but it's possible.

So, how do you beat your disability? You beat it by never letting it define you. I wasn't a 14-year-old who had CP, I was a 14-year-old who loved drums, read every book he could lay his hands on, and probably played his music too loud. As people, we're defined not by our abilities or disabilities—it's our choices, our aspirations, and our attitudes that define us. So go out there and be outrageously passionate about something.

You beat your disability by knowing where you want to be—be that on crutches or walking independently—and then working your ass off to get there. You beat it by never settling for less than what you can achieve. You might have a disability, but don't let the disability have you.

You beat it by setting goals. I could quote life mottos like, "Don't wait for your ship to come in, swim out to meet it," but nobody listens to those. That said, they are rooted in truth. Managing your CP isn't something that's going to fall into your lap as you sit at home moping: you have to work toward it. You beat it with pragmatism. It's true, you'll probably never be a professional footballer. Or an astronaut. Or a stunt double. Or a boxer. You're faced with a choice: let yourself be constantly held back by it, or shrug it off and focus on all the things you can do.

And then, if you manage all that? You'll have beaten it—and, more importantly, you'll have the satisfaction of leading a full life despite your disability. And that's an incredible achievement.

—Tommy

Tommy's book is available at www.GilletteChildrensHealthcarePress .org/sdbook.

Acknowledgments

It takes a village to raise a child
African proverb

It takes a village to raise a child with spastic diplegia—bilateral CP. It takes a village to write a book on the subject.

The village who worked with me on this book included Dr. Tom Novacheck, Jean Stout, Amy Schultz, and Candice Johnson from Gillette. I am forever indebted to each of them for not only sharing the vision and helping to create this resource, but also for the huge amount of hard work that they invested in the project, on top of already very busy work schedules. In addition to editing, Tom's leadership and support for the project deserve special mention. His unwavering belief in the need for this book for families meant that we were able to overcome any obstacle we met along the way. Without Tom's leadership and support, there would be no book today. Jean's vast experience of CP, together with her very detailed editing, helped shape the book that you see before you; thank you to Jean for all those long hours that we worked together. Thank you also to Amy and Candice for their editing and valuable contributions, particularly in the areas of physical therapy and occupational therapy. Many other members of staff at Gillette made important contributions: they included Rachel Wobschall, Janey Faber, Heather Forst, Laura Gueron, Jennifer Klein, Liz Boyer, Dr. Jill Gettings, and Dr. Kevin Sheridan. Thank you also to Dennis Jolley, Paula Montgomery, and Barbara Joers for their vision, continued interest and support.

Thank you to Geraldine, Joseph, Tina, Christine, Aaron, Justin, and Rachel for contributing your personal stories in Chapter 5. Sharing your stories greatly contributes to readers' understanding of this condition.

Writing this book involved reading a large number of research papers and books. I deeply appreciate all those who taught me through their writing. Through this book, they are now teaching others. As a parent, I appreciate the work of those researchers whose names frequently appear in the body of CP literature. Thank you also to participants in studies; without participants, there would be no studies. We families depend on this continued research. Indeed, because of the importance of CP research, and how underfunded it is, all sales proceeds from this book will be donated to this cause. Thank you also to Jacqueline Linn, librarian to Gillette, who kept me supplied in research papers.

The great production team who converted a long manuscript into the book you have before you today included Carra Simpson (project manager), Joan McGarry Moore and Rebecca Hiscott (copy editors), Olwyn Roche (illustrator), Jazmin Welch (cover and interior designer), Ruth Wilson (proofreader), and Stephen Ullstrom (indexer). They worked their various magics! I am deeply appreciative of both their professionalism but also their huge interest in producing the best possible book— they understood the importance of the subject matter. Thank you also to Brianna Wolfson who first introduced me to the world of publishing.

Early readers were very important to me in the writing process. I'm very grateful for the time they took to patiently read through various drafts and for providing me with detailed feedback. They sometimes challenged me and the book is all the better for that. They included Mary Bienek, Máire Buckley, Gerald Dundon, Una Dunne-Shannon, Margaret Harty, Íde Hickey, Sandie McCanny, Darlene Meskell, Geraldine Monaghan, Carmel Murray, Katie O'Brien, Reva Seth, Christine Simpson, Sam Tripodi, Mike Walsh, and Bill Watson.

Thank you to those who took the time to read the final manuscript before publication and to write reviews. I was humbled by their words.

Raising a child with spastic diplegia takes effort. It would be impossible to include all medical professionals who supported us in Tommy's journey to adulthood, but some deserve special mention: Szilvia Czibok, Dr. Jim Gage, Dr. Owen Hensey, Ann Jenkinson, Dr. Susan Keane, Ann Kennedy, Lynn Morrison, Carmel Murray, Dr. Tom Novacheck, the late Prof. Tim O'Brien, and Mike Walsh. Tommy would not be where he is today without their great skill, expertise, and genuine care.

To my friends and extended family, thank you for your patience and support, and for not abandoning me while I withdrew to write this book.

Every day, I continue to be awed by Tommy. His positive attitude, his confidence, his love of life and adventure—he has never let his disability define him. Patrick and John, Tommy's two older brothers, have been amazing siblings from when they were all very young children right through to today. I'm very proud of the adults they have each become. The fact that they now work in the same city in the US is no accident but testament to their closeness as brothers. Finally, thanks to my husband, Denis, who supported me, not just every day in the writing of this book but in the whole adventure of our life together.

Gillette is situated in the twin cities—Minneapolis–Saint Paul. The village that helped raise our son and the village that helped write this book are inextricably linked. Thank you so much to my twin villages.

Appendices

Dealing with a diagnosis

One of the early readers of this book, a nurse and psychotherapist who has a son with spastic diplegia, wrote the following about the different stages of dealing with a diagnosis.

Each individual is unique, and so is each individual's inner emotional landscape. While you navigate your own emotional terrain to come to a place of acceptance of your child's disability, you will likely have to take a detour through the stages of grief. There is no way around this challenge; the only way out is through. You are grieving the loss of the child you thought you would have, not the child who is before you. There is no ordered pattern to these stages; some people don't experience all of these emotions, while others experience many of them at the same time.

The grieving process is cyclical. In addition to the diagnosis it is triggered again and again, often when your child undergoes life-changing events. You will witness your child's peers reaching milestones that your child may or may not achieve and it will hurt like crazy. It's perfectly normal and healthy to allow yourself to feel your feelings and have a good cry or vent.

Dr. Ken Moses, a renowned speaker, author, and psychologist who helps people deal with crisis, trauma, and loss, wrote:

Parents generate core-level dreams for their children even before the child is born. Disability shatters those dreams. Grieving is the process whereby parents separate out from those shattered dreams and begin creating new dreams. To separate from a lost dream one must experience and share denial, anxiety, fear, guilt, depression, and anger in whatever order or manner the feelings surface.

The following are some of the stages one may experience:

Denial

The feelings of sadness and isolation that arise in response to the diagnosis are almost universal among parents of a child with a disability. It can present as a sense of, "Just give the child time, they will be fine." Shock and denial blunt the diagnosis and give you time to gather your inner resources to find the strength you need to navigate the new road ahead.

Anxiety

Your whole world has changed now. Added to your day-to-day routines and responsibilities are appointments and home physiotherapy programs. One parent may need to become a stay-at-home caregiver, which can add myriad new worries, concerns, and fears. This is a time of intense anxiety and exhaustion. It forces you to sharply redefine your priorities as the reality of the diagnosis sinks in and you begin to get the structures in place to meet all of your child's medical and day-to-day care needs.

Depression

You begin to realize that no matter what you do, you can't change the diagnosis. You feel overwhelmed and burdened by the responsibilities of the journey ahead. Over time, these feelings of depression—through many tears and feelings of vulnerability and the acknowledgment that it's normal to feel devastated at this juncture—lead to a redefining of your value system.

Once you allow yourself to feel your despair, a new dawn rises: this too shall pass. You begin to see your child through fresh eyes. You look at what your child can do and you redefine your values and goals to include a child with a disability. You begin to see all the possibilities that still lie ahead. This is a turning point.

Anger

At first, the anger may be very intense, triggered by feelings of grief and terrible loss. "Why me and not you?" You may be angry at your spouse for not being supportive; your spouse may still be in the earlier stages of denial or depression. Angry at professionals for having to wait for appointments and equipment due to long waiting lists. Angry with people who say nothing about your child because they don't know what to say; they know you are hurting and are afraid of upsetting you, so they say nothing. Sometimes we are even angry at ourselves for struggling and feeling down. We judge ourselves harshly: "I should be over it by now."

Guilt

"Did I do something wrong?" "Am I being punished for something I said or did?" "Why me?" "Why my child?" You might feel guilty about your child's siblings not getting enough time and attention, or because you aren't doing enough physiotherapy. It's important to learn to be kind to yourself and to set realistic and achievable goals, otherwise you risk spending all your time feeling guilty. Remember to be a parent first and to know when you need a break or some space. The more you give to yourself, the more you have to give to your child. Find a way to release and express all your feelings of guilt, for example by working with a therapist or journaling. Knowing that neither you nor your child are to blame for your child's condition is a very liberating stage, and it allows you to move forward into acceptance and integration of the diagnosis.

Acceptance and integration

Allowing yourself to acknowledge and experience negative emotions will set you on the path to meeting new challenges. Once the parent accepts their feelings of anger, fear, and guilt as normal and healthy, the heavy emotions of grief will no longer feel so draining. You will be able to become the best advocate and support for your child, and both parent and child will continue to grow and create new dreams and endless possibilities.

You will recognize when you have reached this stage because you will be able to speak about your child without unbidden emotions bubbling beneath the surface. You will feel hopeful again, and you will begin to see the many possibilities ahead for your child. You will come to value and cherish the extraordinariness of your child, who continually amazes you with their inner strength, courage, determination, and acceptance of the path they have had to follow and grow upon from birth.

Conclusion

As a parent you are always trying to do the best for your child and help them along their path. However, one day I realized it was my child who was waiting for me to catch up: he was the one who had always accepted who and where he was.

Gross motor function

The Gross Motor Function Measure (GMFM) is a tool used to measure gross motor function in children and adolescents with CP. The GMFM is valid from ages five months to 16 years. It is suitable for those whose motor skills are at or below the level of a typically developing five-year-old child. It is available in English and other languages.

In the GMFM-66 items are graded by difficulty, whereas in the GMFM-88 all items contribute equally to the overall result regardless of difficulty.

The GMFM-66 is scored 0–100. A confidence interval (CI) is commonly reported with a GMFM-66 score. If the CI is 95 percent, it means one can be 95 percent certain that the child's actual score will fall within a given range of values. For example, a GMFM-66 score of 50.1 with a 95 percent CI of 47.8–52.4 means you can be 95 percent certain that the child's actual score at that time is between 47.8 and 52.4. If there is a change in performance between test dates that falls within the confidence interval, it may not be a real change. In this example, the retest result would need to be above 52.4 to be considered an improvement.

Currently there is no published research on the use of the GMFM in adults.

Measurement tools

Measurement tools must be valid, reliable, accurate, and precise. We reviewed these terms in section 1.6. The following table lists examples of some commonly used measurement tools in CP.

Table A.3.1 Measurement tools

MEASUREMENT TOOL	VARIABLE	COMPLETED BY	ICF DOMAIN	WEB LINK
Goniometer	ROM of joint	PT	Body functions and structure	
GMFM (GMFM-88 and GMFM-66)	Gross motor function	PT	Activity	canchild.ca/system/ tenon/assets/ attachments/000/000/ 218/original/ gmfm-88_and_66_ scoresheet.pdf
10-meter or 6-minute walking tests	Walking	PT	Activity	
Gillette Functional Assessment Questionnaire (FAQ)	Functional mobility	Parent or person with CP	Activity and participation	gillettechildrens.org/ assets/uploads/ general/Forms/ Questionnaire_for_ Returning_Patients_ 2.pdf Scroll down to page 2.
Functional Mobility Scale (FMS)	Functional mobility	Parent or person with CP	Activity and participation	
Gait Outcomes Assessment List (GOAL)	Gait priorities and functional mobility	Parent or person with CP	All domains	

Cont'd.

MEASUREMENT TOOL	VARIABLE	COMPLETED BY	ICF DOMAIN	WEB LINK
Pediatric Outcomes Data Collection Instrument (PODCI)	Pediatric health	Parent	Activity and participation	gillettechildrens.org/assets/uploads/general/Forms/Pediatric_Outcomes_Questionnaire.pdf For children aged 2–10 years

Positioning

Positioning to achieve stretch

Examples include:

- **Long sitting:** This stretches the hamstrings, as the knees are extended while the hips are flexed. For the younger child this can be done without a special seat, though a special seat that promotes the 90-degree angle of the hip and ties the knee in extension can be a great help. See Figure A.4.1.

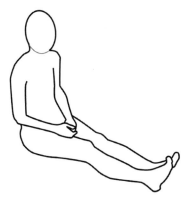

Figure A.4.1 Long sitting

We had a special long sitting seat made for the car so Tommy could get a good stretch on all car journeys. He could tolerate the stretch for long periods of time, but if the journey was really long we would hear him opening the knee straps. If you're using a special car seat, make sure it doesn't compromise safety or affect your car insurance.

If an AFO plus knee immobilizer are worn while the child is positioned in long sitting, stretch of both the calf and hamstring muscles can be achieved.

- **Side sitting:** This gives a nice stretch to the side with the balancing hand. It also stretches the wrist if there is any upper extremity tightness. See Figure A.4.2.

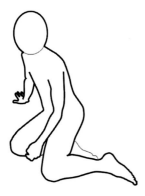

Figure A.4.2 Side sitting

> Tommy had a preference for one side of his body—he always wanted his better hand to be free—so we really had to encourage him to side sit on his less favored side.

- **Tailor sitting:** This stretches the hip adductors but also promotes hip external rotation. See Figure A.4.3.

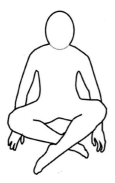

Figure A.4.3 Tailor sitting

- **Prone positioning:** This stretches the hip flexors. Prone propping is a position in which the child lies on their tummy with their feet out behind them and elbows on the floor. In prone lying, the elbows are straight. A triangular wedge is very handy to help promote this position. See Figure A.4.4.

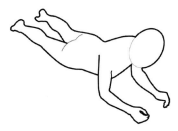

Figure A.4.4 Prone propping

- **Standing:** This stretches the hip flexors, the hamstrings (knee flexors), and the gastrocnemius and soleus muscles. This includes standing while holding on to furniture, standing with orthoses or knee immobilizers, and standing with various standing equipment. Sometimes the equipment allows children to stand on an incline, which helps stretch the gastrocnemius muscle.

Some positions for strengthening

Examples include:
- **Prone positioning** (prone propping; see explanation above): This position promotes shoulder stability and improves trunk control through core strengthening. Crawling involves movement while in a prone position.
- **Tailor sitting:** Promotes the development of trunk control (i.e., trunk strengthening and balance reactions). It also encourages more active play, and because the two hands are free, it encourages crossing the midline (using both sides of the body together).
- **Standing:** Standing strengthens trunk and leg muscles. Playing while standing is also important for developing balance reactions.
- **Side sitting:** Promotes the development of trunk control and balance reactions. It should be practiced evenly on both sides.
- **Sitting on a large roll or bolster with feet supported on the floor:** The child can play at a table in this position. The hips, knees, and ankles are at 90 degrees and both sides of the trunk are straight. This promotes the development of trunk control (i.e., strengthening

the trunk muscles and balance reactions). It also encourages more active play, and because the two hands are free, it encourages crossing the midline. See Figure A.4.5.

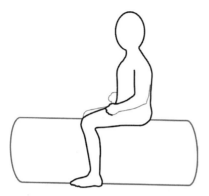

Figure A.4.5 Sitting on a large roll

- **Tall kneeling:** In this position the child is bearing weight on their knees. The child has flexed knees but extended hips and trunk. This position again promotes the development of trunk control and balance reactions, but because it is done in a kneeling rather than a sitting position there is more work being done to oppose gravity. This is a good precursor to standing balance. It is a good play position even if the child has already achieved standing. Some children also practice walking on their knees. See Figure A.4.6.

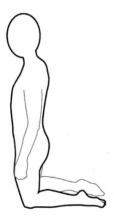

Figure A.4.6 Tall kneeling

Exercise and physical activity

The following are tips gleaned from my own experience, with additional pointers from therapists at Gillette. Your PT or OT can help you develop a targeted and safe exercise program. They will also be able to offer advice on which types of exercise are best for joint preservation.

There's a balance to be struck between preserving joints and playing sports you most enjoy. For example, if playing soccer with friends is what you most enjoy, it is a good sport for you. Swimming is a particularly good sport because of its low impact on the joints.

Exercise and physical activity tips for the younger child

- The typically developing toddler gets their muscle stretching and strengthening exercises through everyday movement: running, climbing, jumping, etc. Since the goal in spastic diplegia is to follow normal development as much as possible (to get normal forces acting on the bones), we need to ensure the young child with spastic diplegia gets their required amount of exercise and physical activity. Movement is essential for the child with spastic diplegia, including moving joints through the entire ROM of which they are capable.
- Incorporating muscle stretching and strengthening into play and other activities the child really enjoys is enormously helpful. For the young child, learning to play and learning through play are very important. Incorporating exercise and stretching into the normal day as much as possible—for example, encouraging the child to use a tricycle to travel short distances—also helps.
- Playgrounds (both outdoor and indoor) are great places for all children to play, but they are especially important for the child with spastic diplegia. Here the child has the opportunity to move in a variety of ways. Playgrounds are also great because they are normal

family settings. Parents of children with limited mobility tend not to bring their children to venues that require lots of movement as often, but in fact the child with spastic diplegia needs such opportunities to move and play even more than the typically developing child. Safety must be a concern, of course, but we cannot be so overzealous about safety that our child misses out on great opportunities for movement.

- Swimming is also great for the young child with spastic diplegia.
- Parents may be reluctant to use adaptive equipment (such as a recumbent bicycle) because they worry it will make the child stand out more. I would advise parents to weigh the perceived costs against the benefits for the child. (I'm not talking about financial costs.) I have also found that children can be very accepting of others; often the prejudice lies with adults, not with our children.

Exercise and physical activity tips for the older child, adolescent, and adult

- For all types of exercise included in Table 3.4.2, a referral to either a PT or OT is recommended, even for just one or two sessions. There are also wonderful athletic trainers who have advanced training in working with people with physical limitations. Trainers who lack this specialized training, however, may advise overexercising, which can lead to injuries. Consider calling the fitness centers or gyms in your area to check if any of their staff have training in adapting exercise programs for people with physical challenges.
- If you're working with weights, consider getting expert guidance on how much weight is safe and how many repetitions to perform.
- Fast walking can achieve many of the same benefits as running and may be safer for some people.
- You have many options when it comes to cycling, including outdoor and indoor (static) bikes. Three-wheeled bikes may be ideal for those with balance issues. You can purchase blocks (trainers) to convert an outdoor bike to an indoor bike when the weather doesn't allow for outdoor mobility.
- A therapist can offer guidance on the appropriate size and type of sports wheelchair to use and can check to see if you are eligible for any funding aid to purchase one.

- A few tips for swimming:
  - Consider scheduling a few sessions with a pool PT or OT to develop an appropriate swimming program.
  - If you use a wheelchair, call around to find a pool with PVC pool chairs and a ramp.
  - A pool temperature of 88–94 degrees Fahrenheit can be very therapeutic and can help reduce pain and stiffness.
  - Nonskid pool shoes are recommended for walking from the changing room to the pool and back to avoid falls on wet pool decks.
  - Swim paddles, kickboards, flippers, etc. can be used to increase resistance for muscle strengthening.
- You can find many excellent videos online (or on DVD) to guide you through adaptive yoga, tai chi, and other such programs. The National Center on Health, Physical Activity and Disability (NCHPAD; nchpad.org) has some.
- Horse riding and dance are not included in Table 3.4.2, but they may be suitable exercises for some people with CP.
- Incorporate as much exercise as you can into the normal day (for example, cycling to school, after-school activities, or work).
- Most school programs include at least a weekly session of physical education. Try to ensure that the program includes the child's or adolescent's needs as much as possible so that they can participate in the sport, even if this means adapting the rules, the equipment, or the mindset of the teacher or coach. Forcing the child or adolescent to sit out their school physical education period is a missed opportunity both in terms of the benefits of exercise and the camaraderie and social experience of teamwork. Research has shown that school-based exercise programs are beneficial for children and adolescents with CP.

Rehabilitation post-selective dorsal rhizotomy (SDR)

Table A.6.1 describes rehabilitation post-selective dorsal rhizotomy (SDR) at Gillette. Rehabilitation protocols vary between centers; your center will provide you with a rehabilitation plan.

Table A.6.1 Rehabilitation post-selective dorsal rhizotomy (SDR)

Acute hospital stay (0–3 days post-surgery)	• Children are on flat bed rest for the first three days after surgery. Doctors/nurses direct pain management. • Children wear knee immobilizers to help manage leg spasms. • Children are monitored for bladder changes in addition to pain in the early days. Bladder changes are relatively uncommon and typically resolve during the hospital stay.
Inpatient rehabilitation (4–6 weeks post-surgery)	• Children are admitted to inpatient rehabilitation (rehab). The inpatient rehab includes PMR physicians, nurses, PT, OT, psychology, therapeutic recreation, social work, and child life. • Children participate in therapies for at least three hours per day. • Children also use equipment (prone cart, wheelchair, mobile prone stander) for positioning and strengthening. • Emphasis is on developing new patterns for movement now that spasticity has been reduced. • At the time of discharge home, children are generally pain-free but may need additional help with mobility. Most children use a wheelchair. • Children are able to return to school full-time at the time of their discharge home.

Cont'd.

Outpatient rehabilitation (up to 1 year)	• PT five times per week for one month and then at decreasing frequency based on the child's progress. • Emphasis is on continued strengthening, gross motor activities, balance, and gait training. • There is a gradual return to independent mobility and baseline walking function. • Children also continue with a home program for functional mobility, strengthening, and positioning. Most children do not have outpatient OT related to SDR.
Follow-up	• Follow-up with PMR, orthopedics, PT, and 3D computerized motion analysis. Recommendations for additional treatment are based on the results of evaluation.

Glossary

I'm afraid I have to disagree with Cato the Elder here. In trying to understand spastic diplegia, the terminology is often one of the first obstacles. The many professionals you will meet will often use medical terms, though most remember to explain them. Having an understanding of key terms is helpful both for speaking with professionals and for reading books and scientific literature about spastic diplegia. The following are key terms you are likely to encounter.

TERM	DEFINITION
Achilles tendon	The Achilles tendon is the cord-like structure which attaches the gastrocnemius and soleus muscles (both calf muscles) to the bone at the ankle joint.
Ankle-foot orthosis (AFO)	An ankle-foot orthosis (AFO) is a type of orthosis (brace) that controls the ankle and foot. See *orthosis*.
Assistive mobility devices	Assistive mobility devices (also termed assistive devices, walking aids, mobility aids, and gait aids) vary in the level of support they provide. Here they are listed in order of least to most support: • Walking sticks (canes) • Crutches • Reverse walker • Gait trainer (a device which is more supportive than a walker but less supportive than a wheelchair) • Wheelchair Walking sticks (canes) may be single or triple-pronged (three-point). Triple-pronged walking sticks provide more support if the person has balance issues. There are also quadruple-pronged (four-point) walking sticks for even greater support. One or two walking sticks or crutches may be used. Wheelchairs may be self-propelled or power-assisted.

Baclofen	Used for tone reduction, baclofen is a medication that can be delivered either orally or using a pump connected to a catheter which delivers the drug directly to the intrathecal area (the space between the spinal cord and the protective sheath surrounding it). The latter is termed intrathecal baclofen (ITB).
Bilateral CP	Both sides of the body are affected.
Body mass index (BMI)	Body mass index (BMI) is a weight-to-height ratio that is calculated by dividing a person's body mass by the square of their body height. Feet/inches and pounds or kilograms and meters can be used (though the US and metric systems cannot be mixed). The CDC offers a guide to BMI at cdc.gov/healthyweight/assessing/index.html.
Botulinum neurotoxin A (BoNT-A)	Botulinum neurotoxin A (BoNT-A) is a treatment used to decrease spasticity. It is delivered as an injection.
Cardiometabolic	Concerning both heart disease and metabolic (biochemical) disorders such as diabetes.
Casting	Casting consists of putting a joint in a plaster of Paris or fiberglass cast (for example, a below-knee cast) for sustained passive stretching of the joint.
Centers for Disease Control and Prevention (CDC)	The Centers for Disease Control and Prevention (CDC) is the national public health institute in the US.
Cerebral	Referring to the cerebrum, the front and upper part of the brain, one of the major areas responsible for the control of movement.
Cohort study	A cohort study is a form of longitudinal study that samples a cohort (a group of people who share a defining characteristic, for example a group of children with spastic diplegia), collecting data at intervals over time.
Conductive education	Conductive education is based on an educational rather than a medical model for the treatment of children with CP. It combines educational and rehabilitation goals into a single program. It was developed in Hungary but is now practiced in centers around the world.
Contracture	A contracture is a limitation of the range of motion (ROM) of a joint. The contracture occurs in the muscle-tendon unit (MTU) and/or capsule of the joint, not just the muscle.

Crouch gait	Crouch gait can be defined as persistent flexed-knee gait. The exact degree of knee flexion that constitutes crouch gait varies in the literature but is typically greater than or equal to 20 degrees. This knee flexion is normally also accompanied by persistent hip flexion. The foot position can be variable; it can either be in plantar flexion (the child is on their toes) or dorsiflexion (the child has flat feet and flexed knees).
Diplegia	Diplegia means affecting the two lower limbs. The lower limbs are much more affected, but the upper limbs usually still have some involvement.
Episode of care (EOC)	An episode of care (EOC) is a period of therapy (at the appropriate frequency) followed by a therapy break.
Fine motor function	Fine motor function (or fine motor skills or fine motor activities) refers to smaller movements that occur in the wrists, hands, fingers, feet, and toes. It involves the control of small muscles. Examples include picking up objects between the thumb and forefinger and writing. These movements typically involve hand-eye coordination and require a high degree of precision of hand and finger movement.
Gait	Gait is a person's manner of walking.
Gait analysis	Gait analysis provides detailed information about a person's manner of walking and how much it deviates from typical walking.
Gross motor function	Gross motor function (or gross motor skills or gross motor activities) refers to the movement of the arms, legs, and other large body parts. It involves the use of large muscles. Examples include sitting, crawling, standing, running, jumping, swimming, throwing, catching, and kicking. These movements involve maintaining balance and changing position.
Gross Motor Function Classification System (GMFCS)	The Gross Motor Function Classification System (GMFCS) is a five-level classification system that describes the functional mobilities of children and adolescents with CP. Level I has the fewest limitations and level V has the greatest. It provides an indication of the severity of CP.
Hemiplegia	Hemiplegia means affecting the upper and lower limbs on one side of the body. The upper limb is usually more affected than the lower limb.
Hypotonia/ hypertonia	See *muscle tone*.

International Classification of Functioning, Disability and Health (ICF)	The International Classification of Functioning, Disability and Health (ICF) is a universal framework for considering any health condition. It helps show the impact of a health condition at different levels and how those levels are interconnected.
Magnetic resonance imaging (MRI)	Magnetic resonance imaging (MRI) is a noninvasive imaging technology that produces detailed three-dimensional anatomical images without the use of radiation.
Moment	In biomechanics, a moment is a turning effect produced by a force (e.g., a muscle contraction) acting on a lever (the bone) about a pivot (the joint).
Muscle-tendon unit (MTU)	A combination of the muscle, tendon, and other structures is collectively known as the muscle-tendon unit (MTU).
Muscle tone	Muscle tone is the resting tension in a person's muscles. A range of "normal" muscle tone exists. Tone is considered "abnormal" when it falls outside the range of normal or typical. It can be too low (hypotonia) or too high (hypertonia). Abnormal muscle tone occurs in all types of CP. In children with spastic diplegia tone is typically too high in the legs and arms due to spasticity, but it can be low in the trunk.
Musculoskeletal	Musculoskeletal refers to both the muscles and the skeleton (i.e., the muscles, bones, and joints).
Neurology	Neurology is the branch of medicine dealing with disorders of the nervous system.
Neurosurgery	Neurosurgery is surgery performed on the nervous system, in particular the brain and spinal cord. Selective dorsal rhizotomy (SDR) and intrathecal baclofen (ITB) are two neurosurgical procedures that may be performed on people with spastic diplegia.
Occupational therapy (OT)	Occupational therapy is therapy that helps people participate in the things they want and need to do through the therapeutic use of everyday activities (occupations).
Orthopedic surgery	Orthopedic surgery is surgery performed on the musculoskeletal system: the bones, joints, muscles, ligaments, and tendons.
Orthosis	An orthosis (or brace) is a device designed to hold specific body parts in position in order to modify their structure and function. It is usually made of lightweight, custom-molded plastic or carbon fiber.
Orthotics	Orthotics is the branch of medicine concerned with the design, manufacture and management of orthoses (braces).

Osteoporosis	Osteoporosis means "porous bones" (i.e., bones with low bone density).
Palsy	Palsy means paralysis, though paralysis by pure definition is not a feature of CP.
Passive stretching	Passive stretching is when another person stretches an individual's muscle.
Pediatrics	Pediatrics is the branch of medicine dealing with children and their conditions.
Physical medicine and rehabilitation (PMR, also termed physiatry)	Physical medicine and rehabilitation (PMR, also termed physiatry) is the branch of medicine that aims to enhance and restore functional ability and quality of life among those with physical disabilities. PMR physicians treat a wide variety of medical conditions affecting the brain, spinal cord, nerves, bones, joints, ligaments, muscles, and tendons.
Physical therapy/ physiotherapy (PT)	Physical therapy is therapy that provides services that develop, maintain, and restore a person's maximum movement and functional ability. Physical therapists have different titles in different countries; in many countries they are called physiotherapists.
Pyramidal tracts	The pyramidal tracts are communication tracts that connect the brain and the spinal cord.
Quadriplegia	Quadriplegia means affecting four limbs: all four limbs and the trunk are affected. This is also known as tetraplegia.
Randomized controlled trial (RCT)	The randomized controlled trial (RCT) is the gold standard in research. An RCT is a scientific experiment that has very strict guidelines to ensure that the only aspect that makes the two groups different is that one receives the treatment and the other does not. In an RCT, people are randomly assigned to either the group receiving the treatment or the non-treatment group (also known as the control group). Comparing the outcome of the two groups allows the researcher to determine whether the treatment was effective.
Range of motion (ROM)	The range of motion (ROM), also called range of movement, of a joint is a measure of the joint's flexibility. The actual ROM through which a joint moves is measured in degrees. An instrument called a goniometer is used to measure the ROM of a joint.
Selective dorsal rhizotomy (SDR)	Selective dorsal rhizotomy (SDR) is an irreversible cutting of nerve rootlets in the spinal cord to reduce spasticity.
Single-event multilevel surgery (SEMLS)	Single-event multilevel surgery (SEMLS) involves multiple orthopedic surgical procedures performed on the lower limbs during a single operation.

Speech and language pathology (SLP, also termed speech and language therapy, SLT)	Speech and language therapy is therapy that supports those with speech, language, and communication needs as well as feeding and swallowing difficulties.
Tendon	The tendon is the cord-like structure that attaches the muscle to the bone; for example, the achilles tendon which attaches the gastrocnemius and soleus muscles (both calf muscles) to the bone at the ankle joint.
Three-dimensional computerized motion analysis (3D computerized motion analysis)	Three-dimensional computerized motion analysis (3D computeried motion analysis) provides a very detailed analysis of gait. Gait is analyzed simultaneously in three planes, hence the term "3D." The three planes are: • From back or front: coronal plane • From the side: sagittal plane • From top or bottom: transverse plane 3D computerized motion analysis is the broader term because it includes other forms of motion, such as upper body motion. Gait is just one form of motion. However, the terms "3D computerized motion analysis" and "3D computerized gait analysis" can be used interchangeably.
Tone	See *muscle tone.*
Unilateral CP	One side of the body is affected.
W-sitting	W-sitting describes the sitting position which the child with spastic diplegia (and other forms of spastic CP) adopts. The child's bottom is on the floor while their feet are out. Looking from the top, the legs form a "W" shape.

References

PREFACE
1. **Graham HK, Rosenbaum P, Paneth N, et al. (2016)** Cerebral palsy. *Nat Rev Dis Primers* 2: 1–24.
2. **Novak I (2014)** Evidence-based diagnosis, health care, and rehabilitation for children with cerebral palsy. *J Child Neurol* 29: 1141–1156.
3. **Franki I, Desloovere K, De Cat J, et al. (2012)** The evidence-base for conceptual approaches and additional therapies targeting lower-limb function in children with cerebral palsy: a systematic review using the ICF as a framework. *J Rehabil Med* 44: 396–405.
4. **Gage JR (1991)** *Gait Analysis in Cerebral Palsy*. London: Mac Keith Press.
5. **Bailes A, Gannotti M, Bellows DM, Shusterman M, Lyman J (2018)** On the journey together translating the GMFCS into practice: clinician and caregiver perspectives. AACPDM 2018 instructional course.
6. **Nieuwenhuijsen C, van der Laar Y, Donkervoort M, Nieuwstraten W, Roebroeck ME, Stam HJ (2008)** Unmet needs and health care utilization in young adults with cerebral palsy. *Disabil Rehabil* 30: 1254–1262.
7. **Murkoff H, Mazel S (1984)** *What to Expect When You're Expecting*. New York: Workman Publishing Co., Inc.
8. **Gross PH, Bailes AF, Horn SD, et al. (2018)** Setting a patient-centered research agenda for cerebral palsy: a participatory action research initiative. *Dev Med Child Neurol* 60: 1278–1284.
9. **Palisano R, Rosenbaum P, Walter S, Russell D, Wood E, Galuppi B (1997)** Development and reliability of a system to classify gross motor function in children with cerebral palsy. *Dev Med Child Neurol* 39: 214–223.
10. **Glader L, Stevenson R (2019)** *Children and Youth with Complex Cerebral Palsy*. London: Mac Keith Press.

CHAPTER 1 CEREBRAL PALSY (CP)
Section 1.1 Introduction
1. **Rosenbaum P, Paneth N, Leviton A, Goldstein M, Bax M (2007)** A report: the definition and classification of cerebral palsy April 2006. *Dev Med Child Neurol* 49 Suppl 2: 8–14.
2. **Graham HK (2014)** Cerebral palsy prevention and cure: vision or mirage? A personal view. *J Paediatr Child Health* 50: 89–90.

Section 1.2 Causes, risk factors, and prevalence
1. **World Health Organization (WHO) (2019)** *Health Topics: Risk Factors*. [online] Available at: <who.int/topics/risk_factors/en/>.

2. **Gillette Children's Specialty Healthcare (2019)** *What Is Cerebral Palsy?* [online] Available at: <gillettechildrens.org/conditions-care/cerebral-palsy/what-is-cerebral-palsy>.

3. **Nelson KB (2008)** Causative factors in cerebral palsy. *Clin Obstet Gynecol* 51: 749–762.

4. **Klebanoff MA (2009)** The collaborative perinatal project: a 50-year prospective. *Pediatr Perinat Epidemiol* 23: 2–8.

5. **Graham HK, Thomason P, Novacheck TF (2014)** Cerebral palsy. In: Weinstein SL, Flynn JM, editors, *Lovell and Winter's Pediatric Orthopedics, Level 1 and 2*. Philadelphia: Lippincott Williams & Wilkins, pp 484–554.

6. **Hadders-Algra M (2014)** Early diagnosis and early intervention in cerebral palsy. *Front Neurol* 5(185): 1–13.

7. **Graham HK, Rosenbaum P, Paneth N, et al. (2016)** Cerebral palsy. *Nat Rev Dis Primers* 2: 1–24.

8. **Rosenbaum P, Rosenbloom L (2012)** *Cerebral Palsy: From Diagnosis to Adulthood*. London: Mac Keith Press.

9. **Oskoui M, Coutinho F, Dykeman J, Jetté N, Pringsheim T (2013)** An update on the prevalence of cerebral palsy: a systematic review and meta-analysis. *Dev Med Child Neurol* 55: 509–519.

10. **Galea C, Mcintyre S, Smithers-Sheedy H, et al. (2019)** Cerebral palsy trends in Australia (1995–2009): a population-based observational study. *Dev Med Child Neurol* 61: 186–193.

11. **Australian Cerebral Palsy Register (ACPR) Group (2013)** *Australian Cerebral Palsy Register Report 2013*. [pdf] Available at: <cerebralpalsy.org.au/wp-content/uploads/2013/04/ACPR-Report_Web_2013.pdf>.

12. **National Institutes of Health (NIH) (2019)** *Estimates of Funding for Various Research, Condition, and Disease Categories (RCDC)*. [online] Available at: <report.nih.gov/categorical_spending.aspx>.

Section 1.3 Diagnosis

1. **McIntyre S, Morgan C, Walker K, Novak I (2011)** Cerebral palsy—don't delay. *Dev Disabil Res Rev* 17: 114–129.

2. **Graham HK, Rosenbaum P, Paneth N, et al. (2016)** Cerebral palsy. *Nat Rev Dis Primers* 2: 1–24.

3. **Campbell SK, Kolobe TH, Osten ET, Lenke M, Girolami GL (1995)** Construct validity of the test of infant motor performance. *Phys Ther* 75: 585–596.

4. **Novak I, Morgan C, Adde L, et al. (2017)** Early, accurate diagnosis and early intervention in cerebral palsy: advances in diagnosis and treatment. *JAMA Pediatr* 171: 897–907.

5. **Novak I (2014)** Evidence-based diagnosis, health care, and rehabilitation for children with cerebral palsy. *J Child Neurol* 29: 1141–1156.

6. **Lach LM, Rosenbaum P, Bailey S, et al. (2014)** Parenting a child with cerebral palsy: family and social issues. In: Dan B, Mayston M, Paneth N, Rosenbloom L, editors, *Cerebral Palsy: Science and Clinical Practice*. London: Mac Keith Press, pp 27–42.

7. **Wittenberg GF (2009)** Neural plasticity and treatment across the lifespan for motor deficits in cerebral palsy. *Dev Med Child Neurol* 51 Suppl 4: 130–133.

8. **Graham HK, Thomason P, Novacheck TF (2014)** Cerebral palsy. In: Weinstein SL, Flynn JM, editors, *Lovell and Winter's Pediatric Orthopedics, Level 1 and 2.* Philadelphia: Lippincott Williams & Wilkins, pp 484–554.

Section 1.4 The International Classification of Functioning, Disability and Health (ICF)

1. **WHO (2001)** *International Classification of Functioning, Disability and Health.* [online]. Available at: <who.int/classifications/icf/en/>.
2. **WHO (2002)** *Towards a Common Language for Functioning, Disability and Health.* [pdf] Available at: <who.int/classifications/icf/icfbeginnersguide.pdf>.
3. **Rosenbaum P, Paneth N, Leviton A, Goldstein M, Bax M (2007)** A report: the definition and classification of cerebral palsy April 2006. *Dev Med Child Neurol* 49 Suppl 2: 8–14.
4. **Holsbeeke L, Ketelaar M, Schoemaker MM, Gorter JW (2009)** Capacity, capability, and performance: different constructs or three of a kind? *Arch Phys Med Rehabil* 90(5): 849–855.
5. **Rosenbaum P, Gorter JW (2012)** The "F-words" in childhood disability: I swear this is how we should think! *Child Care Health Dev* 38(4): 457–463.
6. **Novak I (2014)** Evidence-based diagnosis, health care, and rehabilitation for children with cerebral palsy. *J Child Neurol* 29(8): 1141–1156.

Section 1.5 Motor function, gross motor milestones

1. **WHO Multicentre Growth Reference Study Group (2006)** WHO Motor Development Study: windows of achievement for six gross motor development milestones. *Acta Paediatr Suppl* 450: 86–95.
2. **Rosenbaum P, Rosenbloom L (2012)** *Cerebral Palsy: From Diagnosis to Adulthood.* London: Mac Keith Press.
3. **Damiano DL (2006)** Activity, activity, activity: rethinking our physical therapy approach to cerebral palsy. *Phy Ther* 86(11): 1534–1540.
4. **Russell DJ, Rosenbaum PL, Cadman DT, Gowland C, Hardy S, Jarvis S (1989)** The gross motor function measure: a means to evaluate the effects of physical therapy. *Dev Med Child Neurol* 31(3): 341–352.
5. **Russell D, Rosenbaum PL, Avery L, Lane M (2002)** *The Gross Motor Function Measure (GMFM-66 and GMFM-88) Users' Manual.* London: Mac Keith Press.

Section 1.6 Classification of CP

1. **Rosenbaum P, Rosenbloom L (2012)** *Cerebral Palsy: From Diagnosis to Adulthood.* London: Mac Keith Press.
2. **Graham HK, Rosenbaum P, Paneth N, et al. (2016)** Cerebral palsy. *Nat Rev Dis Primers* 2: 1–24.
3. **Cans C (2000)** Surveillance of cerebral palsy in Europe: a collaboration of cerebral palsy surveys and registers. *Dev Med Child Neurol* 42: 816–824.
4. **Rosenbaum P (2014)** Definition and clinical classification. In: Dan B, Mayston M, Paneth N, Rosenbloom L, editors, *Cerebral Palsy: Science and Clinical Practice.* London: Mac Keith Press, pp 17–26.
5. **Graham HK, Thomason P, Novacheck TF (2014)** Cerebral palsy. In: Weinstein SL, Flynn JM, editors, *Lovell and Winter's Pediatric Orthopedics, Level 1 and 2.* Philadelphia: Lippincott Williams & Wilkins, pp 484–554.

6. **National Institute of Neurological Disorders and Stroke (NINDS) (2019)** *Spasticity Information Page.* [pdf] Available at: <ninds.nih.gov/disorders/all-disorders/spasticity-information-page>.

7. **Lance JW (1980)** Pathophysiology of spasticity and clinical experience with baclofen. In: Feldman RG, Young RR, Koella WP, editors, *Spasticity: Disordered Motor Control.* Chicago: Year Book Medical, pp 183–203.

8. **NINDS (2019)** *Dystonias Information Page.* [pdf] Available at: <ninds.nih.gov/Disorders/All-Disorders/Dystonias-Information-Page>.

9. **NINDS (2019)** *Chorea Information Page.* [pdf] Available at: <ninds.nih.gov/Disorders/All-Disorders/Chorea-Information-Page>.

10. **NINDS (2019)** *Ataxias and Cerebellar or Spinocerebellar Degeneration Information Page.* [pdf] Available at: <ninds.nih.gov/Disorders/All-Disorders/Ataxias-and-Cerebellar-or-Spinocerebellar-Degeneration-Information-Page>.

11. **Palisano R, Rosenbaum P, Walter S, Russell D, Wood E, Galuppi B (1997)** Development and reliability of a system to classify gross motor function in children with cerebral palsy. *Dev Med Child Neurol* 39(4): 214–223.

12. **Palisano RJ, Rosenbaum P, Bartlett D, Livingston MH (2008)** Content validity of the expanded and revised Gross Motor Function Classification System. *Dev Med Child Neurol* 50: 744–750.

13. **Alriksson-Schmidt A, Nordmark E, Czuba T, Westbom L (2017)** Stability of the Gross Motor Function Classification System in children and adolescents with cerebral palsy: a retrospective cohort registry study. *Dev Med Child Neurol* 59: 641–646.

14. **Morris C, Galuppi BE, Rosenbaum PL (2004)** Reliability of family report for the Gross Motor Function Classification System. *Dev Med Child Neurol* 46(7): 455–460.

15. **Kinsner-Ovaskainen A, Lanzoni M, Delobel M, Ehlinger V, Arnaud C, Martin S (2017)** *Surveillance of Cerebral Palsy in Europe: Development of the JRC-SCPE Central Database and Public Health Indicators.* [pdf] Available at: <publications.jrc.ec.europa.eu/repository/bitstream/JRC109418/kjna28935enn.pdf>.

16. **McCormick A, Brien M, Plourde J, et al. (2007)** Stability of the Gross Motor Function Classification System in adults with cerebral palsy. *Dev Med Child Neurol* 49: 265–269.

17. **Gorter JW, Rosenbaum PL, Hanna SE, et al. (2004)** Limb distribution, motor impairment, and functional classification of cerebral palsy. *Dev Med Child Neurol* 46(7): 461–467.

18. **Himmelmann K, Beckung E, Hagberg G, Uvebrant P (2006)** Gross and fine motor function and accompanying impairments in cerebral palsy. *Dev Med Child Neurol* 48(6): 417–523.

19. **Shevell MI, Dagenais L, Hall N; REPACQ Consortium (2009)** The relationship of cerebral palsy subtype and functional motor impairment: a population-based study. *Dev Med Child Neurol* 51(11): 872–877.

20. **Hidecker MJC, Ho NT, Dodge N, et al. (2012)** Inter-relationships of functional status in cerebral palsy: analyzing gross motor function, manual ability, and communication function classification systems in children. *Dev Med Child Neurol* 54: 737–742.

21. **ACPR Group (2013)** *Australian Cerebral Palsy Register Report.* [pdf] Available at: <cerebralpalsy.org.au/wp-content/uploads/2013/04/ACPR-Report_Web_2013.pdf>.

22. **Eliasson AC, Krumlinde-Sundholm L, Rösblad B, et al. (2006)** The Manual Ability Classification System (MACS) for children with cerebral palsy: scale development and evidence of validity and reliability. *Dev Med Child Neurol* 48: 549–554.

23. **Eliasson AC, Ullenhag A, Wahlström U, Krumlinde-Sundholm L (2017)** Mini-MACS: development of the Manual Ability Classification System for children younger than 4 years of age with signs of cerebral palsy. *Dev Med Child Neurol* 59(1): 72–78.

24. **Hidecker MJC, Paneth N, Rosenbaum PL, et al. (2011)** Developing and validating the Communication Function Classification System (CFCS) for individuals with cerebral palsy. *Dev Med Child Neurol* 53(8): 704–710.

25. **Shevell M (2018)** Cerebral palsy to cerebral palsy spectrum disorder: Time for a name change. *Neurology* (epub ahead of print).

26. **Rosenbaum PL, Walter SD, Hanna SE, et al. (2002)** Prognosis for gross motor function in cerebral palsy. *JAMA* 288(11): 1357–1363.

27. **Hanna SE, Bartlett DJ, Rivard LM, Russell DJ (2008)** Reference curves for the Gross Motor Function Measure: percentiles for clinical description and tracking over time among children with cerebral palsy. *Phys Ther* 88(5): 596–607.

CHAPTER 2 SPASTIC DIPLEGIA—BILATERAL CP

Section 2.1 Introduction

1. **Gage JR (1991)** *Gait Analysis in Cerebral Palsy.* London: Mac Keith Press.

2. **Horstmann HM, Bleck EE (2007)** *Orthopedic Management in Cerebral Palsy.* London: Mac Keith Press.

Section 2.2 The brain injury

1. **Gage JR (1991)** *Gait Analysis in Cerebral Palsy.* London: Mac Keith Press.

2. **Hadders-Algra M (2014)** Early diagnosis and early intervention in cerebral palsy. *Front Neurol* 5(185): 1–13.

3. **Graham HK, Rosenbaum P, Paneth N, et al. (2016)** Cerebral palsy. *Nat Rev Dis Primers* 2: 1–24.

4. **Wittenberg GF (2009)** Neural plasticity and treatment across the lifespan for motor deficits in cerebral palsy. *Dev Med Child Neurol* 51 Suppl 4: 130–133.

5. **Novak I, McIntyre S, Morgan C, et al. (2013)** A systematic review of interventions for children with cerebral palsy: state of the evidence. *Dev Med Child Neurol* 55: 885–910.

Section 2.3 Growth

1. **Centers for Disease Control and Prevention (CDC) (2001)** *Birth to 36 Months: Boys.* [pdf] Available at: <cdc.gov/growthcharts/data/set1clinical/cj41l017.pdf>.

2. **Keogh J, Sugden DA (1985)** *Movement Skill Development.* London: Macmillan.

3. **CDC (2015)** *BAM! Body and Mind.* [online] Available at: <cdc.gov/bam/body/body-qa.html#3>.

4. **Day SM, Strauss DJ, Vachon PJ, Rosenbloom L, Shavelle RM, Wu YW (2007)** Growth patterns in a population of children and adolescents with cerebral palsy. *Dev Med Child Neurol* 49: 167–171.

5. **Brooks J, Day S, Shavelle R, Strauss D (2011)** Low weight, morbidity, and mortality in children with cerebral palsy: new clinical growth charts. *Pediatrics* 128(2): e299–307.

6. **CDC (2000)** *2 to 20 Years: Girls.* [pdf] Available at: <u>cdc.gov/growthcharts/data/set2clinical/cj41c072.pdf</u>.

7. **CDC (2001)** *2 to 20 Years: Boys.* [pdf] Available at: <u>cdc.gov/growthcharts/data/set1clinical/cj41l021.pdf</u>.

8. **Wright CM, Reynolds L, Ingram E, Cole TJ, Brooks J (2017)** Validation of US cerebral palsy growth charts using a UK cohort. *Dev Med Child Neurol* 59(9): 933–938.

Section 2.4 Bones, muscles, joints, and movements

1. **Kendall FP, Kendall McCreary E, Provance PG, McIntyre Rodgers M, Romani WA (2005)** *Muscles: Testing and Function, with Posture and Pain.* Baltimore: Lippincott Williams & Wilkins.

2. **Hislop HJ, Montgomery J (1995)** *Daniels and Worthingham's Muscle Testing Techniques of Manual Examination.* Philadelphia: WB Saunders Company.

3. **Khot A, Sloan S, Desai S, Harvey A, Wolfe R, Graham HK (2008)** Adductor release and chemodenervation in children with cerebral palsy: a pilot study in 16 children. *J Child Orthop* 2(4): 293–299.

4. **Stout JL, Novacheck TF, Gage JR, Schwartz MH (2009)** Treatment of crouch gait. In: Gage JR, Schwartz MH, Koop SE, Novacheck TF, editors, *The Identification and Treatment of Gait Problems in Cerebral Palsy.* London: Mac Keith Press, pp 555–578.

5. **Van Campenhout A, Bar-On L, Desloovere K, Huenaerts C, Molenaers G (2015)** Motor endplate-targeted botulinum toxin injections of the gracilis muscle in children with cerebral palsy. *Dev Med Child Neurol* 57(5): 476–483.

Section 2.5 Normal walking

1. **Gage JR, Schwartz MH (2009)** Normal gait. In: Gage JR, Schwartz MH, Koop SE, Novacheck TF, editors, *The Identification and Treatment of Gait Problems in Cerebral Palsy.* London: Mac Keith Press, pp 31–64.

Section 2.6 Primary abnormalities

1. **Gage JR (1991)** *Gait Analysis in Cerebral Palsy.* London: Mac Keith Press.

2. **Gage JR, Novacheck TF (2001)** An update on the treatment of gait problems in cerebral palsy. *J Ped Orthop B* 10: 265–274.

3. **Graham HK, Rosenbaum P, Paneth N, et al. (2016)** Cerebral palsy. *Nat Rev Dis Primers* 2: 1–24.

4. **Gage JR, Schwartz MH (2009)** Consequences of brain injury on musculoskeletal development. In: Gage JR, Schwartz MH, Koop SE, Novacheck TF, editors, *The Identification and Treatment of Gait Problems in Cerebral Palsy.* London: Mac Keith Press, pp 107–129.

5. **Dewar R, Love S, Johnston LM (2015)** Exercise interventions improve postural control in children with cerebral palsy: a systematic review. *Dev Med Child Neurol* 57(6): 504–420.

6. **NINDS (2019)** *Spasticity Information Page.* [pdf] Available at: <u>ninds.nih.gov/disorders/all-disorders/spasticity-information-page</u>.

7. **Lance JW (1980)** Pathophysiology of spasticity and clinical experience with baclofen. In: Feldman RG, Young RR, Koella WP, editors, *Spasticity: Disordered Motor Control.* Chicago: Year Book Medical, pp 183–203.

8. **Khot A, Sloan S, Desai S, Harvey A, Wolfe R, Graham HK (2008)** Adductor release and chemodenervation in children with cerebral palsy: a pilot study in 16 children. *J Child Orthop* 2(4): 293–299.

9. **Stout JL, Novacheck TF, Gage JR, Schwartz MH (2009)** Treatment of crouch gait. In: Gage JR, Schwartz MH, Koop SE, Novacheck TF, editors, *The Identification and Treatment of Gait Problems in Cerebral Palsy.* London: Mac Keith Press, pp 555–578.

10. **Van Campenhout A, Bar-On L, Desloovere K, Huenaerts C, Molenaers G (2015)** Motor endplate-targeted botulinum toxin injections of the gracilis muscle in children with cerebral palsy. *Dev Med Child Neurol* 57(5): 476–483.

11. **NINDS (2019)** *Dystonias Information Page.* [pdf] Available at: <ninds.nih.gov/Disorders/All-Disorders/Dystonias-Information-Page>.

12. **Wiley ME, Damiano DL (1998)** Lower-extremity strength profiles in spastic cerebral palsy. *Dev Med Child Neurol* 40: 100–107.

13. **Pirila S, van der Meere J, Korhonen P, et al. (2004)** A retrospective neurocognitive study in children with spastic diplegia. *Dev Neuropsychol* 26(3): 679–690.

14. **Bottcher L (2010)** Children with spastic cerebral palsy, their cognitive functioning, and social participation: a review. *Child Neuropsychol* 16: 209–228.

15. **Shevell MI, Dagenais L, Hall N; REPACQ Consortium (2009)** Comorbidities in cerebral palsy and their relationship to neurologic subtype and GMFCS level. *Neurology* 72(24): 2090–2096.

16. **Dufresne D, Dagenais L, Shevell MI; REPACQ Consortium (2014)** Spectrum of visual disorders in a population-based cerebral palsy cohort. *Pediatr Neurol* 50(4): 324–328.

17. **Zhang JY, Oskoui M, Shevell M (2015)** A population-based study of communication impairment in cerebral palsy. *J Child Neurol* 30(3): 277–284.

Section 2.7 Secondary abnormalities

1. **Yau KI, Chang MH (1993)** Growth and body composition of preterm, small-for-gestational-age infants at a postmenstrual age of 37–40 weeks. *Early Hum Dev* 33(2): 117–131.

2. **Gough M, Shortland AP (2012)** Could muscle deformity in children with spastic cerebral palsy be related to an impairment of muscle growth and altered adaptation? *Dev Med Child Neurol* 54(6): 495–499.

3. **Gage JR, Novacheck TF (2001)** An update on the treatment of gait problems in cerebral palsy. *J Ped Orthop B* 10: 265–274.

4. **Nordmark E, Hägglund G, Lauge-Pedersen H, Wagner P, Westbom L (2009)** Development of lower limb range of motion from early childhood to adolescence in cerebral palsy: a population-based study. *BMC Med* 28(7): 65.

5. **Graham HK, Rosenbaum P, Paneth N, et al. (2016)** Cerebral palsy. *Nat Rev Dis Primers* 2: 1–24.

6. **Tosi LL, Maher N, Windlow Moore D, Goldstein M, Laisen M (2009)** Adults with cerebral palsy: a workshop to define the challenges of treating and preventing secondary musculoskeletal and neuromuscular complications in this rapidly growing population. *Dev Med Child Neurol* 51 Suppl 4: 2–11.

7. **Barber L, Hastings-Ison T, Baker R, Barrett R, Lichtwark G (2011)** Medial gastrocnemius muscle volume and fascicle length in children aged 2 to 5 years with cerebral palsy. *Dev Med Child Neurol* 53(6): 543–548.

8. **Herskind A, Ritterband-Rosenbaum A, Willerslev-Olsen M, et al. (2016)** Muscle growth is reduced in 15-month-old children with cerebral palsy. *Dev Med Child Neurol* 58(5): 485–491.

9. **Graham HK, Selber P (2003)** Musculoskeletal aspects of cerebral palsy. *J Bone Joint Surg* 85-B(2): 157–166.

10. **Gage JR (1991)** *Gait Analysis in Cerebral Palsy*. London: Mac Keith Press.

11. **American Academy for Cerebral Palsy and Developmental Medicine (AACPDM) (2017)** *Hip Surveillance in Cerebral Palsy*. [online] Available at: <aacpdm.org/publications/care-pathways/hip-surveillance>.

12. **Elkamil AI, Andersen GL, Hägglund G, Lamvik T, Skranes J, Vik T (2011)** Prevalence of hip dislocation among children with cerebral palsy in regions with and without a surveillance programme: a cross sectional study in Sweden and Norway. *BMC Musculoskelet Disord* 12: 284.

13. **Soo B, Howard JJ, Boyd RN, et al. (2006)** Hip displacement in cerebral palsy. *J Bone Joint Surg Am* 88(1): 121–129.

14. **Graham HK, Thomason P, Novacheck TF (2014)** Cerebral palsy. In: Weinstein SL, Flynn JM, editors, *Lovell and Winter's Pediatric Orthopedics, Level 1 and 2*. Philadelphia: Lippincott Williams & Wilkins, pp 484–554.

15. **Walker K (2009)** Radiographic evaluation of the patient with cerebral palsy. In: Gage JR, Schwartz MH, Koop SE, Novacheck TF, editors, *The Identification and Treatment of Gait Problems in Cerebral Palsy*. London: Mac Keith Press, pp 244–259.

16. **Wise (2015)** *Orthopedic Manual Physical Therapy*. Philadelphia: F.A. Davis Company.

17. **Koop SE (2009)** Musculoskeletal growth and development. In: Gage JR, Schwartz MH, Koop SE, Novacheck TF, editors, *The Identification and Treatment of Gait Problems in Cerebral Palsy*. London: Mac Keith Press, pp 21–30.

18. **Inman VT, Ralston HJ, Todd F (1981)** *Human Walking*. Baltimore: Williams & Wilkins.

Section 2.8 Tertiary abnormalities

1. **Gage JR, Novacheck TF (2001)** An update on the treatment of gait problems in cerebral palsy. *J Ped Orthop B* 10: 265–274.

Section 2.9 Walking in individuals with spastic diplegia

1. **Stout JL (2017)** Development and analysis of gait. In: Palisano RJ, Orlin MN, Schreiber J, editors, *Campbell's Physical Therapy for Children*. St. Louis: Elsevier, Chapter 34 (online only).

2. **Palisano RJ, Rosenbaum P, Bartlett D, Livingston MH (2008)** Content validity of the expanded and revised Gross Motor Function Classification System. *Dev Med Child Neurol* 50: 744–750.

3. **Rodda JM, Graham HK, Carson L, Galea MP, Wolfe R (2004)** Sagittal gait patterns in spastic diplegia. *J Bone Joint Surg Br* 86(2): 251–258.

4. **Steele KM, Shuman BR, Schwartz MH (2017)** Crouch severity is a poor predictor of elevated oxygen consumption in cerebral palsy. *J Biomech* 60: 170–174.

5. **Rethlefsen SA, Blumstein G, Kay RM, Dorey F, Wren TAL (2017)** Prevalence of specific gait abnormalities in children with cerebral palsy revisited: influence of age, prior surgery, and Gross Motor Function Classification System level. *Dev Med Child Neurol* 59: 79–88.

6. **Õunpuu S, Gorton G, Bagley A, et al. (2015)** Variation in kinematic and spatiotemporal gait parameters by Gross Motor Function Classification System level in children and adolescents with cerebral palsy. *Dev Med Child Neurol* 57: 955–962.

7. **Johnson DC, Damiano DL, Abel MF (1997)** The evolution of gait in childhood and adolescent cerebral palsy. *J Pediatr Orthop* 17(3): 392–396.

8. **Bell KJ, Õunpuu S, DeLuca PA, Romness MJ (2002)** Natural progression of gait in children with cerebral palsy. *J Pediatr Orthop* 22: 677–682.

9. **Gough M, Eve LC, Robinson RO, Shortland AP (2004)** Short-term outcome of multilevel surgical intervention in spastic diplegic cerebral palsy compared with the natural history. *Dev Med Child Neurol* 46: 91–97.

10. **Stout JL, Novacheck TF, Gage JR, Schwartz MH (2009)** Treatment of crouch gait. In: Gage JR, Schwartz MH, Koop SE, Novacheck TF, editors, *The Identification and Treatment of Gait Problems in Cerebral Palsy*. London: Mac Keith Press, pp 555–578.

11. **Rozumalski A, Schwartz MH (2009)** Crouch gait patterns defined using k-means cluster analysis are related to underlying clinical pathology. *Gait Posture* 30(2): 155–160.

12. **Gage JR (1991)** *Gait Analysis in Cerebral Palsy*. London: Mac Keith Press.

CHAPTER 3 MANAGEMENT AND TREATMENT OF SPASTIC DIPLEGIA—BILATERAL CP TO AGE 20

Section 3.1 Introduction

1. **Rosenbaum P, Rosenbloom L, Mayston M (2012)** Therapists and therapies in cerebral palsy. In: Rosenbaum P, Rosenbloom L, editors, *Cerebral Palsy: From Diagnosis to Adulthood*. London: Mac Keith Press, pp 124–148.

Section 3.2 What does best practice look like?

1. **Gillette Children's Specialty Healthcare (2016a)** *Therapy Care Planning: Episodes of Care*. Unpublished patient leaflet.

2. **Stivers T (2012)** Physician-child interaction: when children answer physicians' questions in routine medical encounters. *Patient Educ Couns* 87(1): 3–9.

3. **Martinek TJ (1996)** Fostering hope in youth: A model for explaining learned helplessness in physical activity. *Quest* 48: 409–421.

4. **Jahnsen R, Villien L, Aamodt G, Stanghelle JK, Holm I (2003)** Physiotherapy and physical activity—experiences of adults with cerebral palsy, with implications for children. *Adv Physiother* 5: 21–32.

5. **CanChild (2019)** *Family-Centred Service*. [online] Available at: <canchild.ca/en/research-in-practice/family-centred-service>.

6. **Sackett DL, Rosenberg WM, Gray JA, Haynes RB, Richardson WS (1996)** Evidence based medicine: what it is and what it is not. *BMJ* 312: 71–72.

7. **Palisano RJ (2006)** A collaborative model of service delivery for children with movement disorders: a framework for evidence-based decision making. *Phys Ther* 86: 1295–1305.

8. **Mayston M (2018)** More studies are needed in paediatric neurodisability. (Editorial) *Dev Med Child Neurol* 60(10): 966.

9. **Morris ZS, Wooding S, Grant J (2011)** The answer is 17 years, what is the question: understanding time lags in translational research. *J R Soc Med* 104(12): 510–520.

10. **Deville C, McEwen I, Arnold SH, Jones M, Zhao YD (2015)** Knowledge translation of the Gross Motor Function Classification System among pediatric physical therapists. *Pediatr Phys Ther* 27(4): 376–384.

11. **Bailes AF, Gannotti M, Bellows DM, Shusterman M, Lyman J, Horn SD (2018)** Caregiver knowledge and preferences for gross motor function information in cerebral palsy. *Dev Med Child Neurol* 60(12): 1264–1270.

12. **Thomason P, Baker R, Dodd K, et al. (2011)** Single-event multilevel surgery in children with spastic diplegia: a pilot randomized controlled trial. *J Bone Joint Surg Am* 93: 451–460.

13. **Gross PH, Bailes AF, Horn SD, et al. (2018)** Setting a patient-centered research agenda for cerebral palsy: a participatory action research initiative. *Dev Med Child Neurol* 60: 1278–1284.

14. **Gillette Children's Specialty Healthcare (2016b)** *Cerebral Palsy Road Map: What to Expect as Your Child Grows.* [pdf] Available at: <gillettechildrens.org/assets/uploads/care-and-conditions/CP_Roadmap.pdf>.

15. **Wallwiener M, Brucker SY, Wallwiener D, Steering Committee (2012)** Multidisciplinary breast centres in Germany: a review and update of quality assurance through benchmarking and certification. *Arch Gynecol Obstet* 285(6): 1671–1683.

16. **Gage JR (1991)** *Gait Analysis in Cerebral Palsy.* London: Mac Keith Press.

17. **Keogh J, Sugden DA (1985)** *Movement Skill Development.* London: Macmillan.

18. **Chiarello L, Catalino T (2017)** Infants, toddlers, and their families: early intervention services under IDEA. In: Palisano RJ, Orlin MN, Schreiber J, editors, *Campbell's Physical Therapy for Children.* St. Louis: Elsevier, pp 703–722.

19. **Löwing K, Bexelius A, Brogren Carlberg E (2009)** Activity focused and goal directed therapy for children with cerebral palsy—do goals make a difference? *Disabil Rehabil* 31(22): 1808–1816.

20. **Phoenix M, Rosenbaum P (2014)** Development and implementation of a pediatric rehabilitation care path for hard-to-reach families: a case report. *Child Care Health Develop* 41 (3): 494–499.

21. **Vroland-Nordstrand K, Eliasson A-C, Jacobsson H, Johansson U, Krumlinde-Sundholm L (2016)** Can children identify and achieve goals for intervention? A randomized trial comparing two goal-setting approaches. *Dev Med Child Neurol* 58: 589–596.

22. **Rosenbaum P, Rosenbloom L (2012)** *Cerebral Palsy: From Diagnosis to Adulthood.* London: Mac Keith Press.

Section 3.3 Therapies

1. **Rosenbaum P, Rosenbloom L, Mayston M (2012)** Therapists and therapies in cerebral palsy. In: Rosenbaum P, Rosenbloom L, editors, *Cerebral Palsy: From Diagnosis to Adulthood*. London: Mac Keith Press, pp 124–148.

2. **World Confederation for Physical Therapy (WCPT) (2019)** [online] Available at: <wcpt.org>.

3. **Damiano DL (2006)** Activity, activity, activity: rethinking our physical therapy approach to cerebral palsy. *Phy Ther* 86(11): 1534–1540.

4. **American Physical Therapy Association (APTA) (2012)** *Intensity of Service in an Outpatient Setting for Children with Chronic Conditions*. [pdf] Available at: <pediatricapta.org/includes/fact-sheets/pdfs/12%20Intensity%20of%20Service.pdf>.

5. **Franki I, Desloovere K, De Cat J, et al. (2012)** The evidence-base for conceptual approaches and additional therapies targeting lower-limb function in children with cerebral palsy: a systematic review using the ICF as a framework. *J Rehabil Med* 44(5): 396–405.

6. **Novak I, McIntyre S, Morgan C, et al. (2013)** A systematic review of interventions for children with cerebral palsy: state of the evidence. *Dev Med Child Neurol* 55: 885–910.

7. **Ziring PR, Brazdziunas D, Cooley WC, et al. (1999)** American Academy of Pediatrics. Committee on Children with Disabilities. The treatment of neurologically impaired children using patterning. *Pediatrics* 104(5 pt1): 1149–1151.

8. **Pin T, Dyke P, Chan M (2006)** The effectiveness of passive stretching in children with cerebral palsy. *Dev Med Child Neurol* 48(10): 855–862.

9. **Graham HK, Rosenbaum P, Paneth N, et al. (2016)** Cerebral palsy. *Nat Rev Dis Primers* 2: 1–24.

10. **Gorter JW, Becher J, Oosterom I, et al. (2007)** To stretch or not to stretch in children with cerebral palsy. *Dev Med Child Neurol* 49(10): 797–800.

11. **Wiley ME, Damiano DL (1998)** Lower-extremity strength profiles in spastic cerebral palsy. *Dev Med Child Neurol* 40: 100–107.

12. **Damiano DL, Arnold AS, Steele KM, Delp SL (2010)** Can strength training predictably improve gait kinematics? A pilot study on the effects of hip and knee extensor strengthening on lower-extremity alignment in cerebral palsy. *Phys Ther* 90(2): 269–279.

13. **Dodd KJ, Taylor NF, Damiano DL (2002)** A systematic review of the effectiveness of strength-training programs for people with cerebral palsy. *Arch Phys Med Rehabil* 83(8): 1157–1164.

14. **Scholtes VA, Becher JG, Janssen-Potten YJ, Dekkers H, Smallenbroek L, Dallmeijer AJ (2012)** Effectiveness of functional progressive resistance exercise training on walking ability in children with cerebral palsy: a randomized controlled trial. *Res Dev Disabil* 33(1): 181–188.

15. **Taylor NF, Dodd KJ, Baker RJ, Willoughby K, Thomason P, Graham HK (2013)** Progressive resistance training and mobility-related function in young people with cerebral palsy: a randomized controlled trial. *Dev Med Child Neurol* 55(9): 806–812.

16. **Stout JL (2017)** Physical fitness during childhood and adolescence. In: Palisano RJ, Orlin MN, Schreiber J, editors, *Campbell's Physical Therapy for Children.* St. Louis: Elsevier, pp 117–144.

17. **Damiano DL (2014)** Progressive resistance.exercise increases strength but does not improve objective measures of mobility in young people with cerebral palsy. *J Physiother* 60: 58.

18. **Orlin MN, Pierce SR, Stackhouse CL, et al. (2005)** Immediate effect of percutaneous intramuscular stimulation during gait in children with cerebral palsy: a feasibility study. *Dev Med Child Neurol* 47(10): 684–690.

19. **Postans NJ, Granat MH (2005)** Effect of functional electrical stimulation, applied during walking, on gait in spastic cerebral palsy. *Dev Med Child Neurol* 47(1): 46–52.

20. **Van der Linden ML, Hazlewood ME, Hillman SJ, Robb JE (2008)** Functional electrical stimulation to the dorsiflexors and quadriceps in children with cerebral palsy. *Pediatr Phys Ther* 20(1): 23–29.

21. **Prosser LA, Curatalo LA, Alter KE, Damiano DL (2012)** Acceptability and potential effectiveness of a foot drop stimulator in children and adolescents with cerebral palsy. *Dev Med Child Neurol* 54(11): 1044–1049.

22. **American Occupational Therapy Association (AOTA) (2019)** *Patients & Clients: Learn about Occupational Therapy.* [online] Available at: <aota.org/About-Occupational-Therapy/Patients-Clients.aspx>.

23. **Royal College of Speech and Language Therapists (RCSLT) (2017)** *Speech and Language Therapy.* [pdf] Available at: <rcslt.org/speech_and_language_therapy/slt_work_settings/justice_slcn/justice_evidence_base2017>.

24. **AACPDM (n.d.)** *Executive Function in Individuals with Cerebral Palsy, Spina Bifida, and Brain Injury.* [pdf] Available at: <aacpdm.org/UserFiles/file/ExecutiveFunctionFactSheet.pdf>.

25. **Bailes AF, Reder R, Burch C (2008)** Development of guidelines for determining frequency of therapy services in a pediatric medical setting. *Pediatr Phys Ther* 20(2): 194–198.

26. **Gillette Children's Specialty Healthcare (2016)** *Rehabilitation Therapies Episodes of Care in Childhood and Adolescence.* [pdf] Available at: <gillettechildrens.org/assets/uploads/care-and-conditions/Episodes_of_Care-English.pdf>.

27. **Lowe A, Schmit J, Wenz A, Harpster K (2015)** *Saddling up for Episodic Care: Presentation Background.* [pdf] Available at: <aacpdm.org/UserFiles/file/BRK7-Lowe.pdf>.

Section 3.4 The home program

1. **Novak I, McIntyre S, Morgan C, et al. (2013)** A systematic review of interventions for children with cerebral palsy: state of the evidence. *Dev Med Child Neurol* 55: 885–910.

2. **Graham HK, Rosenbaum P, Paneth N, et al. (2016)** Cerebral palsy. *Nat Rev Dis Primers* 2: 1–24.

3. **American Council on Exercise (2015)** *Physical Activity vs. Exercise: What's the Difference?* [online] Available at: <acefitness.org/education-and-resources/lifestyle/blog/5460/physical-activity-vs-exercise-what-s-the-difference>.

4.   O'Neil ME, Fragala-Pinkham M, Lennon N, George A, Forman J, Trost SG (2016) Reliability and validity of objective measures of physical activity in youth with cerebral palsy who are ambulatory. *Phys Ther* 96(1): 37–45.

5.   Bjornson K, Fiss A, Avery L, et al. (2019) Longitudinal trajectories of physical activity and walking performance by gross motor function classification system level for children with cerebral palsy. *Disabil Rehabil* (epub ahead of print).

6.   Bjornson KF, Zhou C, Stevenson R, Christakis D, Song K (2014) Walking activity patterns in youth with cerebral palsy and youth developing typically. *Disabil Rehabil* 36(15): 1279–1284.

7.   Obeid J, Balemans AC, Noorduyn SG, Gorter JW, Timmons BW (2014) Objectively measured sedentary time in youth with cerebral palsy compared with age, sex, and season-matched youth who are developing typically: an explorative study. *Phys Ther* 94(8): 1163–1167.

8.   Maltais DB, Pierrynowski MR, Galea VA, Bar-Or O (2005) Physical activity level is associated with the O2 cost of walking in cerebral palsy. *Med Sci Sports Exerc* 37(3): 347–353.

9.   Ryan JM, Hensey O, McLoughlin B, Lyons A, Gormley J (2014) Reduced moderate-to-vigorous physical activity and increased sedentary behavior are associated with elevated blood pressure values in children with cerebral palsy. *Phys Ther* 94(8): 1144–1153.

10. Slaman J, Roebroeck M, Dallmijer A, et al. (2014) Can a lifestyle intervention program improve physical behavior among adolescents and young adults with spastic cerebral palsy? A randomized controlled trial. *Dev Med Child Neurol* 57(2): 159–166.

11. Maher CA, Toohey M, Ferguson M (2016) Physical activity predicts quality of life and happiness in children and adolescents with cerebral palsy. *Disabil Rehabil* 38(9): 865–869.

12. Zwinkels M, Verschuren O, Balemans A, et al. (2018) Effects of a school-based sports program on physical fitness, physical activity, and cardiometabolic health in youth with physical disabilities: data from the Sport-2-Stay-Fit study. *Front Pediatr* 6: 75.

13. Fowler EG, Kolobe TH, Damiano DL, et al. (2007) Promotion of physical fitness and prevention of secondary conditions for children with cerebral palsy: section on pediatrics research summit proceedings. *Phys Ther* 87(11): 1495–1510.

14. Verschuren O, Peterson MD, Balemans AC, Hurvitz EA (2016) Exercise and physical activity recommendations for people with cerebral palsy. *Dev Med Child Neurol* 58(8): 798–808.

15. WHO (2010) *Global Recommendations on Physical Activity for Health.* [pdf] Available at: <who.int/iris/bitstream/handle/10665/44399/9789241599979_eng.pdf;jsessionid=62E6290990EE116CAB15A883B0A96C21?sequence=1>.

16. Tipton CM (2014) The history of "Exercise Is Medicine" in ancient civilizations. *Adv Physiol Educ* 38(2): 109–117.

17. Adolph KE, Vereijken B, Shrout PE (2003) What changes in infant walking and why. *Child Dev* 74(2): 475–497.

18. Loughborough University Peter Harrison Centre for Disability Sport (n.d.) *Fit for Life.* [pdf] Available at: <lboro.ac.uk/media/wwwlboroacuk/content/peterharrison centre/downloads/brochures/pdfs/Cerebral%20Palsy%20guide_Fit_for_Life.pdf>.

19. **Loughborough University Peter Harrison Centre for Disability Sport (n.d.)** *Fit for Sport.* [pdf] Available at: <lboro.ac.uk/media/wwwlboroacuk/content/peterharrisoncentre/downloads/brochures/pdfs/Cerebral%20Palsy%20guide_Fit_for_Sport.pdf>.

20. **O'Sullivan J (2016)** "We all have limits. I am not a disabled athlete, I am a Paralympic athlete." *Irish Times* [online] Available at: <irishtimes.com/sport/we-all-have-limits-i-am-not-a-disabled-athlete-i-am-a-paralympic-athlete-1.2787039>.

21. **de Menezes J (2016)** Paralympics 2016: Four 1500m runners finish faster than Rio Olympics gold medal winning time. *Independent* [online] Available at: <independent.co.uk/sport/olympics/paralympics/paralympics-2016-abdellatif-baka-four-1500m-runners-finish-faster-olympic-gold-medal-winningtime-a7239821.html>.

22. **Shapiro J (2012)** Paralympian's pursuit enables aspiring athletes. *NPR* [online] Available at: <npr.org/2012/09/02/160382788/paralympians-pursuit-enables-aspiring-athletes>.

23. **US Paralympics (2018)** *US Olympic Committee Elevates Investment in US Paralympians.* [online] Available at: <teamusa.org/US-Paralympics/Features/2018/September/21/US-Olympic-Committee-Elevates-Investment-in-US-Paralympians>.

24. **WHO Multicentre Growth Reference Study Group (2006)** WHO Motor Development Study: windows of achievement for six gross motor development milestones. *Acta Paediatr Suppl* 450: 86–95.

25. **van der Heide JC, Hadders-Algra M (2005)** Postural muscle dyscoordination in children with cerebral palsy. *Neural Plast* 12(2-3): 197–203.

26. **Gajdosik CG, Cicirello N (2001)** Secondary conditions of the musculoskeletal system in adolescents and adults with cerebral palsy. *Phys Occup Ther Pediatr* 21(4): 49–68.

Section 3.5 Orthoses

1. **Novacheck TF, Kroll GJ, Gent G, Rozumalski A, Beattie C, Schwartz MH (2009)** Orthoses. In: Gage JR, Schwartz MH, Koop SE, Novacheck TF, editors, *The Identification and Treatment of Gait Problems in Cerebral Palsy.* London: Mac Keith Press, pp 327–348.

2. **Barr M, Dull A, Lenz A, Holtz K, Matousek S (2014)** Influence of different ankle-foot orthosis types on crouch gait: a retrospective review using computerized gait analysis. *Dev Med Child Neurol* 56 Suppl 5: 87–88.

3. **Ries AJ, Schwartz MH (2019)** Ground reaction and solid ankle-foot orthoses are equivalent for the correction of crouch gait in children with cerebral palsy. *Dev Med Child Neurol* 61(2): 219–225.

4. **Novak I, McIntyre S, Morgan C, et al. (2013)** A systematic review of interventions for children with cerebral palsy: state of the evidence. *Dev Med Child Neurol* 55: 885–910.

5. **Ries AJ, Novacheck TF, Schwartz MH (2015)** The efficacy of ankle-foot orthoses on improving the gait of children with diplegic cerebral palsy: a multiple outcome analysis. *PMR* 7(9): 922–929.

6. **Aboutorabi A, Arazpour M, Ahmadi Bani M, Saeedi H, Head JS (2017)** Efficacy of ankle foot orthoses types on walking in children with cerebral palsy: a systematic review. *Ann Phys Rehabil Med* 60(6): 393–402.

Section 3.6 Tone reduction

1. **NINDS (2019)** *Spasticity Information Page.* [pdf] Available at: <ninds.nih.gov/disorders/all-disorders/spasticity-information-page>.

2. **Lance JW (1980)** Pathophysiology of spasticity and clinical experience with baclofen. In: Feldman RG, Young RR, Koella WP, editors, *Spasticity: Disordered Motor Control.* Chicago: Year Book Medical, pp 183–203.

3. **NINDS (2019)** *Dystonias Information Page.* [pdf] Available at: <ninds.nih.gov/Disorders/All-Disorders/Dystonias-Information-Page>.

4. **Grunt S, Graham Fieggen A, Jeroen Vermeulen R, Becher JG, Langerak NG (2014)** Selection criteria for selective dorsal rhizotomy in children with spastic cerebral palsy: a systematic review of the literature. *Dev Med Child Neurol* 56: 302–312.

5. **Nicolini-Panisson RDA, Tedesco AP, Folle MR, Donadio MVF (2018)** Selective dorsal rhizotomy in cerebral palsy: selection criteria and postoperative physical therapy protocols. *Rev Paul Pediatr* 36(1): 100–108.

6. **Wang KK, Munger ME, Chen BP, Novacheck TF (2018)** Selective dorsal rhizotomy in ambulant children with cerebral palsy. *J Child Orthop* 12(5): 413–427.

7. **Ward M (2009)** Pharmacologic treatment with oral medications. In: Gage JR, Schwartz MH, Koop SE, Novacheck TF, editors, *The Identification and Treatment of Gait Problems in Cerebral Palsy.* London: Mac Keith Press, pp 349–362.

8. **Novak I, McIntyre S, Morgan C, et al. (2013)** A systematic review of interventions for children with cerebral palsy: state of the evidence. *Dev Med Child Neurol* 55: 885–910.

9. **Molenaers G, Desloovere K (2009)** Pharmacologic treatment with botulinum toxin. In: Gage JR, Schwartz MH, Koop SE, Novacheck TF, editors, *The Identification and Treatment of Gait Problems in Cerebral Palsy.* London: Mac Keith Press, pp 363–380.

10. **Gillette (2013)** *Managing Spasticity.* Unpublished patient leaflet.

11. **Graham HK, Thomason P, Novacheck TF (2014)** Cerebral palsy. In: Weinstein SL, Flynn JM, editors, *Lovell and Winter's Pediatric Orthopedics, Level 1 and 2.* Philadelphia: Lippincott Williams & Wilkins, pp 484–554.

12. **Love SC, Novak I, Kentish M, et al. (2010)** Botulinum toxin assessment, intervention and after-care for lower-limb spasticity in children with cerebral palsy: international consensus statement. *Eur J Neurol* 17(2): 9–37.

13. **Delgado MR, Hirtz D, Aisen M, et al. (2010)** Practice parameter: pharmacologic treatment of spasticity in children and adolescents with cerebral palsy (an evidence-based review). *Neurol* 74: 336–343.

14. **Molenaers G, Fagard K, Van Campenhout A, Desloovere K (2013)** Botulinum toxin: a treatment of the lower extremities in children with cerebral palsy. *J Child Orthop* 7(5): 383–387.

15. **Williams SA, Elliott C, Valentine J, Gubbay A, Shipman P, Reid S (2013)** Combining strength training and botulinum neurotoxin intervention in children with cerebral palsy: the impact on muscle morphology and strength. *Disabil Rehabil* 35(7): 596–605.

16. **Fortuna R, Horisberger M, Vaz MA, Herzog W (2013)** Do skeletal muscle properties recover following repeat onabotulinum toxin A injections? *J Biomech* 46(14): 2426–2433.

17. **Fortuna R, Vaz MA, Sawatsky A, Hart DA, Herzog W (2015)** A clinically relevant BTX-A injection protocol leads to persistent weakness, contractile material loss, and an altered mRNA expression phenotype in rabbit quadriceps muscles. *J Biomech* 48(10): 1700–1706.

18. **Mathevon L, Michel F, Decavel P, et al. (2015)** Muscle structure and stiffness assessment after botulinum toxin type A injection: a systematic review. *Ann Phys Rehabil Med* 58: 343–350.

19. **Valentine J, Stannage K, Fabian V, et al. (2016)** Muscle histopathology in children with spastic cerebral palsy receiving botulinum toxin type A. *Muscle Nerve* 53(3): 407–414.

20. **Graham HK, Rosenbaum P, Paneth N, et al. (2016)** Cerebral palsy. *Nat Rev Dis Primers* 2: 1–24.

21. **Alexander C, Elliott C, Valentine J, et al. (2018)** Muscle volume alterations after first botulinum neurotoxin A treatment in children with cerebral palsy: a 6-month prospective cohort study. *Dev Med Child Neurol* 60(11): 1165–1171.

22. **Schless SH, Cenni F, Bar-On L, et al. (2019)** Medial gastrocnemius volume and echo-intensity after botulinum neurotoxin A interventions in children with spastic cerebral palsy. *Dev Med Child Neurol* 61(7): 783–790.

23. **Gough M, Fairhurst C, Shortland AP (2005)** Botulinum toxin and cerebral palsy: time for reflection? *Dev Med Child Neurol* 47(10): 709–712.

24. **Barrett RS (2011)** What are the long-term consequences of botulinum toxin injections in spastic cerebral palsy? (Commentary) *Dev Med Child Neurol* 53(6): 485.

25. **Krach LE (2009)** Treatment of spasticity with intrathecal baclofen. In: Gage JR, Schwartz MH, Koop SE, Novacheck TF, editors, *The Identification and Treatment of Gait Problems in Cerebral Palsy*. London: Mac Keith Press, pp 383–396.

26. **Hasnat MJ, Rice JE (2015)** Intrathecal baclofen for treating spasticity in children with cerebral palsy. *Cochrane Database Syst Rev* 11 (CD004552).

27. **Georgiadis AG, Schwartz MH, Walt K, Ward ME, Kim PD, Novacheck TF (2017)** Team approach: single-event multilevel surgery in ambulatory patients with cerebral palsy. *JBJS Rev* 5(8): e10.

28. **Langerak NG, Tam N, Vaughan CL, Graham Fieggen A, Schwartz MH (2012)** Gait status 17–26 years after selective dorsal rhizotomy. *Gait Posture* 35: 244–249.

29. **Bolster EA, van Schie PE, Becher JG, van Ouwerkerk WJ, Strijers RL, Vermeulen RJ (2013)** Long-term effect of selective dorsal rhizotomy on gross motor function in ambulant children with spastic bilateral cerebral palsy, compared with reference centiles. *Dev Med Child Neurol* 55(7): 610–616.

30. **Munger ME, Aldahondo N, Krach LE, Novacheck TF, Schwartz MH (2017)** Long-term outcomes after selective dorsal rhizotomy: a retrospective matched cohort study. *Dev Med Child Neurol* 59(11): 1196–1203.

Section 3.7 Orthopedic surgery

1. **Thomason P, Rodda J, Willoughby K, Graham HK (2014)** Lower limb function. In: Dan B, Mayston M, Paneth N, Rosenbloom L, editors, *Cerebral Palsy: Science and Clinical Practice*. London: Mac Keith Press, pp 461–488.

2. **Molenaers G, Desloovere K (2009)** Pharmacologic treatment with botulinum toxin. In: Gage JR, Schwartz MH, Koop SE, Novacheck TF, editors, *The Identification and Treatment of Gait Problems in Cerebral Palsy.* London: Mac Keith Press, pp 363–380.
3. **Molenaers G, Desloovere K, De Cat J, et al. (2001)** Single event multilevel botulinum toxin type A treatment and surgery: similarities and differences. *Eur J Neurol* 8 Suppl 5: 88–97.
4. **Saraph V, Zwick EB, Zwick G, Steinwender C, Steinwender G, Linhart W (2002)** Multilevel surgery in spastic diplegia: evaluation by physical examination and gait analysis in 25 children. *J Pediatr Orthop* 22(2): 150–157.
5. **Graham HK, Selber P (2003)** Musculoskeletal aspects of cerebral palsy. *J Bone Joint Surg* 85-B(2) 157–166.
6. **Schwartz MH, Viehweger E, Stout J, Novacheck TF, Gage JR (2004)** Comprehensive treatment of ambulatory children with cerebral palsy: an outcome assessment. *J Pediatr Orthop* 24(1): 45–53.
7. **Graham HK, Thomason P, Novacheck TF (2014)** Cerebral palsy. In: Weinstein SL, Flynn JM, editors, *Lovell and Winter's Pediatric Orthopedics, Level 1 and 2.* Philadelphia: Lippincott Williams & Wilkins, 484–554.
8. **Gage JR (1991)** *Gait Analysis in Cerebral Palsy.* London: Mac Keith Press.
9. **Rethlefsen SA, Blumstein G, Kay RM, Dorey F, Wren TAL (2017)** Prevalence of specific gait abnormalities in children with cerebral palsy revisited: influence of age, prior surgery, and Gross Motor Function Classification System level. *Dev Med Child Neurol* 59: 79–88.
10. **Dreher T, Thomason P, Švehlík M, et al. (2018)** Long-term development of gait after multilevel surgery in children with cerebral palsy: a multicentre cohort study. *Dev Med Child Neurol* 60: 88–93.
11. **Rang M (1990)** Cerebral palsy. In: Morrissy R, editor, *Pediatric Orthopedics.* Philadelphia: Lippincott, pp 465–506.
12. **Thomason P, Baker R, Dodd K, et al. (2011)** Single-event multilevel surgery in children with spastic diplegia: a pilot randomized controlled trial. *J Bone Joint Surg Am* 93: 451–460.
13. **Narayanan U, Davidson B, Weir S. (2011)** Gait Outcomes Assessment List (The GOAL): developing a meaningful outcome measure for ambulatory children with cerebral palsy. *Dev Med Child Neurol* 53 Suppl 5: 79.
14. **Thomason P, Tan A, Donnan A, Rodda J, Graham HK, Narayanan U (2018)** The Gait Outcomes Assessment List (GOAL): validation of a new assessment of gait function for children with cerebral palsy. *Dev Med Child Neurol* 60(6): 618–623.
15. **Johnson DC, Damiano DL, Abel MF (1997)** The evolution of gait in childhood and adolescent cerebral palsy. *J Pediatr Orthop* 17(3): 392–396.
16. **Bell KJ, Õunpuu S, DeLuca PA, Romness MJ (2002)** Natural progression of gait in children with cerebral palsy. *J Pediatr Orthop* 22: 677–682.
17. **Gough M, Eve LC, Robinson RO, Shortland AP (2004)** Short-term outcome of multilevel surgical intervention in spastic diplegic cerebral palsy compared with the natural history. *Dev Med Child Neurol* 46: 91–97.
18. **Vuillermin C, Rodda J, Rutz E, Shore BJ, Smith K, Graham HK (2011)** Severe crouch gait in spastic diplegia can be prevented: a population-based study. *J Bone Joint Surg Br* 93(12): 1670–1675.

19. **McGinley JL, Dobson F, Ganeshalingam R, Shore BJ, Rutz E, Graham HK (2012)** Single-event multilevel surgery for children with cerebral palsy: a systematic review. *Dev Med Child Neurol* 54: 117–128.

20. **van Bommel EEH, Arts MME, Jongerius PH, Ratter J, Rameckers EAA (2019)** Physical therapy treatment in children with cerebral palsy after single-event multilevel surgery: a qualitative systematic review. A first step towards a clinical guideline for physical therapy after single-event multilevel surgery. *Ther Adv Chronic Dis* Jul 5: 10 (eCollection 2019).

21. **Colvin, C, Greve, K, Lehn, C, Menner, M, Tally, M, Thomas, M (2018)** *Division of Occupational Therapy and Physical Therapy, Cincinnati Children's Hospital Medical Center: Evidence-Based Clinical Care Guideline for Physical Therapy Management of Single Event Multi-Level Surgeries (SEMLS) for Children, Adolescents, and Young Adults with Cerebral Palsy or Other Similar Neuromotor Conditions.* [pdf] Available at: <cincinnatichildrens.org/service/j/anderson-center/evidence-based-care/recommendations>. (Click "Browse by topic" and look under "SEMLS.")

22. **Gorton GE, Abel MF, Oeffinger DJ, et al. (2009)** A prospective cohort study of the effects of lower extremity orthopedic surgery on outcome measures in ambulatory children with cerebral palsy. *J Pediatr Orthop* 29(8): 903–909.

23. **Thomason P, Selber P, Graham HK (2013)** Single event multilevel surgery in children with bilateral spastic cerebral palsy: a 5 year prospective cohort study. *Gait Posture* 37: 23–28.

24. **Amirmudin NA, Lavelle G, Theologis T, Thompson N, Ryan JM (2019)** Multilevel surgery for children with cerebral palsy: a meta-analysis. *Pediatrics* 143(4) e20183390.

25. **Gillette Children's Specialty Healthcare (2014)** *Gait and Motion Analysis for Treatment Planning and Outcomes Assessment.* [pdf] Available at: <gillettechildrens.org/assets/uploads/care-and-conditions/Gait_Lab_Outcome_Report_-_Final.pdf>.

26. **Delp SL, Statler K, Carroll NC (1995)** Preserving plantar flexion strength after surgical treatment for contracture of the triceps surae: a computer simulation study. *J Orthop Res* 13: 96–104.

27. **Rodda JM, Graham HK, Carson L, Galea MP, Wolfe R (2004)** Sagittal gait patterns in spastic diplegia. *J Bone Joint Surg Br* 86(2): 251–258.

28. **Rodda JM, Graham HK, Nattrass GR, Galea MP, Baker R, Wolfe R (2006)** Correction of severe crouch gait in patients with spastic diplegia with use of multilevel orthopaedic surgery. *J Bone Joint Surg Am* 88(12): 2653–2664.

29. **Stout JL, Gage JR, Schwartz MH, Novacheck TF (2008)** Distal femoral extension osteotomy and patellar tendon advancement to treat persistent crouch gait in cerebral palsy. *J Bone Joint Surg Am* 90: 2470–2484.

30. **Zwick EB, Saraph V, Linhart WE, Steinwender G (2001)** Propulsive function during gait in diplegic children: evaluation after surgery for gait improvement. *J Pediatr Orthop B* 10(3): 226–233.

31. **Gage JR, Novacheck TF (2001)** An update on the treatment of gait problems in cerebral palsy. *J Ped Orthop B* 10: 265–274.

Section 3.8 The overall musculoskeletal management plan to age 20

1. **Thomason P, Rodda J, Willoughby K, Graham HK (2014)** Lower limb function. In: Dan B, Mayston M, Paneth N, Rosenbloom L, editors, *Cerebral Palsy: Science and Clinical Practice*. London: Mac Keith Press, pp 461–488.

2. **Rutz E, Thomason P, Willoughby K, Graham HK (2018)** Integrated management in cerebral palsy: musculoskeletal surgery and rehabilitation in ambulatory patients. In: Panteliadis CP, editor, *Cerebral Palsy: A Multidisciplinary Approach*. Cham: Springer International Publishing AG, pp 229–251.

3. **Graham HK, Thomason P, Novacheck TF (2014)** Cerebral palsy. In: Weinstein SL, Flynn JM, editors, *Lovell and Winter's Pediatric Orthopedics, Level 1 and 2*. Philadelphia: Lippincott Williams & Wilkins, pp 484–554.

4. **Thomason P, Selber P, Graham HK (2013)** Single event multilevel surgery in children with bilateral spastic cerebral palsy: a 5 year prospective cohort study. *Gait Posture* 37: 23–28.

5. **Dreher T, Thomason P, Švehlík M, et al. (2018)** Long-term development of gait after multilevel surgery in children with cerebral palsy: a multicentre cohort study. *Dev Med Child Neurol* 60: 88–93.

Section 3.9 Alternative and complementary treatments

1. **Majnemer A, Shikako-Thomas K, Shevell MI, et al. (2013)** Pursuit of complementary and alternative medicine treatments in adolescents with cerebral palsy. *J Child Neurol* 28(11): 1443–1447.

2. **Novak I, McIntyre S, Morgan C, et al. (2013)** A systematic review of interventions for children with cerebral palsy: state of the evidence. *Dev Med Child Neurol* 55: 885–910.

3. **Franki I, Desloovere K, De Cat J, et al. (2012)** The evidence-base for basic physical therapy techniques targeting lower-limb function in children with cerebral palsy: a systematic review using the International Classification of Functioning, Disability and Health as a conceptual framework. *J Rehabil Med* 44: 385–395.

4. **Beldick S, Fehlings MG (2017)** *Current State of Stem Cell Treatments for Cerebral Palsy: A Guide for Patients, Families, and Service Providers*. [online] Available at: <canchild.ca/en/resources/276-current-state-of-stem-cell-treatments-for-cerebral-palsy-a-guide-for-patients-families-and-service-providers>.

5. **Graham HK, Rosenbaum P, Paneth N, et al. (2016)** Cerebral palsy. *Nat Rev Dis Primers* 2: 1–24.

6. **Dan B (2016)** Stem cell therapy for cerebral palsy. (Editorial) *Dev Med Child Neurol* 58(5): 424.

7. **Novak I, Walker K, Hunt RW, Wallace EM, Fahey M, Badawi N (2016)** Concise review: stem cell interventions for people with cerebral palsy: systematic review with meta-analysis. *Stem Cells Translational Medicine* 5: 1014–1025.

8. **Wagenaar N, Nijboer CH, van Bel F (2017)** Repair of neonatal brain injury: bringing stem cell-based therapy into clinical practice. *Dev Med Child Neurol* 59(10): 997–1003.

9. **Graham HK (2014)** Cerebral palsy prevention and cure: vision or mirage? A personal view. *J Paediatr Child Health* 50(2): 89–90.

Section 3.10 What the parent can do to help the child, what the adolescent can do to help themselves

1. **Lach LM, Rosenbaum P, Bailey S, Bogossian A, MacCulloch R (2014)** Parenting a child with cerebral palsy: family and social issues. In: Dan B, Mayston M, Paneth N, Rosenbloom L, editors, *Cerebral Palsy: Science and Clinical Practice*. London: Mac Keith Press, pp 27–41.

2. **Rosenbaum P, Rosenbloom L (2012)** *Cerebral Palsy: From Diagnosis to Adulthood*. London: Mac Keith Press.

3. **Verschuren O, McPhee P, Rosenbaum P, Gorter JW (2016)** The formula for health and well-being in individuals with cerebral palsy: physical activity, sleep, and nutrition. *Dev Med Child Neurol* 58(9): 989–990.

4. **Mergler S (2018)** Bone status in cerebral palsy. In: Panteliadis CP, editor, *Cerebral Palsy: A Multidisciplinary Approach*. Cham: Springer International Publishing AG, pp 253–257.

5. **Mus-Peters CTR, Huisstede BMA, Noten S, Hitters MWMGC, van der Slot WMA, van den Berg-Emons RJG (2018)** Low bone mineral density in ambulatory persons with cerebral palsy? A systematic review. *Disabil Rehabil* 22: 1–11.

6. **Damiano DL (2006)** Activity, activity, activity: rethinking our physical therapy approach to cerebral palsy. *Phy Ther* 86(11): 1534–1540.

7. **United Nations (1990)** *Convention on the Rights of the Child*. [online] Available at: <ohchr.org/en/professionalinterest/pages/crc.aspx>.

8. **UNESCO (2017)** *School Violence and Bullying Global Status Report*. [online] Available at: <unesdoc.unesco.org/ark:/48223/pf0000246970? posInSet=1&queryId=N-EXPLORE-8864b64c-4b12-445e-a56d-b655a1a86afd>.

9. **Lindsay S, McPherson AC (2012a)** Experiences of social exclusion and bullying at school among children and youth with cerebral palsy. *Disabil Rehabil* 34(2): 101–109.

10. **Lindsay S, McPherson AC (2012b)** Strategies for improving disability awareness and social inclusion of children and young people with cerebral palsy. *Child Care Health Dev* 38(6): 809–816.

11. **Tindal SR (2017)** Students with mild cerebral palsy in the classroom: information and guidelines for teachers. *Papers & Publications: Interdisciplinary Journal of Undergraduate Research* 6(14): 70–78.

12. **Dickinson HO, Parkinson KN, Ravens-Sieberer U, et al. (2007)** Self-reported quality of life of 8-12-year-old children with cerebral palsy: a cross-sectional European study. *Lancet* 369(9580): 2171–2178.

13. **Colver A, Rapp M, Eisemann N, et al. (2015)** Self-reported quality of life of adolescents with cerebral palsy: a cross-sectional and longitudinal analysis. *Lancet* 385(9969): 705–716.

14. **Wehmeyer ML, Palmer SB (2003)** Adult outcomes for students with cognitive disabilities three years after high school: the impact of self-determination. *Educ Train Dev Disabil* 38(2): 131–144.

15. **Thomason P, Graham HK (2013)** Rehabilitation of children with cerebral palsy after single-event multilevel surgery. In: Robert Iansek R, Morris ME, editors, *Rehabilitation in Movement Disorders*. Cambridge: Cambridge University Press, pp 203–217.

16. **King GA, Cathers T, Miller Polgar J, MacKinnon E, Havens L (2000)** Success in life for older adolescents with cerebral palsy. *Qualitative Health Research* 10 (6): 734–749.

CHAPTER 4 THE ADULT WITH SPASTIC DIPLEGIA—BILATERAL CP
Section 4.1 Introduction

1. **Strauss D, Brooks J, Rosenbloom L, Shavelle R (2008)** Life expectancy in cerebral palsy: an update. *Dev Med Child Neurol* 50(7): 487–493.
2. **Graham HK, Rosenbaum P, Paneth N, et al. (2016)** Cerebral palsy. *Nat Rev Dis Primers* 2: 1–24.
3. **Novak I (2014)** Evidence-based diagnosis, health care, and rehabilitation for children with cerebral palsy. *J Child Neurol* 29(8): 1141–1156.
4. **WHO (2013)** *HIV/AIDS: Definition of Key Terms.* [online] Available at: <who.int/hiv/pub/guidelines/arv2013/intro/keyterms/en/>.
5. **Liptak GS (2008)** Health and well being of adults with cerebral palsy. *Curr Opin Neurol* 21: 136–142.
6. **CDC (2018)** *Disability and Health Related Conditions.* [online] Available at: <cdc.gov/ncbddd/disabilityandhealth/relatedconditions.html>.
7. **Novak I, Walker K, Hunt RW, Wallace EM, Fahey M, Badawi N (2016)** Concise review: stem cell interventions for people with cerebral palsy: systematic review with meta-analysis. *Stem Cells Transl Med* 5: 1014–1025.
8. **Wu YW, Mehravari AS, Numis AL, Gross P (2015)** Cerebral palsy research funding from the National Institutes of Health, 2001 to 2013. *Dev Med Child Neurol* 57: 936–941.
9. **NIH (2019)** *Estimates of Funding for Various Research, Condition, and Disease Categories (RCDC).* [online] Available at: <report.nih.gov/categorical_spending.aspx>.
10. **Thorpe D (2009)** The role of fitness in health and disease: status of adults with cerebral palsy. *Dev Med Child Neurol* 51 Suppl 4: 52–58.
11. **Tosi LL, Maher N, Windlow Moore D, Goldstein M, Laisen M (2009)** Adults with cerebral palsy: a workshop to define the challenges of treating and preventing secondary musculoskeletal and neuromuscular complications in this rapidly growing population. *Dev Med Child Neurol* 51 Suppl 4: 2–11.

Section 4.2 Aging in the typical population

1. **Santilli V, Bernetti A, Mangone M, Paoloni M (2014)** Clinical definition of sarcopenia. *Clin Cases Miner Bone Metab* 11(3): 177–180.
2. **Ni Lochlainn M, Bowyer RCE, Steves CJ (2018)** Dietary protein and muscle in aging people: the potential role of the gut microbiome. *Nutrients* 10(7): E929.
3. **Bauer J, Biolo G, Cederholm T, et al. (2013)** Evidence-based recommendations for optimal dietary protein intake in older people: a position paper from the PROT-AGE Study Group. *J Am Med Dir Assoc* 14(8): 542–559.
4. **Karaguzel G, Holick MF (2010)** Diagnosis and treatment of osteopenia. *Rev Endocr Metab Disord* 11(4): 237–251.
5. **National Institute of Arthritis and Musculoskeletal and Skin Diseases (NIAMS) (2016)** *Osteoporosis.* [online] Available at: <niams.nih.gov/health-topics/osteoporosis#tab-overview>.

6. **Mergler S (2018)** Bone status in cerebral palsy. In: Panteliadis CP, editor, *Cerebral Palsy: A Multidisciplinary Approach*. Cham: Springer International Publishing AG, pp 253–257.

7. **WHO (2018)** *Noncommunicable diseases*. [online] Available at: <who.int/news-room/fact-sheets/detail/noncommunicable-diseases>.

8. **WHO (2019)** *Health Topics: Risk Factors*. [online]. Available at: <who.int/topics/risk_factors/en/>.

9. **WHO (2013)** *Global Action Plan for the Prevention and Control of Noncommunicable Diseases 2013–2020*. [pdf] Available at: <who.int/iris/bitstream/handle/10665/94384/9789241506236_eng.pdf>.

10. **WHO (2009)** *Global Health Risks*. [pdf]. Available at: <who.int/healthinfo/global_burden_disease/GlobalHealthRisks_report_full.pdf>.

11. **Crowley C, Lodge HS (2004)** *Younger Next Year*. New York: Workman Publishing Company, Inc.

12. **Rauch J (2018)** *The Happiness Curve: Why Life Gets Better after Midlife*. London: Bloomsbury Publishing.

Section 4.3 Aging with spastic diplegia

1. **Sheridan KJ (2009)** Osteoporosis in adults with cerebral palsy. *Dev Med Child Neurol* 51 Suppl 4: 38–51.

2. **Thomason P, Graham HK (2009)** Consequences of interventions. In: Gage JR, Schwartz MH, Koop SE, Novacheck TF, editors, *The Identification and Treatment of Gait Problems in Cerebral Palsy*. London: Mac Keith Press, pp 605–623.

3. **Nooijen C, Slaman J, van der Slot W, et al. (2014)** Health-related physical fitness of ambulatory adolescents and young adults with spastic cerebral palsy. *J Rehabil Med* 46: 642–647.

4. **Gillett JG, Lichtwark GA, Boyd RN, Barber LA (2018)** Functional capacity in adults with cerebral palsy: lower limb muscle strength matters. *Arch Phys Med Rehabil* 99: 900–906.

5. **Peterson MD, Ryan JM, Hurvitz EA, Mahmoudi E (2015)** Research letter—chronic conditions in adults with cerebral palsy. *JAMA* 14 (21): 2303–2305.

6. **O'Connell NE, Smith KJ, Peterson MD, et al. (2019)** Incidence of osteoarthritis, osteoporosis and inflammatory musculoskeletal diseases in adults with cerebral palsy: A population-based cohort study. *Bone* 125: 30–35.

7. **Morgan P, McGinley J (2014)** Gait function and decline in adults with cerebral palsy: a systematic review. *Disabil Rehabil* 36(1): 1–9.

8. **Thorpe D (2009)** The role of fitness in health and disease: status of adults with cerebral palsy. *Dev Med Child Neurol* 51 Suppl 4: 52–58.

9. **Murphy KP (2010)** The adult with cerebral palsy. *Orthop Clin N Am* 41: 595–605.

10. **Opheim A, Jahnsen R, Olsson E, Stanghelle JK (2012)** Balance in relation to walking deterioration in adults with spastic bilateral cerebral palsy. *Phys Ther* 92(2): 279–288.

11. **Whitney DG, Alford AI, Devlin MJ, Caird MS, Hurvitz EA, Peterson MD (2019)** Adults with cerebral palsy have higher prevalence of fracture compared with adults without cerebral palsy independent of osteoporosis and cardiometabolic diseases. *J Bone Miner Res* (epub ahead of print).

12. Jahnsen R, Villien L, Aamodt G, Stanghelle JK, Holm I (2004) Musculoskeletal pain in adults with cerebral palsy compared with the general population. *J Rehabil Med* 36: 78–84.

13. Van Der Slot WM, Nieuwenhuijsen C, Van Den Berg-Emons RJ, et al. (2012) Chronic pain, fatigue, and depressive symptoms in adults with spastic bilateral cerebral palsy. *Dev Med Child Neurol* 54(9): 836–842.

14. Liptak GS (2008) Health and well being of adults with cerebral palsy. *Curr Opin Neurol* 21: 136–142.

15. Van der Slot WM, Roebroeck ME, Nieuwenhuijsen C, et al. (2013) Cardiovascular disease risk in adults with spastic bilateral cerebral palsy. *J Rehabil Med* 45(9): 866–872.

16. Ryan JM, Crowley VE, Hensey O, Broderick JM, McGahey A, Gormley J (2014) Habitual physical activity and cardiometabolic risk factors in adults with cerebral palsy. *Res Dev Disabil* 35(9): 1995–2002.

17. Cremer N, Hurvitz EA, Peterson MD (2017) Multimorbidity in middle-aged adults with cerebral palsy. *Am J Med* 130(6): 744.e9–744.e15.

18. Ryan JM, Allen E, Gormley J, Hurvitz EA, Peterson MD (2018) The risk, burden, and management of non-communicable diseases in cerebral palsy: a scoping review. *Dev Med Child Neurol* 60: 753–764.

19. Peterson MD, Kamdar N, Hurvitz EA (2019) Age-related trends in cardiometabolic disease among adults with cerebral palsy. *Dev Med Child Neurol* 61(4): 484–489.

20. Heyn PC, Tagawa A, Pan Z, Thomas S, Carollo JJ (2019) Prevalence of metabolic syndrome and cardiovascular disease risk factors in adults with cerebral palsy. *Dev Med Child Neurol* 61(4): 477–483.

21. Ryan JM, Peterson MD, Ryan N, et al. (2019) Mortality due to cardiovascular disease, respiratory disease, and cancer in adults with cerebral palsy. *Dev Med Child Neurol* 61(8): 924–928.

22. McPhee PG, Claridge EA, Noorduyn SG, Gorter JW (2019) Cardiovascular disease and related risk factors in adults with cerebral palsy: a systematic review. *Dev Med Child Neurol* 61(8): 915–923.

23. Jahnsen R, Villien L, Stanghelle JK, Holm I (2003) Fatigue in adults with cerebral palsy in Norway compared with the general population. *Dev Med Child Neurol* 45(5): 296–303.

24. Lundh S, Nasic S, Riad J (2018) Fatigue, quality of life and walking ability in adults with cerebral palsy. *Gait Posture* 61: 1–6.

25. McPhee PG, Brunton LK, Timmons BW, Bentley T, Gorter JW (2017) Fatigue and its relationship with physical activity, age, and body composition in adults with cerebral palsy. *Dev Med Child Neurol* 59(4): 367–373.

26. Jahnsen R, Villien L, Aamodt G, Stanghelle JK, Holm I (2003) Physiotherapy and physical activity—experiences of adults with cerebral palsy, with implications for children. *Adv Physiother* 5: 21–32.

27. Russchen HA, Slaman J, Stam HJ, et al. (2014) Focus on fatigue amongst young adults with spastic cerebral palsy. *J Neuroeng Rehabil* 11: 161.

28. NIH (2018) *Depression*. [online] Available at: <nimh.nih.gov/health/topics/depression/index.shtml>.

29. **Gannotti ME, Gorton GE 3rd, Nahorniak MT, Masso PD (2013)** Gait and participation outcomes in adults with cerebral palsy: a series of case studies using mixed methods. *Disabil Health J* 6(3): 244–252.

30. **NIH (2018)** *Anxiety Disorders.* [online] Available at: <nimh.nih.gov/health/topics/anxiety-disorders/index.shtml>.

31. **Smith KJ, Peterson MD, O'Connell NE, et al. (2019)** Risk of depression and anxiety in adults with cerebral palsy. *JAMA Neurol* 76(3): 294–300.

32. **The World Health Organization Quality of Life (WHOQOL) (1995)** The World Health Organization Quality of Life assessment: position paper from the World Health Organization. *Soc Sci Med* 41(10): 1403–1409.

33. **Rosenbaum P, Rosenbloom L (2012)** *Cerebral Palsy: From Diagnosis to Adulthood.* London: Mac Keith Press.

34. **Munger ME, Aldahondo N, Krach LE, Novacheck TF, Schwartz MH (2017)** Long-term outcomes after selective dorsal rhizotomy: a retrospective matched cohort study. *Dev Med Child Neurol* 59(11): 1196–1203.

35. **Boyer ER, Stout JL, Laine JC, et al. (2018)** Long-term outcomes of distal femoral extension osteotomy and patellar tendon advancement in individuals with cerebral palsy. *J Bone Joint Surg Am*100(1): 31–41.

36. **Van der Slot WM, Nieuwenhuijsen C, van den Berg-Emons RJ, et al. (2010)** Participation and health-related quality of life in adults with spastic bilateral cerebral palsy and the role of self-efficacy. *J Rehabil Med* 42(6): 528–535.

37. **Verhoef JA, Bramsen I, Miedema HS, Stam HJ, Roebroeck ME; Transition and Lifespan Research Group South West Netherlands (2014)** Development of work participation in young adults with cerebral palsy: a longitudinal study. *J Rehabil Med* 46(7): 648–655.

38. **Opheim A, Jahnsen R, Olsson E, Stanghelle JK (2011)** Physical and mental components of health-related quality of life and musculoskeletal pain sites over seven years in adults with spastic cerebral palsy. *J Rehabil Med* 43(5): 382–387.

39. **Boucher N, Dumas F, Maltais DB, Richards CL (2010)** The influence of selected personal and environmental factors on leisure activities in adults with cerebral palsy. *Disabil Rehabil* 32(16): 1328–1338.

40. **National Center for Health Statistics (2012)** *Healthy People 2010 Final Review.* [pdf] Available at: <cdc.gov/nchs/data/hpdata2010/hp2010_final_review.pdf>.

41. **Wiegerink DJ, Roebroeck ME, van der Slot WM, Stam HJ, Cohen-Kettenis PT; South West Netherlands Transition Research Group (2010)** Importance of peers and dating in the development of romantic relationships and sexual activity of young adults with cerebral palsy. *Dev Med Child Neurol* 52(6): 576–582.

42. **Wiegerink D, Roebroeck M, Bender J, Stam H, Cohen-Kettenis P, Transition Research Group South West Netherlands (2011)** Sexuality of young adults with cerebral palsy: experienced limitations and needs. *Sex Disabil* 29(2): 119–128.

43. **Nieuwenhuijsen C, van der Laar Y, Donkervoort M, Nieuwstraten W, Roebroeck ME, Stam HJ (2008)** Unmet needs and health care utilization in young adults with cerebral palsy. *Disabil Rehabil* 30(17): 1254–1262.

44. **Freeman M, Stewart D, Cunningham CE, Gorter JW (2018)** "If I had been given that information back then": an interpretive description exploring the information needs of adults with cerebral palsy looking back on their transition to adulthood. *Child Care Health Dev* 44(5): 689–696.

45. **O'Brien G, Bass A, Rosenbloom L (2009)** Cerebral palsy and aging. In: O'Brien G, Rosenbloom L, editors, *Developmental Disability and Aging*. London: Mac Keith Press, pp 39–52.

Section 4.4 Management and treatment of spastic diplegia in adulthood

1. **Jahnsen R, Villien L, Aamodt G, Stanghelle JK, Holm I (2003)** Physiotherapy and physical activity—experiences of adults with cerebral palsy, with implications for children. *Adv Physiother* 5: 21–32.

2. **Hilberink SR, Roebroeck ME, Nieuwstraten W, Jalink L, Verheijden JM, Stam HJ (2007)** Health issues in young adults with cerebral palsy: towards a life-span perspective. *J Rehabil Med* 39(8): 605–611.

3. **Liptak GS (2008)** Health and well being of adults with cerebral palsy. *Curr Opin Neurol* 21: 136–142.

4. **Ryan JM, Crowley VE, Hensey O, McGahey A, Gormley J (2014)** Waist circumference provides an indication of numerous cardiometabolic risk factors in adults with cerebral palsy. *Arch Phys Med Rehabil* 95(8): 1540–1546.

5. **Putz C, Döderlein L, Mertens EM, et al. (2016)** Multilevel surgery in adults with cerebral palsy. *Bone Joint J* 98-B(2): 282–288.

6. **Cassidy C, Campbell N, Madady M, Payne M (2016)** Bridging the gap: the role of physiatrists in caring for adults with cerebral palsy. *Disabil Rehabil* 38(5): 493–498.

7. **Tosi LL, Maher N, Windlow Moore D, Goldstein M, Laisen M (2009)** Adults with cerebral palsy: a workshop to define the challenges of treating and preventing secondary musculoskeletal and neuromuscular complications in this rapidly growing population. *Dev Med Child Neurol* 51 Suppl 4: 2–11.

8. **Gajdosik CG, Cicirello N (2001)** Secondary conditions of the musculoskeletal system in adolescents and adults with cerebral palsy. *Phys Occup Ther Pediatr* 21(4): 49–68.

9. **Murphy KP (2018)** Cerebral palsy, non-communicable diseases, and lifespan care. (Commentary) *Dev Med Child Neurol* 60(8): 733.

10. **Rosenbaum P (2019)** Diagnosis in developmental disability: a perennial challenge, and a proposed middle ground. (Editorial) *Dev Med Child Neurol* 61(6): 620.

11. **Imms C, Dodd KJ (2010)** What is cerebral palsy? In: Dodd KJ, Imms C, Taylor NF, editors, *Physiotherapy and Occupational Therapy for People with Cerebral Palsy: A Problem-Based Approach to Assessment and Management*. London: Mac Keith Press, pp 7–30.

12. **Ryan JM, Allen E, Gormley J, Hurvitz EA, Peterson MD (2018)** The risk, burden, and management of non-communicable diseases in cerebral palsy: a scoping review. *Dev Med Child Neurol* 60: 753–764.

13. **Sheridan (2019)** Personal communication.

14. **Rosenbaum P, Rosenbloom L, Mayston M (2012)** Therapists and therapies in cerebral palsy. In: Rosenbaum P, Rosenbloom L, editors, *Cerebral Palsy: From Diagnosis to Adulthood*. London: Mac Keith Press, pp 124–148.

15. **Louw A, Diener I, Butler DS, Puentedura EJ (2011)** The effect of neuroscience education on pain, disability, anxiety, and stress in chronic musculoskeletal pain. *Arch Phys Med Rehabil* 92(12): 2041–2056.

16. **Moseley GL, Butler DS (2015)** Fifteen years of experiencing pain: the past, present, and future. *J Pain* 16(9): 807–813.
17. **O'Brien G, Bass A, Rosenbloom L (2009)** Cerebral palsy and aging. In: O'Brien G, Rosenbloom L, editors, *Developmental Disability and Aging*. London: Mac Keith Press, pp 39–52.
18. **Maanum G, Jahnsen R, Stanghelle JK, Sandvik L, Keller A (2011)** Effects of botulinum toxin A in ambulant adults with spastic cerebral palsy: a randomized double-blind placebo controlled-trial. *J Rehabil Med* 43(4): 338–347.
19. **Reynolds MR, Ray WZ, Strom RG, Blackburn SL, Lee A, Park TS (2011)** Clinical outcomes after selective dorsal rhizotomy in an adult population. *World Neurosurg* 75(1): 138–144.
20. **Thomason P, Graham HK (2013)** Rehabilitation of children with cerebral palsy after single-event multilevel surgery. In: Robert Iansek R, Morris ME, editors, *Rehabilitation in Movement Disorders*. Cambridge: Cambridge University Press, pp 203–217.
21. **Murphy KP (2010)** The adult with cerebral palsy. *Orthop Clin N Am* 41: 595–605.
22. **Gannotti ME, Gorton GE 3rd, Nahorniak MT, Masso PD (2013)** Gait and participation outcomes in adults with cerebral palsy: a series of case studies using mixed methods. *Disabil Health J* 6(3): 244–252.
23. **WHO (2010)** *Global Recommendations on Physical Activity for Health*. [pdf] Available at: <who.int/iris/bitstream/handle/10665/44399/9789241599979_eng.pdf;jsessionid=62E6290990EE116CAB15A883B0A96C21?sequence=1>.
24. **Peterson MD, Gordon PM, Hurvitz EA (2013)** Chronic disease risk among adults with cerebral palsy: the role of premature sarcopoenia, obesity and sedentary behavior. *Obes Rev* 14(2): 171–182.
25. **Morgan P, McGinley J (2014)** Gait function and decline in adults with cerebral palsy: a systematic review. *Disabil Rehabil* 36(1): 1–9.
26. **Verschuren O, Peterson MD, Balemans AC, Hurvitz EA (2016)** Exercise and physical activity recommendations for people with cerebral palsy. *Dev Med Child Neurol* 58(8): 798–808.
27. **Garber CE, Blissmer B, Deschenes MR, et al. (2011)** American College of Sports Medicine position stand. Quantity and quality of exercise for developing and maintaining cardiorespiratory, musculoskeletal, and neuromotor fitness in apparently healthy adults: guidance for prescribing exercise. *Med Sci Sports Exerc* 43(7): 1334–1359.

Index

Abbreviations used in index: CP cerebral palsy, AFO ankle-foot orthosis
Figures and tables indicated by page numbers in italics

A

abducted forefoot, *50, 92, 92*

Achilles tendon, 64–65, 186–87

active movement, 84, 129. *See also* exercise and physical activity

activity and activity limitation, 18, 25, 83. *See also* exercise and physical activity; International Classification of Functioning, Disability and Health (ICF); physical therapy (PT)/physiotherapy

acupuncture, *198*

aerobic (cardiorespiratory) exercise, *149*, 249

aging, spastic diplegia, 228–39; introduction, 228–30; areas of unmet need, 238–39; civil status, 237; employment, 237; falls, 232; fatigue, depression, and anxiety, 235–36; fractures, 233; having children, 238; health-related quality of life (HRQoL), 236; mobility, 231–32; musculoskeletal decline, 230–31; noncommunicable diseases (NCDs), 233–34, *234*; osteoarthritis, 231; osteoporosis, 231, 242; pain, 233; participation, 236–38; quality of life (QoL), 236; sarcopenia, 230–31

aging, typical population, 222–27; introduction, 222–23; healthy aging, 226–27; noncommunicable diseases (NCDs), 225–26; osteoporosis, *224*, 224–25; sarcopenia, 223

alternative and complementary treatments, 197–200, *198–99*

ankle dorsiflexion (ankle dorsiflexors), 67

ankle-foot orthosis (AFO), 161–64

ankle plantar flexion (ankle plantar flexors), 66

anterior pelvic tilt, *49*

anxiety, 235–36

articulated AFO, 161–62

assistive mobility devices, 98, 131, 244–45

ataxic CP (ataxia), 30, *31*

B

baclofen: intrathecal baclofen (ITB), *167*, 171–72, 245; oral baclofen, *167*, 168–69

balance: dogs for, 245; poor balance, 75, 82; posterior balance, *49*

bilateral CP, 29, 30, *30, 31*, 37. *See also* spastic diplegia

body mass index (BMI), 226n107

botulinum neurotoxin A (BoNT-A) injection, *167*, 169–70, 194, 245

brain injury, 4–5, 53–55, *54*. *See also* periventricular leukomalacia (PVL)

C

cardiometabolic risk factors, 226

cardiorespiratory (aerobic) exercise, *149*, 249

cardiovascular disease, 223, 225–26, 233–34

case series, 271

casting, 84, 128–29

cerebral palsy (CP), 1–45; introduction, 2–6; causes and risk factors, 7–10; classification, 27–43; definition, 2–3, *3–4*, 239; diagnosis, 12–15; gender and, 11; prevalence, 10–11; research and funding, 11, 220–21, 247

children, having, 238

chondromalacia, 100

chorco-athetotic CP (choreo-athetosis), *31*

civil status, 237

clonus, 76

cohort study, 271

Communication Function Classification System (CFCS), 38–40, *38–39*

complementary and alternative treatments, 197–200, *198–99*

constraint-induced movement therapy (CIMT), 55

contractures: abnormal bone development and, 86; abnormal muscle growth and, 81–84; in adulthood, 231; crouch gait and, 99, 100, 102; growth and, 58; management and treatment, 109, 193; orthopedic surgery and, 186; orthoses and, 158, 159, 163; selective dorsal rhizotomy (SDR) and, 174; stretching for, 127
cranial osteopathy, *198*
crouch gait, 97, 99–103, 164, 186–87, 235

D

dantrolene sodium, 168–69
decision-making, data-driven, 115–16
depression, 235
diagnosis, for CP, 12–15
diazepam, 168–69
diplegia. *See* spastic diplegia
dogs, balance, 245
driving, 243
dynamic AFO (DAFO), 164
dyskinetic CP (dyskinesia), 30, *31*
dystonic CP (dystonia): definition, *31*, 77; tone reduction and, 172, 174, 194

E

early intervention, 13, 23, 78n44, 118
electrical stimulation, neuromuscular (NMES), 132–33
employment, 237
episodes of care (EOC), 136, *137, 243*
equinus, *50, 97, 99, 164*
evidence-based medicine, 113–15, 270–71
excessive femoral anteversion, 88–90, *90*
executive function, 134–35
exercise and physical activity, 147–53; in adulthood, 247, 248–49; athletes with CP, 153, 249; benefits, 148, 231–32, 235; definition, 147; recommendations, 148, *149–50*; types of exercise for people with CP, *150–52*

F

falls, 225, 231, 232, 243, 244, 249. *See also* balance
family-centered care, 112–13
fatigue, 235
femoral anteversion, excessive, 88–90, *90*
femoral torsion, 88, 90, 91
fine motor function, 22–23. *See also* gross motor function
floor reaction AFO, 163

foot orthosis (FO), 160
fractures, 224, 225, 231, 233, 242
functional mobility, 131. *See also* Gross Motor Function Classification System
Functional Mobility Scale (FMS), *291*

G

gait: classification of gait patterns, 97; crouch gait, 97, 99–103; definition, 69, 96; energy expenditure, 97–98; gait analysis, 179–82; gait cycle, 70, *71*; Gait Outcomes Assessment List (GOAL), 183–84, *291*; gait training, 131–32; GMFCS level and, 98; three-dimensional (3D) computerized motion analysis, 98, 120, 180–81; treatment importance, 99. *See also* walking
gait analysis, 95, 167–68, 179–82, 186, 229, Appendix 7 (online)
Gait Outcomes Assessment List (GOAL), 183–84, *291*
gender, 11, 59–60, *60*
Gillette Functional Assessment Questionnaire (FAQ), 120, *291*
goal-setting, 118–20
goniometer, *65, 291*
gross motor function: classification of CP on basis of, 32–40; definition, 22; development of, 23; gross motor development curves, 40–41, *41*; measurement of, 24–25, 290. *See also* fine motor function
Gross Motor Function Classification System (GMFCS), 32–40; introduction, 32–33; adoption in clinical practice, 114; assessment process, 34; femoral anteversion and, 90; gross motor development curves and, 40–41, *41*; hip displacement and, 88; level descriptions, 32, *35–36*; and manual ability and communication function classification systems, 37–40, *38–39*; spastic diplegia and, 34, 37, *37, 39,* 39–40; stability of, 33; treatment and, 109, 193; walking and, 33, 98
Gross Motor Function Measure (GMFM), 24–25, 290, *291*
gross motor milestones, 23–24
ground reaction AFO (GRAFO), 163
ground reaction force (GRF), *101,* 101–2, 164
growth, 56–61

H

health-related quality of life (HRQoL), 236
health services, for adults, 109, 219–20, 238–39, 240–42
hemiplegia, 28, *29*, 34, *37*, *55*, 78
hip: abduction (hip abductors), *67*; adduction (hip adductors), *50*, *66*; displacement (subluxation/dislocation), *87*, 87–88, 194, 199; dysplasia, 88; extension (hip extensors), *67*; external rotation, *67*; flexion (hip flexors), *50*, *66*; internal rotation, *50*, *66*; replacement surgery, 246, 247
home program, for adults, 247–49
home program, to age 20, 144–57; introduction, 144–46; exercise and physical activity, 147–53; homework from therapies, 146; orthoses, 146; postural management, 154–55; stretching, 146–47
hyperactive stretch reflex, 76
hyperbaric oxygen, *198*, 200
hypotonia/hypertonia, 76

I

International Classification of Functioning, Disability and Health (ICF), 16–21
intrathecal baclofen (ITB), *167*, 171–72, 245

K

knee: extension (knee extensors), *67*; flexion (knee flexors), *50*, *66*; hyperextended knees, *50*
kneeling, tall, 296

L

learned helplessness, 112
lever-arm dysfunction, 86–93; introduction, 86; excessive femoral anteversion, 88–90, *90*; femoral torsion, 88, 90, 91; hip displacement, *87*, 87–88; pes valgus, 91–93, *92*; tibial torsion, 90–91, *91*
long sitting, 68, 293
lumbar lordosis, *49*

M

management and treatment, best practice, 111–22; introduction, 111; data-driven decision-making, 115–16; early intervention, 118; evidence-based medicine, 113–15; family-centered care and patient-centered care, 112–13; goal-setting, 118–20; measuring outcome, 120–21; multidisciplinary team approach, 116–17; specialist centers, 117

management and treatment, in adulthood, 240–52; introduction, 240; exercise and physical activity, 231–32, 247, 248–49; health services, 109, 219–20, 238–39, 240–42; home program, 247–49; orthopedic surgery, 246–47; physical therapy and occupational therapy, 243–45; tone reduction, 245; treatments, 242–47
management and treatment, to age 20, 108–215; introduction, 108–10; alternative and complementary treatments, 197–200; best practice, 111–22; home program, 144–57; musculoskeletal management plan, 193–96, *195*; orthopedic surgery, 178–92; orthoses, 158–65; therapies, 123–43; tone reduction, 166–77
Manual Ability Classification System (MACS), 37–40, *38–39*
massage, *198*, 200
measurement tools, 120, *121*, 138, 291–92
measuring outcome, 120–21
migration percentage (MP)/migration index (MI), 88
Mini-MACS, 37, 38, 40. *See also* Manual Ability Classification System (MACS)
mixed CP, *31*
mobility: in adulthood, 231–32; assessment and training, 244; assistive mobility devices, 98, 131, 244–45; functional mobility training, 131. *See also* gait; walking
moment, 64, 86, 186
monoplegia, *29*
motor capability, 19
motor capacity, 18–19
motor function. *See* fine motor function; gross motor function
motor learning theory, 125
motor performance, 18–19
multidisciplinary team approach, 116, 117, 240
muscles: abnormal growth, 81–84; abnormal tone, 76–77; contractions, types of, 64; key movements and lower limb muscles, 66–67, 68; sarcopenia, 223, 230–31; strength vs. power, 65; weakness in, 77–78, 82, 83, 129. *See also* strengthening; stretching; tone reduction
muscle-tendon unit (MTU), 64–65, 82n46, 127, 159
musculoskeletal decline, 230–31

N

neuromotor exercise, 249
neuromuscular electrical stimulation (NMES), 132–33
neuroplasticity, 13n25, 55, 118, 125
night splints, 128
noncommunicable diseases (NCDs), 223, 225–26, 233–34, 234

O

obesity, 226n107
occupational therapy (OT), 126, 133, 134, 243–45. See also rehabilitation, after surgery; therapies
oral medications, for tone reduction, 167, 168–69, 245
orthopedic surgery, 178–92; introduction, 178–79; for adults, 246–47; gait analysis and, 179–82; in management plan to age 20, 194–96, 195; plantar flexor lengthening, 186–87; single-event multilevel surgery (SEMLS), 182–86; tone reduction and, 174–75. See also single-event multilevel surgery (SEMLS)
orthoses, 158–65; introduction, 158–59; for adults, 247; in home program, 146; for stretching, 84, 128; types of, 160–64
osteoarthritis, 231
osteopathy, cranial, 198
osteopenia, 224–25
osteoporosis, 224, 224–25, 231, 242
overuse injuries, 244
oxygen, hyperbaric, 198, 200

P

pain, 76, 100, 231, 233, 234, 243
Paralympians, with spastic diplegia, 153, 249
participation, 18, 98, 109, 133, 193, 236–38, 242, 244
passive stretching, 84, 127
patient-centered care, 112–13
Pediatric Outcomes Data Collection Instrument (PODCI), 292
pelvis: anterior pelvic tilt, 49; pelvic obliquity, 94; retracted pelvis, 94
periventricular leukomalacia (PVL), 53–54, 54, 73, 174
pes valgus, 91–93, 92
phenol injection, 167, 170–71, 245
physical activity. See exercise and physical activity

physical therapy (PT)/physiotherapy, 124–33; introduction, 124–26; for adults, 243–45; electrical stimulation (ES), 132–33; functional mobility training, 125–26, 131; gait training, 131–32; strengthening, 129–30; stretching, 126–29. See also rehabilitation, after surgery; therapies
positioning: for sitting, standing, and sleeping, 154, 154–55; for strengthening, 130, 295–96; for stretching, 127–28, 293–95
posterior leaf-spring AFO (PLS AFO), 162
postural management, 154, 154–55, 243, 247–48
Prechtl's General Movements Assessment, 13
preterm birth, 7, 8, 10, 13n22, 53, 81, 174
primary abnormalities, 72–79; introduction, 72–73; abnormal tone, 76–77; loss of selective motor control, 74; muscle weakness, 77–78; poor balance, 75; sensory and other problems, 78
pronation of the midfoot, 92, 92
prone positioning, 294–95
puberty, 58n40, 59, 89, 185, 194

Q

quadriplegia, 28, 29, 34, 37, 37
quality of life (QoL), 236

R

randomized controlled trial (RCT), 114n59, 271
range of motion (ROM), 65, 66–67, 68, 81–84, 126–29, 167, 248, 291
rehabilitation, after surgery: in adulthood, 245, 246–47; selective dorsal rhizotomy (SDR), 174, 175, 300–301; single-event multilevel surgery (SEMLS), 184–85
retracted pelvis, 94
romantic and sexual relationships, 238

S

sarcopenia, 223, 230–31
secondary abnormalities, 80–93; introduction and conclusion, 72, 80, 93; abnormal bone development, 85–93; abnormal muscle growth, 81–84; excessive femoral anteversion, 88–90, 90; femoral torsion, 88, 90, 91; hip displacement, 87, 87–88; pes valgus, 91–93, 92; tibial torsion, 90–91, 91
secondary conditions, 219–21, 239, 241–42
selective dorsal rhizotomy (SDR), 167, 168, 172–75, 194–96, 195, 245, 300–301

selective motor control, loss of, 74, 82
sensory problems, 78, 82
service dogs, 245
sexual and romantic relationships, 238
shoes, 159, 160
side sitting, 294, 295
single-event multilevel surgery (SEMLS), 182–86; for adults, 246–47; "birthday syndrome" vs., 182–83, 229; data-driven decision-making, 115–16; evidence supporting, 114, 115, 185, 271; gait analysis and, 179–82, 186; in management plan to age 20, 194–96, 195
sitting, good posture for, 154, 154
sitting positions: on large roll or bolster, 295–96; long sitting, 68, 293; side sitting, 294, 295; tailor sitting, 294, 295; W-sitting, 128
sleeping, good posture for, 154, 155
solid AFO (SAFO), 162–63
spastic CP, 30, 31
spastic diplegia, 47–105; introduction, 48–51; bones, muscles, joints, and movements, 62–68; brain injury, 53–55; growth, 56–61; normal walking and, 69–71; primary abnormalities, 72–79; secondary abnormalities, 80–93; tertiary abnormalities, 94–95; walking in individuals with, 96–103
spasticity, 31, 76–77, 82, 166
specialist centers, 117, 176
speech and language pathology (SLP) (speech and language therapy [SLT]), 134–35. See also therapies
standing: good posture for, 154, 154; positioning, 295
stem cell therapy, 199, 199
strengthening, 129–30, 149, 295–96
stretching, 68, 126–29, 146–47, 185, 293–95
supramalleolar orthosis (SMO), 161
systematic review, 271

T
tailor sitting, 294, 294, 295
tertiary abnormalities, 73, 94–95
Test of Infant Motor Performance (TIMP), 13
therapies, 123–43; introduction, 123–24; in adulthood, 243–45; delivery guidelines, 135–38, 137; episodes of care (EOC), 136, 137, 243; homework from, 146, 247; life span overview, 138–40; neuroplasticity and, 13n25, 55, 118, 125; occupational

therapy (OT), 126, 133, 134, 243–45; physical therapy (PT)/physiotherapy, 124–33, 243–45; speech and language pathology (SLP) (speech and language therapy [SLT]), 134–35
three-dimensional (3D) computerized motion analysis, 98, 120, 180–81
tibial torsion, 90–91, 91
tizanidine, 168–69
tone: abnormal, 76–77; classification of CP on basis of motor impairment, 30, 31
tone reduction, 166–77; introduction and conclusion, 166–68, 167, 176; for adults, 245; botulinum neurotoxin A (BoNT-A) injection, 169–70, 245; intrathecal baclofen (ITB), 171–72, 245; oral medications, 168–69, 245; phenol injection, 170–71, 245; selective dorsal rhizotomy (SDR), 172–75, 245, 300–301
transitional care units (TCUs), 246
treatment. See management and treatment
triplegia, 29
truncal sway, 94, 95

U
unilateral CP, 29, 30, 30, 31, 37, 78
University of California Biomechanics Lab (UCBL) orthosis, 160

V
valgus hindfoot, 50, 92, 92
vaulting, 94, 95
visual impairments, 78
visual perception, 78

W
walking: introduction, 69; adulthood mobility, 231–32; assistive mobility devices, 98, 131, 244–45; balance, 75; delayed in individuals with spastic diplegia, 33; gross motor milestones and, 23–24; measurement tools, 291–92; normal walking, 69–71; orthoses assistance, 164. See also gait; mobility
W-sitting, 128

Made in the USA
Middletown, DE
18 December 2020

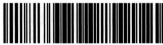

29047594R00206